T0329553

Cognition and Behavior in Multiple Sclerosis

Cognition and Behavior in Multiple Sclerosis

EDITED BY

John DeLuca and
Brian M. Sandroff

AMERICAN PSYCHOLOGICAL ASSOCIATION
Washington, DC

Published by
American Psychological Association
750 First Street, NE
Washington, DC 20002
www.apa.org

APA Order Department
P.O. Box 92984
Washington, DC 20090-2984
Phone: (800) 374-2721; Direct: (202) 336-5510
Fax: (202) 336-5502; TDD/TTY: (202) 336-6123
Online: http://www.apa.org/pubs/books
E-mail: order@apa.org

In the U.K., Europe, Africa, and the Middle East, copies may be ordered from
Eurospan Group
c/o Turpin Distribution
Pegasus Drive
Stratton Business Park
Biggleswade, Bedfordshire
SG18 8TQ United Kingdom
Phone: +44 (0) 1767 604972
Fax: +44 (0) 1767 601640
Online: https://www.eurospanbookstore.com/apa
E-mail: eurospan@turpin-distribution.com

Typeset in Goudy by Circle Graphics, Inc., Columbia, MD

Printer: Sheridan Books, Chelsea, MI
Cover Designer: Beth Schlenoff Design, Bethesda, MD
Cover Art: Photographs by Bing Yao, PhD; courtesy of the Kessler Foundation

Library of Congress Cataloging-in-Publication Data

Names: DeLuca, John, 1956- editor. | Sandroff, Brian M., editor.
Title: Cognition and behavior in multiple sclerosis / edited by John DeLuca
    and Brian M. Sandroff.
Description: Washington, DC : American Psychological Association, 2018. |
    Includes bibliographical references and index.
Identifiers: LCCN 2018003584| ISBN 9781433829321 | ISBN 1433829320
Subjects: LCSH: Multiple sclerosis—Complications. | Cognition disorders.
Classification: LCC RC377 .C53 2018 | DDC 616.8/34—dc23 LC record available at
https://lccn.loc.gov/2018003584

British Library Cataloguing-in-Publication Data
A CIP record is available from the British Library.

Printed in the United States of America
First Edition

http://dx.doi.org/10.1037/0000097-000

10 9 8 7 6 5 4 3 2 1

CONTENTS

CONTRIBUTORS

Nadine Akbar, PhD, Postdoctoral Research Fellow, Adjunct Professor, School of Rehabilitation Therapy, Queen's University, Kingston, Ontario, Canada

Maria Pia Amato, MD, Full Professor of Neurology, Department NEURO-FARBA, Neurosciences Section, University of Florence, Florence, Italy

Ornella Argento, Research Fellow, IRCCS "Santa Lucia" Foundation, Rome, Italy

Peter A. Arnett, PhD, Professor and Director, Neuropsychology of Sports Concussion and MS Programs, Psychology Department, Pennsylvania State University, University Park

Brenda Banwell, MD, Professor, Division of Neurology, Children's Hospital of Philadelphia, Philadelphia, PA

Ralph H. B. Benedict, Professor of Neurology and Psychiatry, University at Buffalo, State University of New York, Buffalo

Bruno Brochet, MD, Professor of Clinical Neurology, University of Bordeaux, France; Head, Department of Neurology, University Hospital of Bordeaux, France

Margaret Cadden, MS, Doctoral Candidate, Department of Psychology, Pennsylvania State University, University Park

Massimiliano Calabrese, MD, Professor of Neurology, Multiple Sclerosis Center, Neurology B, Department of Neurosciences, Biomedicine and Movement Sciences, University of Verona, Verona, Italy

Nancy D. Chiaravalloti, PhD, Director, Neuropsychology & Neuroscience and Traumatic Brain Injury Research, Kessler Foundation, West Orange, NJ; Research Professor, Department of Physical Medicine & Rehabilitation, Rutgers New Jersey Medical School, Newark

John DeLuca, PhD, Senior Vice President for Research and Training, Kessler Foundation, West Orange, NJ; Professor, Department of Physical Medicine & Rehabilitation, and Department of Neurology, Rutgers New Jersey Medical School, Newark

Ekaterina Dobryakova, PhD, Traumatic Brain Injury Research, Kessler Foundation, West Orange, NJ; Department of Physical Medicine & Rehabilitation, Rutgers New Jersey Medical School, Newark

Anthony Feinstein, MPhil, PhD, FRCP, Professor, Department of Psychiatry, University of Toronto; Sunnybrook Health Sciences Centre, Toronto, Ontario, Canada

Massimo Filippi, MD, Neuroimaging Research Unit and Department of Neurology, Institute of Experimental Neurology, Division of Neuroscience, San Raffaele Scientific Institute; Vita-Salute San Raffaele University, Milan, Italy

Sten Fredrikson, MD, PhD, Professor of Neurology, Department of Clinical Neuroscience, Karolinska Institutet, Stockholm, Sweden

Quinten van Geest, MSc, Doctoral Candidate, Department of Anatomy & Neurosciences, Amsterdam Neuroscience, MS Center Amsterdam, VU University Medical Center, Amsterdam, the Netherlands

Jeroen J. G. Geurts, PhD, Professor of Translational Neurosciences, Department of Anatomy & Neurosciences, Amsterdam Neuroscience, MS Center Amsterdam, VU University Medical Center, Amsterdam, the Netherlands

Benedetta Goretti, PhD, Specialist in Neuropsychology, Department NEUROFARBA, Section Neurosciences, University of Florence, Florence, Italy

Yael Goverover, PhD, OT, Associate Professor, Department of Occupational Therapy, Steinhardt School of Culture, Education, and Human Development, New York University, New York

Erin Guty, MS, Doctoral Candidate, Department of Psychology, Pennsylvania State University, University Park

Hanneke E. Hulst, PhD, Assistant Professor, Department of Anatomy & Neurosciences, Amsterdam Neuroscience, MS Center Amsterdam, VU University Medical Center, Amsterdam, the Netherlands

Chiara Concetta Incerti, Research Fellow, IRCCS "Santa Lucia" Foundation, Rome, Italy

Kim A. Meijer, MSc, Doctoral Candidate, Department of Anatomy & Neurosciences, Amsterdam Neuroscience, MS Center Amsterdam, VU University Medical Center, Amsterdam, the Netherlands

Robert W. Motl, PhD, Professor, Department of Physical Therapy, University of Alabama at Birmingham

Ugo Nocentini, MD, Senior Researcher, University of Rome "Tor Vergata"; IRCCS "Santa Lucia" Foundation, Rome, Italy

Bennis Pavisian, BAH, Department of Psychiatry, University of Toronto; Sunnybrook Health Sciences Centre, Toronto, Ontario, Canada

Marco Pitteri, PhD, Postdoctoral Research Fellow, Multiple Sclerosis Center, Neurology B, Department of Neurosciences, Biomedicine and Movement Sciences, University of Verona, Verona, Italy

Maria Assunta Rocca, MD, Neuroimaging Research Unit and Department of Neurology, Institute of Experimental Neurology, Division of Neuroscience, San Raffaele Scientific Institute, Vita-Salute San Raffaele University, Milan, Italy

Cristina Roman, MS, Doctoral Candidate, Department of Psychology, Pennsylvania State University, University Park

Shumita Roy, PhD, Department of Neurology, Jacobs School of Medicine and Biomedical Sciences, University at Buffalo, The State University of New York, Buffalo

Brian M. Sandroff, PhD, Assistant Professor, Department of Physical Therapy, University of Alabama at Birmingham

Lauren B. Strober, PhD, Senior Research Scientist, Neuropsychology and Neuroscience Laboratory, Kessler Foundation; Assistant Research Professor, Department of Physical Medicine & Rehabilitation, Rutgers New Jersey Medical School, Newark

Christine Till, PhD, Associate Professor, Department of Psychology, York University, Toronto, Ontario, Canada

Cognition
and
Behavior
in Multiple
Sclerosis

INTRODUCTION

JOHN DeLUCA AND BRIAN M. SANDROFF

Multiple sclerosis (MS) is a nontraumatic, immune-mediated, and neuro-degenerative disease of the central nervous system that afflicts persons in the prime of their lives and can have devastating personal, social, vocational, family, and financial consequences. MS was first recognized by Charcot in 1868 as a progressive neurologic disease involving multiple lesions distributed throughout the central nervous system. MS is one of the most common neurological diseases worldwide, with global prevalence estimates exceeding 2 million cases. It has been reported to have the highest prevalence estimates in Western Europe and North America, followed by areas in central and eastern Europe, the Balkans, and Australia/New Zealand.

Currently, MS is typically characterized by initial episodes of acute inflammation (i.e., acute demyelinating lesions) in the central nervous system, damaging myelinated axons and neurons. After an episodic period of acute central nervous system inflammation, during a remission phase, trophic

http://dx.doi.org/10.1037/0000097-001
Cognition and Behavior in Multiple Sclerosis, J. DeLuca and B. M. Sandroff (Editors)

factors promote remyelination of damaged axons in the central nervous system; these axons undergoing remyelination can regain their conduction capacity, although often at a diminished capacity. The ability for growth factors to remyelinate damaged axons after a relapse decreases over time, resulting in neuronal degeneration and eventually irreversible neurological disability (i.e., disease progression). Collectively, this central nervous system damage is associated with physical and cognitive impairments.

Cognitive impairment is a common and debilitating symptom of MS. Although Charcot identified that MS patients demonstrate cognitive symptoms, including slowed information processing and impaired memory, focal research on cognitive impairment in MS started only in the 1980s. The presence of cognitive impairment as part of the disease was hotly debated for the first half of the 20th century, but it is now recognized that 45% to 70% of individuals with MS experience some degree of cognitive impairment based on objective neuropsychological testing. This cognitive impairment is associated with brain atrophy and altered brain activation/functional connectivity based on neuroimaging. Indeed, MS-related cognitive impairment is further associated with high personal and societal economic costs, as well as many mental health consequences, including depression, fatigue, reduced quality of life, unemployment, and reduced ability to perform activities of daily living. Importantly, pharmacological and behavioral treatment approaches for managing MS-related cognitive impairment have largely been unsuccessful.

There is a dearth of existing volumes that have comprehensively addressed cognition and its correlates, consequences, and treatment in persons with MS. Indeed, this first edition of *Cognition and Behavior in Multiple Sclerosis* will provide a comprehensive compilation of the effects of MS on cognition in a single volume. Its purpose is to uniquely advance the science on understanding and managing the cognitive consequences of the disease by bringing together world-renowned, international experts in this area. This book aims to be the definitive text for clinicians and researchers, as well as to serve as a primary resource for students and other professionals (e.g., government officials, attorneys, public policy experts).

This volume consists of 15 stand-alone chapters that each address an important area pertaining to cognition and behavior in persons with MS. The first section of this textbook involves the latest characterization of MS-related cognitive impairment, with chapters on assessment and neuroimaging (i.e., structural and functional neuroimaging). The second section primarily involves the latest research on the mental health/behavioral correlates and consequences of MS-related cognitive impairment. This includes chapters on depression, neuropsychiatric disorders, fatigue, personality problems, activities of daily living, employment, and economic impact, respectively, and cognition in MS. The third section involves a chapter on pediatric-onset MS. This textbook concludes with a section on treatment approaches for MS-related cognitive impairment. This includes separate chapters on pharmacology, cognitive rehabilitation, exercise and physical activity, and cognitive reserve.

The first edition of *Cognition and Behavior in Multiple Sclerosis* provides readers with a collection of the latest research by top scientists, pertaining to a largely understudied aspect of MS. By comprehensively addressing the correlates, consequences, and treatment of cognitive impairment in MS, it is our hope that this volume inspires new lines of clinical and behavioral research to improve the lives of those living with the disease, considering the common, burdensome, and challenging nature of cognitive impairment.

1

ASSESSMENT OF COGNITIVE IMPAIRMENT IN MULTIPLE SCLEROSIS

SHUMITA ROY AND RALPH H. B. BENEDICT

Cognitive impairment is now recognized as a common feature of multiple sclerosis (MS), affecting between 40% and 70% of patients (Chiaravalloti & DeLuca, 2008). Due to the heterogeneity of cerebral pathology in MS, impairments can be found in multiple domains, but those most typically affected are information processing speed and episodic memory (Benedict et al., 2006; Rao, Leo, Bernardin, & Unverzagt, 1991). These deficits adversely affect daily function (Benedict et al., 2005), ultimately compromising employment status (Frndak et al., 2015) and social functioning (e.g., Rao, Leo, Ellington, et al., 1991). Cognitive impairment is also associated with poor treatment adherence, leading to suboptimal clinical management (Bruce, Hancock, Arnett, & Lynch, 2010).

Despite the high prevalence of cognitive dysfunction among MS patients, detecting and assessing deficits can be challenging. Patients are not always accurate in reporting on the presence or severity of cognitive dysfunction because their perception is influenced by psychological factors,

http://dx.doi.org/10.1037/0000097-002
Cognition and Behavior in Multiple Sclerosis, J. DeLuca and B. M. Sandroff (Editors)

such as depression (Carone, Benedict, Munschauer, Fishman, & Weinstock-Guttman, 2005). A recent study showed that even neurologists are inaccurate in identifying cognitive impairment during a standard neurological examination (Romero, Shammi, & Feinstein, 2015).

Suspected cognitive impairment, based on patient self-report, informant or caregiver report, or clinician observation should trigger psychometric evaluation. However, because there is no well-validated screen, one should expect frequent false-positive referrals. Hence, it is essential that the formal assessment process be as brief as possible, affordable, and focused on the most essential cognitive domains. Neuropsychological assessments can be costly and time-consuming, require staff with specialized training, and may be unavailable in the patient's location. In this chapter, we present current approaches in the assessment of cognitive functioning in MS and discuss future directions in this area.

CONVENTIONAL PSYCHOMETRIC ASSESSMENT TECHNIQUES

Comprehensive neuropsychological assessment typically uses standardized tests covering many spheres of cognition, such as intelligence, language, visual perception and construction, learning, memory, attention, processing speed, and executive function. Before pursuing cognitive evaluation, the MS clinician must determine whether the goal is to quantify current abilities in a clearly diagnosed MS patient or if comprehensive testing is needed for differential diagnosis. Most often we are dealing with the former purpose, and this chapter is therefore focused on assessment of those domains known to be commonly affected in MS.

MS Cognitive Assessments Based on the Work of Stephen Rao, PhD

The seminal work of Stephen Rao and colleagues greatly influenced the recognition of cognitive dysfunction in MS (Rao, Leo, Bernardin, & Unverzagt, 1991). Before then, many clinicians dismissed cognitive impairment as either infrequent or not relevant to medical care or quality of life. Rao's research team applied a comprehensive battery of cognitive tests, lasting several hours, to 102 MS patients. A matched sample of 100 healthy control participants was also assessed. The results revealed a 43% frequency of MS-associated cognitive impairment. The investigators also found that the most sensitive tests in discriminating MS from healthy subjects were those emphasizing the speed of information processing and episodic memory.

With this in mind, the team whinnied down the extensive battery to the key tests, giving rise to the Neuropsychological Screening Battery and the Brief Repeatable Battery for MS (BRB; Rao, 1991a, 1991b).

The BRB includes measures of cognitive processing speed, working memory, language, verbal memory, and visual memory (see Table 1.1). Although not included in the original publication, an adapted version of the Symbol Digit Modalities Test (SDMT; Smith, 1982) was included in the BRB as a measure of cognitive processing speed. The SDMT requires patients to view a key depicting numbers paired with symbols. Below the key are symbols without the paired numbers, and the task is to provide the associated number for each symbol as quickly as possible. In the original SDMT form, examinees first responded by writing the numbers and then, in the next trial, voicing the numbers. The primary outcome is the total number of correctly coded items. Rao's group omitted the first trial to reduce demand for upper-extremity motor function. As will be seen subsequently, this test proved to be very reliable and sensitive in future work.

The memory tests in the BRB included adapted versions of the Selective Reminding Test (SRT; Buschke & Fuld, 1974), and the 7/24 Spatial Recall Test (Barbizet & Cany, 1968). The SRT is a verbal learning test in which a word list containing 12 words is initially presented and only words not recalled by patients are provided on each successive learning trial. The 7/24 presents a checkerboard on which seven stimuli are presented. Patients view the stimulus for 10 seconds and then place checkers in the right location after the stimulus is removed. To have a larger stimulus matrix from which to develop alternate test forms, the 7/24 Spatial Recall Test was replaced by the 10/36 Spatial Recall Test; the larger stimulus matrix permitted more opportunity to develop alternate forms.

Subsequent studies demonstrated that the BRB tests are sensitive (Huijbregts, Kalkers, de Sonneville, de Groot, & Polman, 2006) and correlate well with brain magnetic resonance imaging (MRI) measures such as ventricle enlargement (Christodoulou et al., 2003) and neocortical volume (Amato et al., 2004). It is still a core test battery used throughout Europe (Sepulcre et al., 2006), and it reveals longitudinal changes in the neuropsychological status of MS patients (Amato et al., 1995; Amato, Ponziani, Siracusa, & Sorbi, 2001). Because the battery is brief, requiring only 40 to 45 minutes to administer, large samples in excess of 250 patients have been studied (Patti et al., 2009). Previous studies are primarily based on North American and European patient samples. Caceres and colleagues recently conducted a large multicenter study in Latin America in which they implemented a Spanish translation of the BRB (Caceres, Vanotti, Benedict, & the RELACCEM Work Group, 2014). This was the first study to report on the prevalence of cognitive and neuropsychiatric functioning in a large, multinational, Latin

TABLE 1.1
Conventional Test Batteries Used to Assess Cognitive
Functioning in Multiple Sclerosis

Domains measured	BRNB (1991)	MSFC (1999)	MACFIMS (2002)	BICAMS (2012)	NINDS–CDE (2012)	MS–COG (2014)
Walking speed		25-foot Walk				
Motor dexterity		9HPT				
Cognitive speed	SDMT		SDMT	SDMT	SDMT	SDMT
Working memory	PASAT	PASAT	PASAT		PASAT	PASAT
Language	COWAT		COWAT		COWAT	
Visual perception			JLO			
Verbal memory	SRT		CVLT–II	CVLT–II	CVLT–II	SRT
Visual memory	10/36 Spatial Recall		BVMT–R	BVMT–R	BVMT–R	BVMT–R
Executive functioning			DKEFS Sorting		DKEFS Sorting	

Note. 9HPT = Nine Hole Peg Test; BICAMS = Brief International Cognitive Assessment for MS; BRNB = Brief Repeatable Neuropsychological Battery; BVMT–R = Brief Visuospatial Memory Test—Revised; COWAT = Controlled Oral Word Association Test; CVLT–II = California Verbal Learning Test—Second Edition; JLO = Judgment of Line Orientation; MACFIMS = Minimal Assessment of Cognitive Function in MS; MSFC = Multiple Sclerosis Functional Composite; MS–COG = Multiple Sclerosis Cognition Assessment Battery; NINDS–CDE = National Institute of Neurological Disorders and Stroke—Common Data Elements; PASAT = Paced Serial Addition Test; SDMT = Symbol Digit Modalities Test; SRT = Selective Reminding Test.

American MS sample. The study included 110 MS patients and 34 healthy control participants. MS patients performed worse than control participants on all measures. Similar to other prevalence studies performed in Europe and North America, results with the Spanish BRB showed large effect sizes, ranging from 0.6 to 1.9, with the largest effect sizes for SRT delayed recall and Brief Visuospatial Memory Test—Revised (BVMT–R) delayed recall. The study also found a similar prevalence rate of cognitive impairment (35%), demonstrating cross-cultural utility of the BRB.

The Minimal Assessment of Cognitive Function in MS

In 2001, it was formally acknowledged that the Rao batteries did not cover some domains thought to be important in neuropsychological studies of MS, particularly visual–spatial processing and higher executive function. In addition, there was limited understanding of the psychometric aspects of the BRB—for example, unknown test–retest and alternate-form reliability. With this in mind, a consensus conference was convened to determine an optimal "minimal record" for cognitive function research and clinical application (Benedict et al., 2002). This approach is widely known as the Minimal Assessment of Cognitive Function in MS (MACFIMS). This neuropsychological battery is more comprehensive than the BRB (see Table 1.1) but still emphasizes only domains regarded as commonly involved in MS patients, and thus is useful for research and clinical purposes (Benedict et al., 2002).

The Rao approach and MACFIMS both remain gold standard conventional approaches to neuropsychological assessment in MS. The Rao revisions of the SDMT (Smith, 1982) and the Paced Auditory Serial Addition Test (PASAT; Gronwall, 1977) appear in both batteries, as does the Controlled Oral Word Association Test (COWAT; Benton & Hamsher, 1989). These tests measure information processing speed, working memory, and verbal fluency, respectively.

The memory tests differ, however. Rather than the SRT and 10/36, the MACFIMS includes the California Verbal Learning Test—Second Edition (CVLT–II; Delis, Kramer, Kaplan, & Ober, 2000) and the BVMT–R (Benedict, 1997; Benedict, Schretlen, Groninger, Dobraski, & Shpritz, 1996). Out of the potential memory measures, the expert panel ranked the CVLT–II and BVMT–R most highly because these measures were shown to be psychometrically superior to the SRT and 10/36 Spatial Recall Test, have alternate forms, and are considered to be easier to administer (Benedict et al., 2002). Strober and colleagues (2009) compared these tests in the same sample when discriminating MS patients from control participants. The 65 MS patients and 46 control participants were well matched on demographic characteristics. This study included samples of MS patients with mixed clinical disease courses as defined by Lublin, Reingold, and the National Multiple Sclerosis Society (USA) Advisory Committee on Clinical Trials of New Agents in Multiple Sclerosis (1996; i.e., relapsing remitting [72%], secondary progressive [22%], primary progressive [3%], relapsing progressive [1.5%], clinically isolated syndrome [1.5%]). The mean Expanded Disability Status Scale (EDSS; Kurtzke, 1983) was 3.3 ± 1.7. The data showed similar sensitivity effects for the auditory–verbal memory tests, whereas the BVMT–R better separated the groups compared with the 10/36 Spatial Recall Test. These findings comparing memory measures between the batteries were recently replicated in two separate studies. In a 2015 study (Niccolai et al., 2015), effect sizes were of similar strength for verbal memory tests including the SRT long-term storage ($d = 0.55$), SRT consistent long-term retrieval ($d = 0.61$), and the CVLT–II total learning ($d = 0.61$). The BVMT–R ($d = 0.60$) was again found to have a larger effect size compared with the Spatial Recall Test ($d = 0.38$). In another study, the effect size of BVMT–R Total Learning ($d = 1.1$) was higher than the 7/24 Total Learning ($d = 0.6$), and the BVMT–R Delayed Recall ($d = 1.9$) was also higher than the 7/24 Delayed Recall ($d = 1.0$; Caceres et al., 2014).

To address aforementioned limitations of the BRB, the MACFIMS also includes a test of higher executive function called the Delis–Kaplan Executive Functioning System Sorting Test (DKEFS; Delis, Kaplan, & Kramer, 2001). The DKEFS has similar sensitivity to MS as other, more traditional measures of executive function but is particularly advantageous because it has alternate forms (Parmenter, Zivadinov, et al., 2007). Another unique feature of the MACFIMS is the inclusion of the Judgment of Line Orientation Test (JLO; Benton, Sivan, Hamsher, Varney, & Spreen, 1994), for the assessment of visual–spatial processing.

Much work has been done since the 2001 meeting evaluating the reliability and validity of the MACFIMS. In one study (Benedict, 2005), after separating patients into two groups, several MACFIMS tests were administered twice to assess test–retest reliability. Patients were randomly divided into same form (SF) or alternate form (AF) conditions and were examined at baseline and 1 week later. Patients in the SF condition received the same version of tests at both baseline and follow-up, and patients in the AF condition received different versions at baseline and follow-up. The reliability of the MACFIMS tests ranged from good to excellent, provided that alternate forms were used at follow-up testing.

We also studied the validity of the MACFIMS in a large sample of 291 patients. The demographics and disease characteristics of this sample closely paralleled natural history studies of MS (Jacobs et al., 1999). Like Rao's group, we found that tests emphasizing cognitive processing speed and episodic memory were most sensitive, this time characterized mainly by two visual processing tests, the SDMT (Smith, 1982) and the BVMT–R (Benedict, 1997). Large-sample cross-sectional studies have also shown that the MACFIMS has good construct validity (Benedict et al., 2006) and predicts vocational outcomes (Benedict et al., 2006; Morrow et al., 2010; Parmenter, Zivadinov, et al., 2007). A recent study also validated an Italian version of the MACFIMS (Migliore et al., 2016). The study included 130 MS patients and 60 healthy control participants. All measures discriminated between patients and control participants and approximately 71% of the patient sample was found to be cognitively impaired.

Other consensus standard cognitive test batteries developed for assessing cognitive function in MS include those developed by the National Institute of Neurological Disorders and Stroke-Common Data Elements (Benedict, Krupp, et al., 2012) and the Multiple Sclerosis Cognition Assessment Battery (Erlanger et al., 2014). Table 1.1 provides a summary of these batteries. Note the considerable overlap and, in particular, that three batteries published since 2011 have included exclusively tests in these batteries, in various combinations. Recent reviews of the literature have borne out the general impression that neuropsychological tests involving processing speed, working memory, and episodic memory are most useful in the evaluation of MS patients (Chiaravalloti & DeLuca, 2008).

COMPUTER-ASSISTED TESTING

Conventional in-house neuropsychological assessment may not always be feasible. As such, automated or semiautomated testing using a computer is a viable alternative (Schlegel & Gilliland, 2007). Computerized neuropsychological assessment devices (CNAD) may also enhance accessibility to cognitive assessment for patients receiving care at facilities or in areas without the resources to support a full-time neuropsychology staff (Bauer et al., 2012).

Existing CNAD batteries share a general format of visual and verbal recognition memory assessed via a learning task, followed by various processing speed and attention tests, concluding with delayed recognition memory. Patients are directed to the computer and instructed to follow the on-screen instructions. The extent to which a proctor, technician, or clinician should be involved varies and is not always explicitly indicated. In general, these batteries are regarded as stand-alone, fully automated procedures, and a technician is not deemed necessary. The Cognitive Stability Index was developed to be administered online, which means the patient may take the test while sitting at home, in an uncontrolled setting. Intuitively, these automated approaches would seem to raise questions about validity when outside the confines of a planned, well-controlled study.

Anthony Feinstein's group at the University of Toronto has adopted an intermediary approach by using the advantages of computer-administered stimuli but retaining the involvement of a technician (Akbar, Honarmand, Kou, & Feinstein, 2011; Lapshin et al., 2012). In their study, 96 MS patients and 98 healthy control participants underwent computer-administered versions of the SDMT (C–SDMT) and visual versions of the 2-s and 4-s PASAT (PVSAT). The results were compared with the MACFIMS. A subsample of patients was retested a mean of 71.7 days later to assess reliability. These tests were all successful in discriminating cognitively impaired patients from cognitively intact patients and from healthy control participants. The combination of the three measures had a sensitivity of 82.5% and specificity of 87.5%. Each of the new measures also had good retest reliability (Lapshin, Lanctôt, O'Connor, & Feinstein, 2013). In a follow-up study, this group sought to determine whether performance based on computerized cognitive tests could discriminate between MS disease courses (Lapshin, Audet, & Feinstein, 2014). The cognitive tasks included a computerized STROOP Color–Word Test, the C–SDMT, the PVSAT 4-s and 2-s trials, and a speed of cognition index. Aside from the PVSAT 2 s, there were significant group differences on all measures. Clinically isolated syndrome (CIS) patients were the least impaired, and secondary progressive MS were the most impaired. Relapsing–remitting MS and primary progressive MS patients generally had a similar cognitive profile and were more impaired than the CIS patients but less so than the secondary progressive MS patients.

Our group is also examining this area because we believe that it is simply a matter of time before the psychometric research necessary to confidently apply such methods will be published, followed by wider acceptance in the clinical and research settings. We are currently evaluating the degree to which performance is affected by the presence of a technician in a prospective study. Most data have been published on self-administered batteries including Cognitive Drug Research (CDR) Computerized Assessment System (Edgar et al., 2011), MindStreams, also known as Neurotrax (Achiron et al., 2007), the Headminder Cognitive Stability Index (Younes et al., 2007), and the Automated Neuropsychological Assessment Metrics (ANAM; Wilken et al., 2003). We will also cover a new approach to administer conventional tests in a semiautomated manner, using computer-administered stimuli (Lapshin et al., 2013).

For the moment, let us consider two basic requirements, test–retest reliability and discriminant validity. In a review article, Lapshin et al. (2012) concluded that there are only limited data on the reliability and validity of many computerized measures and that many of these batteries are lacking research specifically in the MS population. Only the CDR and ANAM batteries present test–retest reliability in MS samples. The median (depending on delay length) for the CDR, ranged from 0.58 for numeric and spatial tasks to 0.93 for reaction time tasks (Edgar et al., 2011). For ANAM, mean scores from a third and fourth testing session were compared to establish stability, but a test–retest reliability coefficient was not included (Wilken et al., 2003). These psychometric data are presented in Table 1.2.

Multiple CDR subtests discriminate MS from healthy control participants with *d* values generally ranging from 0.6 for the Continuity of Attention subtest to 1.4 for the Power of Attention subtest (Edgar et al., 2011). MindStreams also shows good discriminant validity (Achiron et al., 2007), as does the Cognitive Stability Index, especially where processing speed measures are emphasized (Younes et al., 2007). Although individual subtests were not examined, using the ANAM, logistic regression indicated 95.8% of subjects were accurately classified as cognitively impaired (Wilken et al., 2003).

As noted, the use of self-administered computerized testing introduces the possibility of remote testing. However, it remains unclear how remote testing compares with traditional in-person clinic testing. In a recent study, researchers compared performance on the ANAM and SDMT of patients tested live-in-office, remote-in-office, and remote-in-home (Settle, Robinson, Kane, Maloni, & Wallin, 2015). In the live-in-office condition, the examiner initiated the computerized ANAM and then administered the paper-based SDMT. In the remote-in-office condition, the examiner left the room after explaining how to use the ANAM program. The SDMT was conducted over a webcam. Finally, the remote-in-home condition was similar to the remote-in-office condition. The only difference was that the examiner communicated with the patient through telehealth technology and was never in the room. Results showed that the ANAM scores were equivalent across all three conditions. However, the live-in-office SDMT scores were significantly higher than both remote administration conditions. These results raise concerns over the accuracy of remote and computerized SDMT administration.

As computer technology advances, it can lead to more adaptive approaches to cognitive assessment. The Multiple Sclerosis Processing Speed Test (MSPT) is an example of this modern form of computerized clinical evaluation (Rudick et al., 2014). The MSPT is an iPAD-based tool that assesses balance, walking speed, manual dexterity, visual function, and cognition. It was developed as an extension to the existing MS Functional Composite (MSFC; Cutter et al., 1999) to assess MS disability and can be used either at the clinical site or remotely in the patient's home. With respect to the cognitive component of the program, the creators developed a computerized task called the Processing Speed Test (PST), which is a coding test similar to the SDMT. It should be noted that although the PASAT, not the SDMT, is in the MSFC, it has been proposed that the SDMT should replace the PASAT (Drake et al., 2010). This is discussed later in the chapter. As part of the validation process, the MSPT was administered to 51 MS patients and

TABLE 1.2
Reliability and Discriminative Validity of Computerized Tests Compared With the SDMT

| | Publication | Test–retest reliability | | Concurrent validity r value | Discriminative validity Cohen's d |
		Low r value	High r value		
SDMT (manual version)	Benedict et al., 2005 Benedict, Smerbeck, et al., 2012	.82	.97	N/A	1.3
PVSAT				.76	0.6
C–SDMT		.75		.86	0.9
CRT	Lapshin et al., 2013	.93			
SRT		.85			
Stroop		.95			
		.81			
CogState	Edgar et al., 2011	.35	.94	.61	1.4
Cognitive Stability Index	Younes et al., 2007	N/R	N/R	.76	N/R
ANAM	Wilken et al., 2003	N/R	N/R	.62	N/R

Note. ANAM = Automated Neuropsychological Assessment Metric; CRT = Choice Reaction Time; C–SDMT = Computerized Symbol Digit Modalities Test; PVSAT = Paced Visual Serial Addition Test; SDMT = Symbol Digit Modalities Test; SRT = Simple Reaction Time.

49 healthy control participants. Test–retest reproducibility was calculated between morning and afternoon administrations for both original technician-based measures and analogous MSPT measures. The concordance correlation coefficient was 0.853 for the technician-based SDMT and 0.867 for PST. Correlation coefficients were greater than 0.90 for both technician and MSPT versions of all other measures. Concurrent validity of the MSPT was also good. That is, Pearson correlation coefficients between MSPT tests and standard technician-based measures were greater than 0.80 for most domains for both MS patients and healthy control participants. Cohen's d values were calculated to determine how well the MSPT could discriminate between patients and control participants. Cohen's d for the technician-based SDMT ranged from 0.50 to 0.78 for two time points and ranged from 0.73 to 0.80 for PST, indicating medium to large effect sizes. The MSPT was also found to be good in discriminating between mild and severe MS disability, with Cohen's d values greater than 0.50 on the majority of its measures. Thus, while these results are promising, further research is needed before the MSPT can be implemented in clinical settings.

In addition to computer-based tasks, virtual reality (VR) is also being explored as a means of cognitive assessment in MS. VR-based tasks have been studied in various neurological patient populations such as epilepsy (Grewe et al., 2014), mild cognitive impairment (Werner, Rabinowitz, Klinger, Korczyn, & Josman, 2009), and traumatic brain injury (Zhang et al., 2003). However, we are aware of only one study that has investigated the application of VR in cognitive evaluation of MS patients (Lamargue-Hamel et al., 2015). Lamargue-Hamel and colleagues (2015) tested 30 MS patients with at least a moderate degree of cognitive impairment on two in-house VR tasks, the Urban DailyCog and the Driving Simulator Dual Task (DSDT). Both tasks were developed to detect attentional deficits and working memory impairments in the context of driving simulation tasks. They also administered a battery of traditional neuropsychological measures to characterize the sample. Results showed that 52% of the patients failed the DSDT and 80% failed the Urban DailyCog task. However, neither of the VR tasks were significantly correlated with performance on any of the traditional cognitive measures in any domains. Thus, although VR technology may be useful in evaluating cognitive dysfunction in MS in the future, existing tasks are not ready for clinical use.

In summary, computerized cognitive assessment has many practical advantages, including convenient access, ease of administration, and cost-effectiveness. However, although initial findings are encouraging, this research must be considered preliminary at this time because the psychometric properties of these tasks are yet to be determined.

SCREENING METHODS

Screening refers to a brief, cost-saving assessment that identifies patients who would benefit from further evaluation or treatment with minimal probability of false positives. For example, there are methods to screen for HIV with nearly 100% sensitivity and high specificity (Kelen, Shahan, & Quinn, 1999). Such nearly perfect screens are rare in medicine, however. The polymerase chain reaction test used to screen for syphilis, for example, has a sensitivity of 83% and specificity of 95% (Gayet-Ageron, Lautenschlager, Ninet, Perneger, & Combescure, 2013). When screening tests produce continuous instead of binary outputs, the cut score can be adjusted to further minimize the chance of a false negative while accepting more false positives, the assumption being that the false-positive patients will merely go on to more accurate evaluation.

As noted, comprehensive cognitive evaluations are time-consuming, costly, and require specialized expertise. Given these limitations, there has been a clear need for some form of brief cognitive screening that could be performed by MS clinicians. In 2002, we set out to find a screening instrument for cognitive impairment in MS. Our thought was to develop a questionnaire that could be completed in a few minutes by either a patient or family member to gain information about the frequency and disruptiveness of various cognitive symptoms. The definitive study was published in 2004, showing marginally acceptable sensitivity and specificity for the informant-report version of the MS Neuropsychological Screening Questionnaire; lower values were obtained for the self-report version (Benedict et al., 2004). Our sample consisted of a mixed clinical sample of patients, many of whom were cognitively impaired. However, such a screen is necessary in situations where patients are less impaired and need to be identified early. Most astute clinicians can detect frank dementia in MS patients; in more mildly affected samples, where a screen is more needed, this method has not proven useful (O'Brien et al., 2007).

Perhaps more efficient screening might be possible using brief performance-based tests rather than surveys. The SDMT would seem to be a good candidate. When patients were defined as cognitively impaired or unimpaired on the basis of other cognitive tests (Parmenter, Weinstock-Guttman, Garg, Munschauer, & Benedict, 2007), SDMT accurately categorized 72% of patients, yielding sensitivity of 0.82 and specificity of 0.60. On the surface, this may seem satisfactory, but consider that 28% of patients were misclassified, which is not really cost-saving or informative. Part of the problem may lie in the fact that SDMT does not require higher executive function or memory, which are commonly involved spheres of cognition in MS.

These results are not surprising considering that MS is a very heterogenous disease affecting cerebral integrity in many ways, in many regions, to varying degrees across patients (Benedict & Zivadinov, 2011). In addition, cognitive reserve exerts a significant influence of cognitive capacity, and this influence varies by the degree of cerebral pathology (Benedict et al., 2010; Roy, Schwartz, et al., 2016). With this in mind, it seems far-fetched to envisage any single, brief test that will detect cognitive impairment with sufficient sensitivity and specificity. Efforts are continuing to validate such a task, but considering the wide heterogeneity of cerebral pathology in MS, it may make more sense to abandon the idea of screening per se and focus on monitoring a few specific cognitive functions in many, if not all, MS patients.

MONITORING AND BRIEF MEASURES
FOR CLINICAL TRIALS

The purpose of monitoring is to target core cognitive domains affected in the majority of MS patients. These domains are information processing speed (IPS) and episodic memory. Recently, an international committee of neurology and neuropsychology experts gathered to discuss this very topic (Langdon et al., 2012). The goal was to determine optimal measures that could be used to monitor many, if not all, patients for impairment or change in these domains.

The process began with a detailed literature review emphasizing both psychometric (reliability, validity, and sensitivity) and pragmatic standards (international applicability, ease of administration, feasibility in the specified context and acceptability to patients) of commonly used neuropsychological tests. Ratings of candidate tests were collated and presented to the full committee for discussion. Next, consensus was achieved regarding the qualitative aspects of the battery. From the outset, it was agreed that for a new monitoring tool to be widely applied, it should not require specialized psychologist training. The panel then agreed that the maximum time limit for the assessment should be 15 minutes. Also, because some centers may not have access to computer technology, the panel decided that the assessment should not require special equipment, other than paper, writing utensils, and a timer.

The result of this meeting was the Brief International Cognitive Assessment for MS or BICAMS (Langdon et al., 2012). The IPS component is the SDMT, specifically Rao's oral adaptation (Rao, 1991a, 1991b). For the domain of memory, the selected tests were the learning trials of the CVLT–II (Delis et al., 2000) and the BVMT–R (Benedict, 1997; Benedict et al., 1996). The rationale for these selections exceeds the scope of this chapter, but in brief, the SDMT and BVMT–R were judged to have superior sensitivity compared with other candidate tests and, in the case of the SDMT, very high reliability (Caceres et al., 2014; Niccolai et al., 2015). For IPS, the PASAT was considered, but SDMT was deemed to be more acceptable to patients and clinicians. The choice between the CVLT–II and SRT was debated more extensively because their sensitivity is roughly equal (Strober et al., 2009). A key factor in the ultimate decision was that the administration of the SRT was deemed to require more advanced testing skill.

The BICAMS panel placed greater emphasis on the use of the SDMT as a monitoring tool and even argued that it could be used in isolation. It is easier to administer than the memory tests, and the primary goal of the committee was to facilitate wide implementation across countries and cultures, rather than multidomain assessment. The abstract of the BICAMS publication includes this summary statement:

> The committee recommended the Symbol Digit Modalities Test, if only 5 minutes was available, with the addition of the learning trials of the California Verbal Learning Test—Second Edition and the Brief Visuospatial Memory Test—Revised if a further 10 minutes could be allocated for testing. (p. 891)

The inclusion of SDMT in BICAMS is timely because there has been increasing endorsement of this test among other groups seeking optimal outcomes for clinical trials. The PASAT, although a component of the highly regarded MSFC (Cutter et al., 1999), is a difficult test for both the patient and the administrator. In 2010, we asked whether supplanting the PASAT with SDMT would come with any cost to reliability or validity (Drake et al., 2010). We found similar validity coefficients for MSFC scores using the SDMT and PASAT. Also, in 115 patients tested twice over 2 years, 27.6% of patients showed decline on the PASAT, whereas 46.6% showed decline on the SDMT, suggesting that SDMT is more sensitive to decline over time. This and other research has led to an emerging consensus that SDMT will play a major role in future neurological composite metrics (Benedict, Krupp, et al., 2012; Cohen, Reingold, Polman, Wolinsky, & the International Advisory Committee on Clinical Trials in Multiple Sclerosis, 2012; Ontaneda, LaRocca, Coetzee, & Rudick, 2012).

Since the initial consensus conference, two groups (Dusankova, Kalincik, Havrdova, & Benedict, 2012; Eshaghi et al., 2012) have undertaken validation of BICAMS in a non-English setting, either explicitly or implicitly by validating the MACFIMS, which includes the BICAMS (see Table 1.1). Cross-cultural validation is an arduous process, and the BICAMS committee recently published consensus psychometric standards for this purpose (Benedict, Amato, et al., 2012). Several international validation studies are currently underway, and a website offering normalization of BICAMS data for clinicians can be accessed at https://www.bicams.net.

In addition to cross-cultural validation, the BICAMS continues to undergo validation in comparison to other conventional MS batteries. The BICAMS was recently compared with the BRB in a sample of 192 MS patients (Niccolai et al., 2015). Of these 192 patients, 45 were classified as being cognitively impaired and 48 were classified as unimpaired on both batteries when SDMT was included. There was moderate agreement between performance on the two batteries, as indicated by a Cohen's K value of 0.46. When the SDMT, the only common measure between the two batteries, was excluded from analysis, 37 patients were classified as impaired and 57 as unimpaired. Without the SDMT, concordance decreased to a Cohen's K value of 0.3. Of all the individual measures in these two batteries, Cohen's d values showing discrimination of patients and control participants, were highest for SDMT (0.83), PASAT 3 s (0.65), and PASAT 2 s (0.84). These results show that, as a whole, the BICAMS is an appropriate tool for evaluating cognitive function in MS patients. This study also further emphasizes the strength of the SDMT as a sensitive and reliable measure.

In addition to the BICAMS, researchers are working on developing other brief cognitive batteries. A brief version of the BRB has been proposed that takes approximately 30 minutes to administer and includes the SDMT, PASAT, and SRT (Hansen et al., 2015). Researchers administered this abbreviated BRB to 127 MS patients and found that sensitivity ranged from 38% to 44% and specificity ranged from 81% to 94% for individual subtests. When combined into a composite score, sensitivity improved to 75% but specificity decreased to 65%. Thus, the brief BRB may be a valid tool to use, but only when all subtests are administered. Another research group selected four measures from the MACFIMS—the BVMT–R, SDMT, DKEFS Card Sorting, and the COWAT—and assessed criterion validity of abbreviated versions of these tests (Gromisch et al., 2016). They reported that BVMT–R Trial 1, a 30 second administration of SDMT, DKEFS Card Sort 1, and letter "F" of the COWAT all had acceptable criterion validity in identifying impairment at −1.5 SD and −2.0 SD on the original versions of these tests. The authors proposed that these four abbreviated measures, along with the first two learning trials of the CVLT–II, could be developed into a brief cognitive battery.

There is a general agreement among experts that there should be ongoing monitoring of cognitive status for MS patients. The next question to ask is: How frequently do we conduct follow-up cognitive assessments? The National Institute for Health and Care Excellence in the United Kingdom recently recommended a routine annual cognitive assessment for MS patients (National Clinical Guideline, 2014). Annual assessments were deemed to be feasible and could potentially be incorporated into the neurological clinic visit. Specifically, annual BICAMS assessments have been recommended as the most efficient and reliable approach to monitoring cognitive status of MS patients (Langdon, 2016).

INTERPRETING COGNITIVE TEST SCORES AND STATISTICAL AND CLINICALLY MEANINGFUL FINDINGS

In 2010, we applied multiple regression analysis to derive regression-based norms for interpreting the MACFIMS (Parmenter, Testa, Schretlen, Weinstock-Guttman, & Benedict, 2010). In brief, the approach first uses a normative sample to develop regression models predicting cognitive test scores on the bases of demographic characteristics. The beta weights from these formulas are then used to demarcate predicted scores, where patient scores would be expected to lie on the basis of the same predictor variables. One tends to find, of course, that MS patients' actual scores tend to differ from the predicted scores, a difference that can be compared to the residuals from the normal group models. In this way, we developed regression-based norms for all of the MACFIMS tests, controlling for standard demographic variables (i.e., age, sex, education). This regression-based approach identified higher rates of impairment than manual-based norms for many of the individual MACFIMS measures. In the future, we intend to use this procedure to help clinicians interpret the BICAMS tests. It is conceivable that a clinician could log on to a website, enter patient demographics and an SDMT score, and instantly receive a z-score equivalent.

A final point concerns our confidence in the ability to detect clinically relevant change using neuropsychological tests. The SDMT may be reliable (Benedict, Smerbeck, et al., 2012), correlated with brain MRI metrics (Benedict & Zivadinov, 2011), and associated with activities of daily living (Benedict et al., 2005), but unless an individual's change on the outcome has inherent or obvious meaning, the result lacks importance (Benedict & Walton, 2012). We have thus endeavored to shed light on the problem by searching for increments of change on SDMT that are associated with marked, easily recognized effects on clinical presentation and work status. In one study (Morrow et al., 2010), 97 employed MS patients were followed over 3.5 years. The core MACFIMS battery covering six domains of cognitive function was used at the start and end of this time period. Deterioration in employment status at follow-up was assigned to patients with paid disability benefits (conservative definition) or reported reduction in hours/work responsibilities (liberal definition). Multiple tests distinguished deteriorating from stable patients. SDMT, however, was most sensitive, and after controlling for demographics and MS disease features, the odds ratio of a deterioration based on a change of 4.0 points was 4.2, 95% confidence interval

[1.2–14.8]. Thus, we might argue that a change of 4 points on SDMT is, in fact, "clinically meaningful." More recently, we established benchmark scores on neuropsychological measures from the MSFC and the BICAMS that are associated with degree of work-related functional impairment in MS patients (Benedict et al., 2016). When evaluated in combination, the Timed 25-Foot Walk and the SDMT were found to be the most robust predictors of functional decline. This is consistent with a previous study that identified benchmark scores on the 25-Foot Walk that were associated with occupational disability, use of a walking cane, and trouble with instrumental activities of daily living (Goldman et al., 2013).

CONCLUSIONS AND FUTURE DIRECTIONS

The process of cognitive evaluation in MS has undergone many changes over the years and continues to evolve. As described in this chapter, the aim of clinicians and researchers is to develop approaches to neuropsychological testing that are readily accessible, cost-effective, and clinically meaningful. In some cases, this may involve a departure from traditional, comprehensive, neuropsychological evaluation, to brief monitoring tools or even remote-access procedures. In our center, we use a brief neuroperformance battery in most patients, for both clinical or research purposes (see Exhibit 1.1). In brief, we evaluate capacity to learn verbal and nonverbal information and then to retain said information over a 25- to 30-minute interval. Between the learning and delayed recall tasks are interspersed measures of ambulation, hand dexterity, and information processing speed, as well as self-report scales assessing fatigue, depression, and employment status. Future work in this area will continue to focus on examining the role of neuropsychological testing in informing clinical management, predicting negative outcomes, and improving quality of life of people with MS.

EXHIBIT 1.1
Brief Neuroperformance Battery Used by Benedict and Colleagues

CVLT–II Learning Trials 1–5	SDMT
CVLT–II Delayed Recall	PASAT 3 s
BVMT–R Learning Trials 1–3	BDI–FS
BVMT–R Delayed Recall	FSS
Timed 25-Foot Walk	MSNQ
Nine Hole Peg Test	Employment Status

Note. BDI–FS = Beck Depression Inventory—Fast Screen; CVLT–II = California Verbal Learning Test—Second Edition; BVMT–R = Brief Visuospatial Memory Test—Revised; FSS = Fatigue Severity Scale; MSNQ = Multiple Sclerosis Neuropsychological Questionnaire; PASAT = Paced Serial Addition Test; SDMT = Symbol Digit Modalities Test.

REFERENCES

Achiron, A., Doniger, G. M., Harel, Y., Appleboim-Gavish, N., Lavie, M., & Simon, E. S. (2007). Prolonged response times characterize cognitive performance in multiple sclerosis. *European Journal of Neurology, 14*, 1102–1108. http://dx.doi.org/10.1111/j.1468-1331.2007.01909.x

Akbar, N., Honarmand, K., Kou, N., & Feinstein, A. (2011). Validity of a computerized version of the symbol digit modalities test in multiple sclerosis. *Journal of Neurology, 258*, 373–379. http://dx.doi.org/10.1007/s00415-010-5760-8

Amato, M. P., Bartolozzi, M. L., Zipoli, V., Portaccio, E., Mortilla, M., Guidi, L., . . . De Stefano, N. (2004). Neocortical volume decrease in relapsing–remitting MS patients with mild cognitive impairment. *Neurology, 63*, 89–93. http://dx.doi.org/10.1212/01.WNL.0000129544.79539.D5

Amato, M. P., Ponziani, G., Pracucci, G., Bracco, L., Siracusa, G., & Amaducci, L. (1995). Cognitive impairment in early-onset multiple sclerosis: Pattern, predictors, and impact on everyday life in a 4-year follow-up. *Archives of Neurology, 52*, 168–172. http://dx.doi.org/10.1001/archneur.1995.00540260072019

Amato, M. P., Ponziani, G., Siracusa, G., & Sorbi, S. (2001). Cognitive dysfunction in early-onset multiple sclerosis: A reappraisal after 10 years. *Archives of Neurology, 58*, 1602–1606. http://dx.doi.org/10.1001/archneur.58.10.1602

Barbizet, J., & Cany, E. (1968). Clinical and psychometrical study of a patient with memory disturbances. *International Journal of Neurology, 7*, 44–54.

Bauer, R. M., Iverson, G. L., Cernich, A. N., Binder, L. M., Ruff, R. M., & Naugle, R. I. (2012). Computerized neuropsychological assessment devices: Joint position paper of the American Academy of Clinical Neuropsychology and the National Academy of Neuropsychology. *The Clinical Neuropsychologist, 26*, 177–196. http://dx.doi.org/10.1080/13854046.2012.663001

Benedict, R. H. B. (1997). *Brief Visuospatial Memory Test—Revised: Professional Manual*. Odessa, FL: Psychological Assessment Resources.

Benedict, R. H. B. (2005). Effects of using same- versus alternate-form memory tests during short-interval repeated assessments in multiple sclerosis. *Journal of the International Neuropsychological Society, 11*, 727–736. http://dx.doi.org/10.1017/S1355617705050782

Benedict, R. H. B., Amato, M. P., Boringa, J., Brochet, B., Foley, F., Fredrikson, S., . . . Langdon, D. (2012). Brief International Cognitive Assessment for MS (BICAMS): International standards for validation. *BMC Neurology, 12*, 55. http://dx.doi.org/10.1186/1471-2377-12-55

Benedict, R. H. B., Cookfair, D., Gavett, R., Gunther, M., Munschauer, F., Garg, N., & Weinstock-Guttman, B. (2006). Validity of the minimal assessment of cognitive function in multiple sclerosis (MACFIMS). *Journal of the International Neuropsychological Society, 12*, 549–558. http://dx.doi.org/10.1017/S1355617706060723

Benedict, R. H. B., Cox, D., Thompson, L. L., Foley, F., Weinstock-Guttman, B., & Munschauer, F. (2004). Reliable screening for neuropsychological impairment in multiple sclerosis. *Multiple Sclerosis, 10*, 675–678. http://dx.doi.org/10.1191/1352458504ms1098oa

Benedict, R. H. B., Drake, A. S., Irwin, L. N., Frndak, S. E., Kunker, K. A., Khan, A. L., . . . Weinstock-Guttman, B. (2016). Benchmarks of meaningful impairment on the MSFC and BICAMS. *Multiple Sclerosis, 22*, 1874–1882. http://dx.doi.org/10.1177/1352458516633517

Benedict, R. H. B., Fischer, J. S., Archibald, C. J., Arnett, P. A., Beatty, W. W., Bobholz, J., . . . Munschauer, F. (2002). Minimal neuropsychological assessment of MS patients: A consensus approach. *The Clinical Neuropsychologist, 16*, 381–397. http://dx.doi.org/10.1076/clin.16.3.381.13859

Benedict, R. H. B., Krupp, L., Francis, G., Rao, S., LaRocca, N., & Langdon, D. (2012). *NINDS common data elements, multiple sclerosis, neuropsychology/cognition recommendations* (MCW Group, Ed.). Washington, DC: National Institute for Neurological Diseases and Stroke.

Benedict, R. H. B., Morrow, S. A., Weinstock Guttman, B., Cookfair, D., & Schretlen, D. J. (2010). Cognitive reserve moderates decline in information processing speed in multiple sclerosis patients. *Journal of the International Neuropsychological Society, 16*, 829–835. http://dx.doi.org/10.1017/S1355617710000688

Benedict, R. H. B., Schretlen, D., Groninger, L., Dobraski, M., & Shpritz, B. (1996). Revision of the Brief Visuospatial Memory Test: Studies of normal performance, reliability, and validity. *Psychological Assessment, 8*, 145–153. http://dx.doi.org/10.1037/1040-3590.8.2.145

Benedict, R. H. B., Smerbeck, A., Parikh, R., Rodgers, J., Cadavid, D., & Erlanger, D. (2012). Reliability and equivalence of alternate forms for the Symbol Digit Modalities Test: Implications for multiple sclerosis clinical trials. *Multiple Sclerosis, 18*, 1320–1325. http://dx.doi.org/10.1177/1352458511435717

Benedict, R. H. B., Wahlig, E., Bakshi, R., Fishman, I., Munschauer, F., Zivadinov, R., & Weinstock-Guttman, B. (2005). Predicting quality of life in multiple sclerosis: Accounting for physical disability, fatigue, cognition, mood disorder, personality, and behavior change. *Journal of the Neurological Sciences, 231*, 29–34. http://dx.doi.org/10.1016/j.jns.2004.12.009

Benedict, R. H. B., & Walton, M. K. (2012). Evaluating cognitive outcome measures for MS clinical trials: What is a clinically meaningful change? *Multiple Sclerosis, 18*, 1673–1679. http://dx.doi.org/10.1177/1352458512454774

Benedict, R. H. B., & Zivadinov, R. (2011). Risk factors for and management of cognitive dysfunction in multiple sclerosis. *Nature Reviews Neurology, 7*, 332–342. http://dx.doi.org/10.1038/nrneurol.2011.61

Benton, A. L., & Hamsher, K. (1989). *Multilingual Aphasia Examination*. Iowa City, IA: AJA Associates.

Benton, A. L., Sivan, A. B., Hamsher, K., Varney, N. R., & Spreen, O. (1994). *Contributions to neuropsychological assessment* (2nd ed.). New York, NY: Oxford University Press.

Bruce, J. M., Hancock, L. M., Arnett, P., & Lynch, S. (2010). Treatment adherence in multiple sclerosis: Association with emotional status, personality, and cognition. *Journal of Behavioral Medicine, 33,* 219–227. http://dx.doi.org/10.1007/s10865-010-9247-y

Buschke, H., & Fuld, P. A. (1974). Evaluating storage, retention, and retrieval in disordered memory and learning. *Neurology, 24,* 1019–1025. http://dx.doi.org/10.1212/WNL.24.11.1019

Caceres, F., Vanotti, S., Benedict, R. H. B., & the RELACCEM Work Group. (2014). Cognitive and neuropsychiatric disorders among multiple sclerosis patients from Latin America: Results of the RELACCEM study. *Multiple Sclerosis and Related Disorders, 3,* 335–340. http://dx.doi.org/10.1016/j.msard.2013.10.007

Carone, D. A., Benedict, R. H. B., Munschauer, F. E., III, Fishman, I., & Weinstock-Guttman, B. (2005). Interpreting patient/informant discrepancies of reported cognitive symptoms in MS. *Journal of the International Neuropsychological Society, 11,* 574–583. http://dx.doi.org/10.1017/S135561770505068X

Chiaravalloti, N. D., & DeLuca, J. (2008). Cognitive impairment in multiple sclerosis. *The Lancet Neurology, 7,* 1139–1151. http://dx.doi.org/10.1016/S1474-4422(08)70259-X

Christodoulou, C., Krupp, L. B., Liang, Z., Huang, W., Melville, P., Roque, C., . . . Peyster, R. (2003). Cognitive performance and MR markers of cerebral injury in cognitively impaired MS patients. *Neurology, 60,* 1793–1798. http://dx.doi.org/10.1212/01.WNL.0000072264.75989.B8

Cohen, J. A., Reingold, S. C., Polman, C. H., Wolinsky, J. S., & the International Advisory Committee on Clinical Trials in Multiple Sclerosis. (2012). Disability outcome measures in multiple sclerosis clinical trials: Current status and future prospects. *The Lancet Neurology, 11,* 467–476. http://dx.doi.org/10.1016/S1474-4422(12)70059-5

Cutter, G. R., Baier, M. L., Rudick, R. A., Cookfair, D. L., Fischer, J. S., Petkau, J., . . . Willoughby, E. (1999). Development of a multiple sclerosis functional composite as a clinical trial outcome measure. *Brain: A Journal of Neurology, 122,* 871–882. http://dx.doi.org/10.1093/brain/122.5.871

Delis, D. C., Kaplan, E., & Kramer, J. H. (2001). *Delis–Kaplan Executive Function System.* San Antonio, TX: The Psychological Corporation.

Delis, D. C., Kramer, J. H., Kaplan, E., & Ober, B. A. (2000). *California Verbal Learning Test* (2nd ed.). San Antonio, TX: The Psychological Corporation.

Drake, A. S., Weinstock-Guttman, B., Morrow, S. A., Hojnacki, D., Munschauer, F. E., & Benedict, R. H. B. (2010). Psychometrics and normative data for the Multiple Sclerosis Functional Composite: Replacing the PASAT with the Symbol Digit Modalities Test. *Multiple Sclerosis, 16,* 228–237. http://dx.doi.org/10.1177/1352458509354552

Dusankova, J. B., Kalincik, T., Havrdova, E., & Benedict, R. H. B. (2012). Cross cultural validation of the Minimal Assessment of Cognitive Function in Multiple Sclerosis (MACFIMS) and the Brief International Cognitive Assessment for Multiple Sclerosis (BICAMS). *The Clinical Neuropsychologist, 26,* 1186–1200. http://dx.doi.org/10.1080/13854046.2012.725101

Edgar, C., Jongen, P. J., Sanders, E., Sindic, C., Goffette, S., Dupuis, M., . . . Wesnes, K. (2011). Cognitive performance in relapsing remitting multiple sclerosis: A longitudinal study in daily practice using a brief computerized cognitive battery. *BMC Neurology, 11,* 68. http://dx.doi.org/10.1186/1471-2377-11-68

Erlanger, D. M., Kaushik, T., Caruso, L. S., Benedict, R. H. B., Foley, F. W., Wilken, J., . . . Deluca, J. (2014). Reliability of a cognitive endpoint for use in a multiple sclerosis pharmaceutical trial. *Journal of the Neurological Sciences, 340,* 123–129. http://dx.doi.org/10.1016/j.jns.2014.03.009

Eshaghi, A., Riyahi-Alam, S., Roostaei, T., Haeri, G., Aghsaei, A., Aidi, M. R., . . . Sahraian, M. A. (2012). Validity and reliability of a Persian translation of the Minimal Assessment of Cognitive Function in Multiple Sclerosis (MACFIMS). *The Clinical Neuropsychologist, 26,* 975–984. http://dx.doi.org/10.1080/13854046.2012.694912

Frndak, S. E., Irwin, L. N., Kordovski, V. M., Milleville, K., Fisher, C., Drake, A. S., & Benedict, R. H. B. (2015). Negative work events reported online precede job loss in multiple sclerosis. *Journal of the Neurological Sciences, 357,* 209–214. http://dx.doi.org/10.1016/j.jns.2015.07.032

Gayet-Ageron, A., Lautenschlager, S., Ninet, B., Perneger, T. V., & Combescure, C. (2013). Sensitivity, specificity and likelihood ratios of PCR in the diagnosis of syphilis: A systematic review and meta-analysis. *Sexually Transmitted Infections, 89,* 251–256. http://dx.doi.org/10.1136/sextrans-2012-050622

Goldman, M. D., Motl, R. W., Scagnelli, J., Pula, J. H., Sosnoff, J. J., & Cadavid, D. (2013). Clinically meaningful performance benchmarks in MS: Timed 25-Foot Walk and the real world. *Neurology, 81,* 1856–1863. http://dx.doi.org/10.1212/01.wnl.0000436065.97642.d2

Grewe, P., Lahr, D., Kohsik, A., Dyck, E., Markowitsch, H. J., Bien, C. G., . . . Piefke, M. (2014). Real-life memory and spatial navigation in patients with focal epilepsy: Ecological validity of a virtual reality supermarket task. *Epilepsy & Behavior, 31,* 57–66. http://dx.doi.org/10.1016/j.yebeh.2013.11.014

Gromisch, E. S., Zemon, V., Holtzer, R., Chiaravalloti, N. D., DeLuca, J., Beier, M., . . . Foley, F. W. (2016). Assessing the criterion validity of four highly abbreviated measures from the Minimal Assessment of Cognitive Function in Multiple Sclerosis (MACFIMS). *The Clinical Neuropsychologist, 30,* 1032–1049. http://dx.doi.org/10.1080/13854046.2016.1189597

Gronwall, D. M. A. (1977). Paced auditory serial-addition task: A measure of recovery from concussion. *Perceptual and Motor Skills, 44,* 367–373. http://dx.doi.org/10.2466/pms.1977.44.2.367

Hansen, S., Muenssinger, J., Kronhofmann, S., Lautenbacher, S., Oschmann, P., & Keune, P. M. (2015). Cognitive screening tools in multiple sclerosis revisited:

Sensitivity and specificity of a short version of Rao's Brief Repeatable Battery. *BMC Neurology, 15,* 246. http://dx.doi.org/10.1186/s12883-015-0497-8

Huijbregts, S. C., Kalkers, N. F., de Sonneville, L. M., de Groot, V., & Polman, C. H. (2006). Cognitive impairment and decline in different MS subtypes. *Journal of the Neurological Sciences, 245,* 187–194. http://dx.doi.org/10.1016/j.jns.2005.07.018

Jacobs, L. D., Wende, K. E., Brownscheidle, C. M., Apatoff, B., Coyle, P. K., Goodman, A., . . . Snyder, D. H. (1999). A profile of multiple sclerosis: The New York State Multiple Sclerosis Consortium. *Multiple Sclerosis, 5,* 369–376. http://dx.doi.org/10.1191/135245899678846302

Kelen, G. D., Shahan, J. B., & Quinn, T. C. (1999). Emergency department-based HIV screening and counseling: Experience with rapid and standard serologic testing. *Annals of Emergency Medicine, 33,* 147–155. http://dx.doi.org/10.1016/S0196-0644(99)70387-2

Kurtzke, J. F. (1983). Rating neurologic impairment in multiple sclerosis: An expanded disability status scale (EDSS). *Annals of Neurology, 33,* 1444–1453.

Lamargue-Hamel, D., Deloire, M., Saubusse, A., Ruet, A., Taillard, J., Philip, P., & Brochet, B. (2015). Cognitive evaluation by tasks in a virtual reality environment in multiple sclerosis. *Journal of the Neurological Sciences, 359,* 94–99. http://dx.doi.org/10.1016/j.jns.2015.10.039

Langdon, D. W. (2016). A useful annual review of cognition in relapsing MS is beyond most neurologists—NO. *Multiple Sclerosis, 22,* 728–730. http://dx.doi.org/10.1177/1352458516640610

Langdon, D. W., Amato, M. P., Boringa, J., Brochet, B., Foley, F., Fredrikson, S., . . . Benedict, R. H. B. (2012). Recommendations for a Brief International Cognitive Assessment for Multiple Sclerosis (BICAMS). *Multiple Sclerosis, 18,* 891–898. http://dx.doi.org/10.1177/1352458511431076

Lapshin, H., Audet, B., & Feinstein, A. (2014). Detecting cognitive dysfunction in a busy multiple sclerosis clinical setting: A computer generated approach. *European Journal of Neurology, 21,* 281–286. http://dx.doi.org/10.1111/ene.12292

Lapshin, H., Lanctôt, K. L., O'Connor, P., & Feinstein, A. (2013). Assessing the validity of a computer-generated cognitive screening instrument for patients with multiple sclerosis. *Multiple Sclerosis, 19,* 1905–1912. http://dx.doi.org/10.1177/1352458513488841

Lapshin, H., O'Connor, P., Lanctôt, K. L., & Feinstein, A. (2012). Computerized cognitive testing for patients with multiple sclerosis. *Multiple Sclerosis and Related Disorders, 1,* 196–201. http://dx.doi.org/10.1016/j.msard.2012.05.001

Lublin, F. D., Reingold, S. C., & National Multiple Sclerosis Society (USA) Advisory Committee on Clinical Trials of New Agents in Multiple Sclerosis. (1996). Defining the clinical course of multiple sclerosis: Results of an international survey. *Neurology, 46,* 907–911. http://dx.doi.org/10.1212/WNL.46.4.907

Migliore, S., Ghazaryan, A., Simonelli, I., Pasqualetti, P., Landi, D., Palmieri, M. G., . . . Filippi, M. M. (2016). Validity of the minimal assessment of cognitive function in multiple sclerosis (MACFIMS) in the Italian population. *Neurological Sciences, 37*, 1261–1270. http://dx.doi.org/10.1007/s10072-016-2578-x

Morrow, S. A., Drake, A., Zivadinov, R., Munschauer, F., Weinstock-Guttman, B., & Benedict, R. H. B. (2010). Predicting loss of employment over three years in multiple sclerosis: Clinically meaningful cognitive decline. *The Clinical Neuropsychologist, 24*, 1131–1145. http://dx.doi.org/10.1080/13854046.2010.511272

National Clinical Guideline. C. (2014). *Multiple sclerosis: Management of multiple sclerosis in primary and secondary care* (National Institute for Health and Care Excellence: Clinical Guidelines). London, England: National Institute for Health and Care Excellence.

Niccolai, C., Portaccio, E., Goretti, B., Hakiki, B., Giannini, M., Pastò, L., . . . Amato, M. P. (2015). A comparison of the brief international cognitive assessment for multiple sclerosis and the brief repeatable battery in multiple sclerosis patients. *BMC Neurology, 15*, 204. http://dx.doi.org/10.1186/s12883-015-0460-8

O'Brien, A., Gaudino-Goering, E., Shawaryn, M., Komaroff, E., Moore, N. B., & DeLuca, J. (2007). Relationship of the Multiple Sclerosis Neuropsychological Questionnaire (MSNQ) to functional, emotional, and neuropsychological outcomes. *Archives of Clinical Neuropsychology, 22*, 933–948. http://dx.doi.org/10.1016/j.acn.2007.07.002

Ontaneda, D., LaRocca, N., Coetzee, T., & Rudick, R. (2012). Revisiting the multiple sclerosis functional composite: Proceedings from the National Multiple Sclerosis Society (NMSS) Task Force on Clinical Disability Measures. *Multiple Sclerosis, 18*, 1074–1080. http://dx.doi.org/10.1177/1352458512451512

Parmenter, B. A., Testa, S. M., Schretlen, D. J., Weinstock-Guttman, B., & Benedict, R. H. B. (2010). The utility of regression-based norms in interpreting the minimal assessment of cognitive function in multiple sclerosis (MACFIMS). *Journal of the International Neuropsychological Society, 16*, 6–16. http://dx.doi.org/10.1017/S1355617709990750

Parmenter, B. A., Weinstock-Guttman, B., Garg, N., Munschauer, F., & Benedict, R. H. B. (2007). Screening for cognitive impairment in multiple sclerosis using the Symbol Digit Modalities Test. *Multiple Sclerosis, 13*, 52–57. http://dx.doi.org/10.1177/1352458506070750

Parmenter, B. A., Zivadinov, R., Kerenyi, L., Gavett, R., Weinstock-Guttman, B., Dwyer, M. G., . . . Benedict, R. H. B. (2007). Validity of the Wisconsin Card Sorting and Delis–Kaplan Executive Function System (DKEFS) Sorting Tests in multiple sclerosis. *Journal of Clinical and Experimental Neuropsychology, 29*, 215–223. http://dx.doi.org/10.1080/13803390600672163

Patti, F., Amato, M. P., Trojano, M., Bastianello, S., Tola, M. R., Goretti, B., . . . the COGIMUS Study Group. (2009). Cognitive impairment and its relation with disease measures in mildly disabled patients with relapsing-remitting multiple sclerosis: Baseline results from the Cognitive Impairment in Multiple Sclerosis (COGIMUS) study. *Multiple Sclerosis, 15,* 779–788. http://dx.doi.org/10.1177/1352458509105544

Rao, S. M. (1991a). *A manual for the Brief, Repeatable Battery of Neuropsychological Tests in Multiple Sclerosis.* Denver, CO: National Multiple Sclerosis Society.

Rao, S. M. (1991b). *Neuropsychological Screening Battery for Multiple Sclerosis.* Denver, CO: National Multiple Sclerosis Society.

Rao, S. M., Leo, G. J., Bernardin, L., & Unverzagt, F. (1991). Cognitive dysfunction in multiple sclerosis. I. Frequency, patterns, and prediction. *Neurology, 41,* 685–691. http://dx.doi.org/10.1212/WNL.41.5.685

Rao, S. M., Leo, G. J., Ellington, L., Nauertz, T., Bernardin, L., & Unverzagt, F. (1991). Cognitive dysfunction in multiple sclerosis. II. Impact on employment and social functioning. *Neurology, 41,* 692–696. http://dx.doi.org/10.1212/WNL.41.5.692

Romero, K., Shammi, P., & Feinstein, A. (2015). Neurologists' accuracy in predicting cognitive impairment in multiple sclerosis. *Multiple Sclerosis and Related Disorders, 4,* 291–295. http://dx.doi.org/10.1016/j.msard.2015.05.009

Roy, S., Schwartz, C. E., Duberstein, P., Dwyer, M. G., Zivadinov, R., Bergsland, N., . . . Benedict, R. H. B. (2016). Synergistic effects of reserve and adaptive personality in multiple sclerosis. *Journal of the International Neuropsychological Society, 22,* 920–927. http://dx.doi.org/10.1017/S1355617716000333

Rudick, R. A., Miller, D., Bethoux, F., Rao, S. M., Lee, J. C., Stough, D., . . . Alberts, J. (2014). The Multiple Sclerosis Performance Test (MSPT): An iPad-based disability assessment tool. *Journal of Visualized Experiments, 88,* e51318.

Schlegel, R. E., & Gilliland, K. (2007). Development and quality assurance of computer-based assessment batteries. *Archives of Clinical Neuropsychology, 22*(Suppl. 1), S49–S61. http://dx.doi.org/10.1016/j.acn.2006.10.005

Sepulcre, J., Vanotti, S., Hernández, R., Sandoval, G., Cáceres, F., Garcea, O., & Villoslada, P. (2006). Cognitive impairment in patients with multiple sclerosis using the Brief Repeatable Battery-Neuropsychology test. *Multiple Sclerosis, 12,* 187–195. http://dx.doi.org/10.1191/1352458506ms1258oa

Settle, J. R., Robinson, S. A., Kane, R., Maloni, H. W., & Wallin, M. T. (2015). Remote cognitive assessments for patients with multiple sclerosis: A feasibility study. *Multiple Sclerosis, 21,* 1072–1079. http://dx.doi.org/10.1177/1352458514559296

Smith, A. (1982). *Symbol Digit Modalities Test: Manual.* Los Angeles, CA: Western Psychological Services.

Strober, L., Englert, J., Munschauer, F., Weinstock-Guttman, B., Rao, S., & Benedict, R. H. B. (2009). Sensitivity of conventional memory tests in multiple sclerosis: Comparing the Rao Brief Repeatable Neuropsychological Battery and the Minimal Assessment of Cognitive Function in MS. *Multiple Sclerosis, 15,* 1077–1084. http://dx.doi.org/10.1177/1352458509106615

Werner, P., Rabinowitz, S., Klinger, E., Korczyn, A. D., & Josman, N. (2009). Use of the virtual action planning supermarket for the diagnosis of mild cognitive impairment: A preliminary study. *Dementia and Geriatric Cognitive Disorders, 27*, 301–309. http://dx.doi.org/10.1159/000204915

Wilken, J. A., Kane, R., Sullivan, C. L., Wallin, M., Usiskin, J. B., Quig, M. E., . . . Keller, M. (2003). The utility of computerized neuropsychological assessment of cognitive dysfunction in patients with relapsing-remitting multiple sclerosis. *Multiple Sclerosis, 9*, 119–127. http://dx.doi.org/10.1191/1352458503ms893oa

Younes, M., Hill, J., Quinless, J., Kilduff, M., Peng, B., Cook, S. D., & Cadavid, D. (2007). Internet-based cognitive testing in multiple sclerosis. *Multiple Sclerosis, 13*, 1011–1019. http://dx.doi.org/10.1177/1352458507077626

Zhang, L., Abreu, B. C., Seale, G. S., Masel, B., Christiansen, C. H., & Ottenbacher, K. J. (2003). A virtual reality environment for evaluation of a daily living skill in brain injury rehabilitation: Reliability and validity. *Archives of Physical Medicine and Rehabilitation, 84*, 1118–1124. http://dx.doi.org/10.1016/S0003-9993(03)00203-X

2

COGNITION AND MULTIPLE SCLEROSIS: THE ROLE OF MAGNETIC RESONANCE IMAGING

QUINTEN VAN GEEST, KIM A. MEIJER, JEROEN J. G. GEURTS, AND HANNEKE E. HULST

Neuroimaging is the most important tool for diagnosing multiple sclerosis (MS; Filippi et al., 2016). Additionally, it allows us to relate neuropsychological changes to in vivo pathological findings in the brain to gain a better understanding of the underlying neurobiological mechanism(s) of cognitive impairment in MS. That is, what changes in brain structure and function relate to cognitive problems? In this chapter, we discuss the most common and promising magnetic resonance imaging (MRI) applications, starting with an elaboration on structural neuroimaging techniques that have been used in the context of cognitive functioning in MS. We then discuss the role of functional neuroimaging techniques.

http://dx.doi.org/10.1037/0000097-003
Cognition and Behavior in Multiple Sclerosis, J. DeLuca and B. M. Sandroff (Editors)

STRUCTURAL BRAIN IMAGING

White Matter Lesions

Demyelination of the white matter (WM; i.e., *lesions*) is the classical pathological hallmark of MS. Since the 1980s, MRI (see Exhibit 2.1 for more information on this technique; see also Table 2.1) has been frequently used to visualize these WM abnormalities in vivo and relate them to physical and cognitive disability. Various conventional MRI sequences can be used to visualize WM lesions (Figure 2.1).

One of the first questions raised was whether WM lesions explained (part of) the cognitive problems frequently seen in MS. Although it was shown that MS patients with moderate to severe cognitive problems had more T2-weighted lesions on MRI than patients with normal cognitive functioning (Medaer et al., 1987), more recent work, based on previous studies, suggested only a weak to moderate relationship between the number of WM lesions and cognitive functioning (Rovaris, Comi, & Filippi, 2006). When lesion location is taken into account, a stronger relationship with specific cognitive dysfunction can be observed than with whole-brain lesion load (i.e., total lesion volume). For example, lesions in the frontal lobe have been related to problems with executive functioning (Wisconsin Card Sorting Test; Arnett et al., 1994). The moderate (at most) correlation between WM lesions and cognitive problems (correlation coefficient [r] of approximately 0.1–0.4) suggests that other brain abnormalities also play an important role in explaining cognitive dysfunction in MS.

Gray Matter Lesions

In addition to lesions in the WM, observations of gray matter (GM) lesions in the post mortem tissue of MS patients has led to the development of specialized MRI sequences to optimally visualize the brain's GM in vivo. One of the most often-used MRI techniques to detect such GM lesions is *double inversion recovery* (DIR; see Exhibit 2.1; Geurts et al., 2005). When a DIR scan is combined with a *phase-sensitive inversion recovery* (PSIR) scan, even more lesions can be detected because the PSIR scan has a higher WM–GM contrast (Nelson et al., 2007). Various studies have linked GM lesions in the cortex and subcortical structures to cognitive problems, which usually results in slightly stronger correlations (approximately 0.4–0.8) than between WM lesions and cognition.

Cortical lesion load and cortical GM volume (discussed in more detail in the next section) have been found to be independent predictors of overall cognitive functioning in MS patients (Calabrese et al., 2009). Also, an

EXHIBIT 2.1
Conventional and Advanced Structural MRI Methods

Conventional MRI techniques

The term *conventional* refers to "standard" magnetic resonance imaging (MRI) sequences, such as T1- and T2-weighted scans, either two- or three-dimensional (see Table 2.1 for an overview of the various MRI techniques and their application in multiple sclerosis [MS]). On a T2-weighted MRI scan, all lesions that have been acquired during the entire life of an MS patient can be seen as hyperintense (i.e., white) "spots" (see Figure 2.1). The volume of all lesions together is often referred to as *lesion load*. These T2-weighted lesions are, however, rather unspecific in terms of underlying pathology. On a T1-weighted MRI scan, the anatomy of the brain (i.e., different brain regions) can be optimally visualized. However, this sequence does not show all white matter (WM) lesions. A subset of the lesions can appear as hypointensities, also known as *black holes*, indicating axonal loss. Furthermore, it is possible to visualize acute inflammatory processes by administration of a contrast agent (gadolinium). Gadolinium (or a related contrast agent) can "leak" into the brain at these areas where the blood–brain barrier is disrupted due to inflammatory processes. Gadolinium is hyperintense on a T1-weighted MRI scan due to iron particles and, in a healthy condition, cannot enter the brain.

Because of the clear anatomical representation of T1-weighted scans, they are used to segment and calculate the volume of specific tissue types to estimate the severity of atrophy (see Color Plate 1). Atrophy of the cortex can be expressed in changes in volume (measured in milliliters) and cortical thickness (measured in millimeters). Cortical thickness can be measured by the automated detection of the WM and gray matter (GM) border and the outside of the brain, on which vertices are placed. Next, the distance between these vertices can be calculated as a measure of cortical thickness. Subcortical atrophy can be measured by calculating the volume of (specific) GM structures after (automated) segmentation.

Advanced MRI techniques

Double Inversion Recovery

The double inversion recovery (DIR) technique is an MRI sequence that suppresses signals from both the WM and cerebrospinal fluid (CSF), resulting in high-contrast images in which GM is optimally visualized (Geurts et al., 2005). Abnormalities in the GM of MS patients, such as cortical lesions, can be visualized as hyperintense spots on a DIR scan (see Figure 2.1).

Phase-Sensitive Inversion Recovery

The phase-sensitive inversion recovery (PSIR) scan is a high-contrast T1-weighted image. Because of the better delineation of GM and WM compared with conventional T1-weighted scans, it can be used to detect GM abnormalities, such as lesions (Hou, Hasan, Sitton, Wolinsky, & Narayana, 2005). Moreover, it has been suggested that PSIR is more sensitive than DIR in detecting new cortical lesions in primary progressive MS patients over time (Harel et al., 2016).

Diffusion Tensor Imaging

Diffusion tensor imaging (DTI) is an MRI technique that measures diffusion of water molecules in the brain and is mostly used to investigate the integrity of the WM (although it can also be used to investigate GM). The diffusivity of the water molecules can be quantified for each voxel and expressed in four measures: *axial diffusivity* (i.e., diffusivity along the axon), *radial diffusivity* (i.e., diffusivity perpendicular

(continues)

EXHIBIT 2.1
Conventional and Advanced Structural MRI Methods *(Continued)*

to the axon), *mean diffusivity* (i.e., average diffusion), and *fractional anisotropy* (FA; i.e., a summary measure that quantifies the degree of anisotropy [directionality] of diffusion). Intact WM restricts the diffusion of water along the axons, resulting in high directionality of water diffusion. However, in MS, diffusion of water also occurs in other directions (e.g., perpendicular on the axon) because of damage to the WM, resulting in decreased directionality of water diffusion.

Magnetic Resonance Spectroscopy

Magnetic resonance spectroscopy (MRS) can detect metabolites in (brain) tissue and its changes due to pathology. Different metabolites (e.g., N-acetylaspartate, creatine, glutamate, gamma-aminobutyric acid) show different magnetic properties that can be picked up by MRS and expressed in a spectrum. This spectrum displays peaks indicating certain brain metabolites and can be used to calculate (relative) levels of metabolites of interest (e.g., glutamate/creatine ratio).

increase in GM lesions over a period of 3 years has been associated with worse cognitive performance in patients with MS (Roosendaal et al., 2009). When differentiating cognitively preserved from cognitively impaired patients, based on performance on a neuropsychological test battery, differences in the number of cortical lesions, but not in WM and contrast-enhanced lesions, can be observed (Calabrese et al., 2009). That is, cognitively impaired patients had a higher cortical lesion load and more cortical atrophy than cognitively preserved patients. Zooming in, lesions in the hippocampus, a structure important for verbal and visuospatial memory, were related ($r = .68$) to impaired visuospatial memory (Location Learning Test; LLT; Roosendaal et al., 2009).

TABLE 2.1
Summary of MRI Techniques and Their Application in Multiple Sclerosis

Technique	Based on	Used for
T2-weighted MRI	T2 relaxation time (hydrogen spin)	Detection of WM lesions
T1-weighted MRI	T1 relaxation time (hydrogen spin)	Detection of black holes and atrophy measures
Double inversion recovery	Suppression of WM and cerebrospinal fluid	Detection of GM lesions
Phase-sensitive inversion recovery	T1 relaxation time (hydrogen spin)	Detection of GM lesions
Diffusion tensor imaging (DTI)	Diffusion of water molecules	Quantification of WM integrity
Magnetic resonance spectroscopy (MRS)	Different magnetic properties of metabolites	Quantification of brain metabolites

Note. GM = gray matter; MRI = magnetic resonance imaging; WM = white matter.

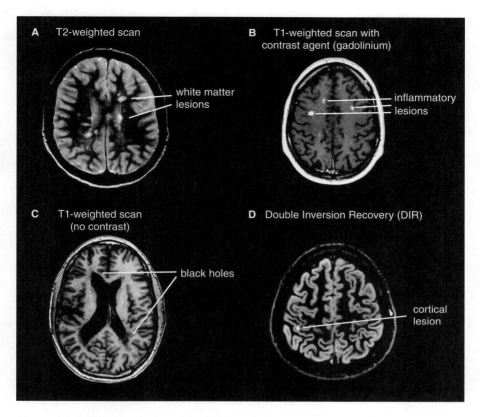

Figure 2.1. MS lesions in the white (WM) and gray matter (GM). Different magnetic resonance imaging (MRI) sequences can be used to visualize lesions in the white and gray matter. (A) A T2-weighted scan that shows WM lesions as areas with hyperintense signal. (B) A T1-weighted scan with intravenous gadolinium (contrast agent) to visualize acute inflammatory lesions in the WM. These inflammatory lesions can be seen due to disruption of the blood–brain barrier that allows contrast agent to leak in. This will be visible as hyperintensity. (C) Another T1-weighted MRI scan, but now without intravenous contrast. Part of the WM lesions are visible on this scan as hypointensity, which are termed *black holes*. Black holes can reflect edema (associated with acute inflammation), which will resolve eventually, or neuronal loss when persistently present. Note that not all WM lesions on a T2-weighted scan will be visible as black holes on a T1-weighted scan because not all T2-weighted lesions show signs of axonal loss. (D) A double inversion recovery sequence on which GM lesions (in this case, in the cortex) can be seen as hyperintensities.

Other studies have found similar results concerning the relationship between GM lesions and cognitive functioning (Mike et al., 2011). Therefore, cortical lesions seem to be a better predictor for cognitive impairment than WM lesions, although it also depends on the cognitive domain that is being investigated. For example, WM lesions, but not cortical lesions, have been related to problems in information processing speed (Symbol Digit Modalities Test

[SDMT]; Rao et al., 2014). Technical advances in hardware and image analysis software have enabled us to better investigate GM lesions in MS. That is, ultra-high-field MRI (7 Tesla) can detect relatively small lesions in the GM because of its higher spatial resolution than 1.5 and 3 Tesla. However, on ultra-high-field MRI, the relationship between cortical lesions and cognitive functioning remains moderate (Harrison et al., 2015). Hence, one can question whether visualizing more GM lesions will make a substantial difference in terms of a better understanding of cognitive decline. That is, the tip of the iceberg, which can be visualized with techniques currently available, might be a good representative for the whole iceberg (Seewann et al., 2012). This suggests that being able to detect more cortical lesions does not necessarily mean that we better understand cognitive problems in MS.

To summarize, lesions characteristic for MS (both in the WM and GM) generally show weak to modest correlations with cognitive functioning. This suggests that other disease-specific changes might be more informative in understanding the underlying mechanisms of cognitive problems.

Brain Atrophy

Brain atrophy is a central hallmark of neurodegenerative diseases. In the late 1970s, several studies used *computerized tomography* (CT; consecutive X-ray scans) to investigate brain atrophy in MS (Cala, Mastaglia, & Black, 1978). At that time, atrophy was usually defined as increased ventricular width, which correlated with worse performance on a neuropsychological test battery measuring verbal intelligence and memory (Rao et al., 1985). The widening of ventricles can occur when WM volume decreases, thereby "pulling" the ventricular walls in an outward (lateral) direction. This process is also termed *central atrophy*. However, it has to be taken into account that ventricular width is not a direct measure of pure WM atrophy because volume loss of deep GM may also play a role. MRI soon replaced CT because it provides a better spatial resolution and higher signal-to-noise ratio and therefore can measure atrophy more accurately (Runge et al., 2015). At first, ventricular width was still used in MRI as a measure of atrophy, but advances in image analysis techniques enabled (semi)-automatic segmentation of WM, GM, and cerebrospinal fluid, allowing calculation of their volumes. This offered opportunities for scientists to zoom in on tissue loss specific to the GM and WM and its effect on cognitive functioning.

In MS, the annualized whole-brain atrophy rate is approximately 3 times higher than in the normal (healthy) aging population (Vollmer et al., 2015). On average, patients show 0.7% brain loss per year, compared with 0.1% to 0.3% brain loss per year in healthy individuals (Vollmer et al., 2015). Atrophy can already be observed during the early phases of MS (Brex et al.,

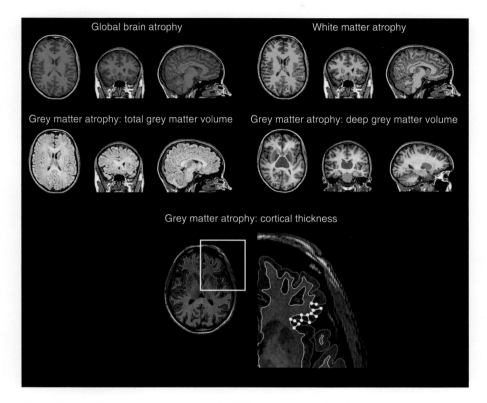

Color Plate 1. Brain atrophy measures. Different types of brain atrophy measures can be calculated by (semi)automatic tissue segmentation software. (a) Segmentation of the entire brain (red), indicating whole-brain atrophy. (b) Segmentation of the white matter (WM; blue), enabling the quantification of WM atrophy. (c) Segmentation of the cortical and subcortical grey matter (GM; yellow), enabling measurement of GM atrophy. (d) Segmentation of deep GM structures, enabling calculation of the volume of GM structures separately. Each color indicates a different subcortical brain region from which the volume can be obtained. (e) Cortical thickness measure. The WM/GM border (yellow line), as well as the outside of the brain (red line), is automatically delineated. Next, vertices are placed on these boundaries, and the distance between vertices is measured to calculate the thickness of the cortex.

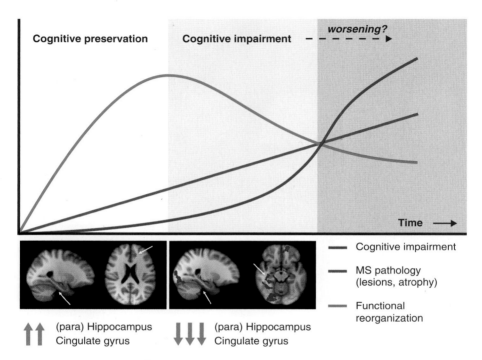

Color Plate 2. The proposed cognitive effects of functional reorganization. Cognitively preserved patients (lightest gray box, left) show only limited structural damage (blue line). It is hypothesized that "functional reorganization" is initially triggered by the presence of multiple sclerosis pathology to maintain cognitive functions. Over time, the degree of structural damage is accumulating. This increase in structural damage limits the possibility for functional reorganization and leads to cognitive impairment (middle and right gray box).

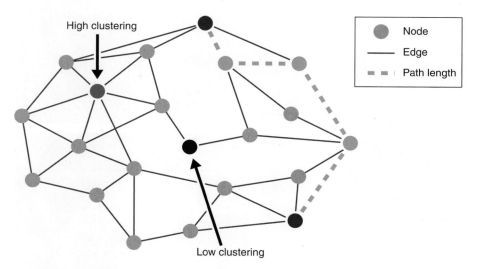

Color Plate 3. Graphical representation of a network (i.e., graph). Network measures are shown in a graph with nodes (gray dots) and edges (gray lines). Some of the nodes are characterized by a high level of clustering (red) and others by a low level of clustering (blue). The distance between two nodes is referred to as the path length (green dotted line).

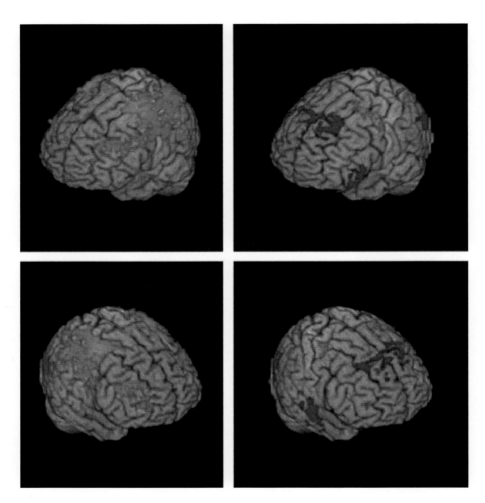

Color Plate 4. Activation map during modified Symbol Digit Modalities Test showing reduced activation in individuals with multiple sclerosis compared with healthy control subjects. From "Examination of Processing Speed Deficits in Multiple Sclerosis Using Functional Magnetic Resonance Imaging," by H. M. Genova, F. G. Hillary, G. Wylie, B. Rypma, and J. Deluca, 2009, *Journal of International Neuropsychological Society, 15*, p. 387. Copyright 2009 by Cambridge University Press. Reprinted with permission.

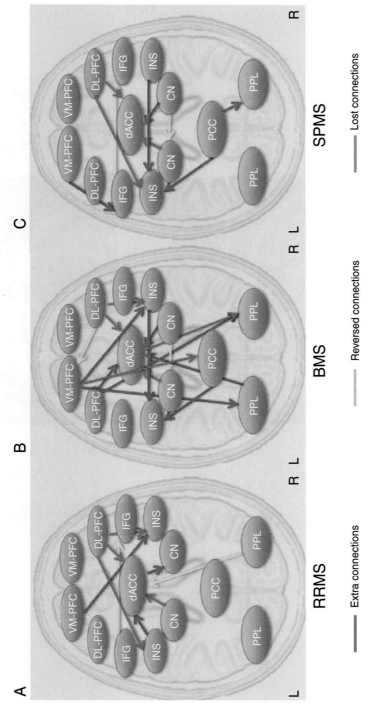

Color Plate 5. A depiction of extra (red), reversed (yellow), and lost (gray) connections in the three groups of participants with multiple sclerosis. From "Abnormalities of the Executive Control Network in Multiple Sclerosis Phenotypes: An fMRI Effective Connectivity Study," by E. Dobryakova, M. A. Rocca, P. Valsasina, A. Ghezzi, B. Colombo, V. Martinelli, . . . M. Filippi, 2016, *Human Brain Mapping Journal, 37,* p. 8. Copyright 2016 by John Wiley and Sons. Reprinted with permission.

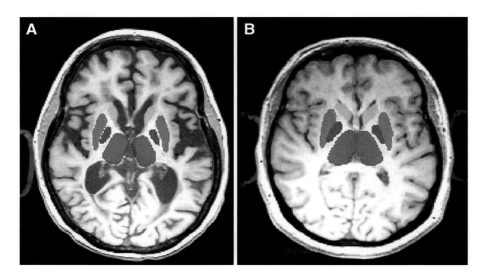

Color Plate 6. Representative image of deep gray matter structures (A) in a patient with relapsing–remitting multiple sclerosis and (B) in an age- and sex-matched healthy control subject. From "Basal Ganglia, Thalamus and Neocortical Atrophy Predicting Slowed Cognitive Processing in Multiple Sclerosis," by S. Batista, R. Zivadinov, M. Hoogs, N. Bergsland, M. Heininen-Brown, M. G. Dwyer, . . . R. H. B. Benedict, 2012, *Journal of Neurology*, *259*, p. 141. Copyright 2012 by Springer. Reprinted with permission.

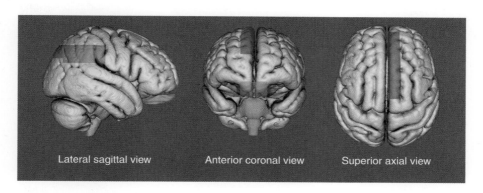

Lateral sagittal view   Anterior coronal view   Superior axial view

Color Plate 7. Brain regions implicated in the neural circuitry of pseudobulbar affect. Blue = inferior parietal; green = medial inferior frontal; red = medial superior frontal; pink = brain stem.

2000) and can predict conversion from clinically isolated syndrome (prestage of MS) to definite MS (Dalton et al., 2004). Furthermore, different "types" of brain atrophy can be distinguished and observed in MS (Color Plate 1), including *global brain atrophy* (i.e., loss of total amount of brain tissue), *WM atrophy* (i.e., loss of WM, sometimes denoted as widening of the ventricles; central atrophy), and GM *atrophy* (i.e., loss of cortical and subcortical GM).

Global Brain Atrophy

Measures of whole-brain volume and brain parenchymal fraction (i.e., ratio of brain tissue to the total volume within the brain surface contour) are relatively gross measures of atrophy because one cannot distinguish between specific loss of WM and GM. Nevertheless, cross-sectional studies in MS have related lower total brain volume to worse performance on various cognitive domains, including visuospatial memory (Spatial Recall Test), information processing speed (SDMT), sustained attention and working memory (Paced Auditory Serial Addition Test [PASAT]), verbal fluency (Word List Generation), abstract reasoning (Standard Raven Progressive Matrices), verbal memory (California Verbal Learning Test [CVLT]) and attention and inhibition (Stroop), with correlation coefficients ranging from 0.3 to 0.8 (Locatelli, Zivadinov, Grop, & Zorzon, 2004; Vollmer et al., 2016). Similar to lesion load, the strength of the correlations between atrophy and cognitive functioning does not differ between 1.5 or 3 Tesla MRI (Chu et al., 2016).

A large downside of cross-sectional studies on brain volume loss is that atrophy is not fully captured because this is, per definition, a process over time. Therefore, longitudinal studies provide a more accurate view on the relationship between atrophy and cognitive functioning. In general, atrophy correlates more strongly with cognitive functioning than, for example, lesion load, a phenomenon that is already present early in the disease (Zivadinov et al., 2001).

Although a reduction in global brain volume over time correlates with cognitive functioning, one can argue that, especially for cognitive functioning, preferential loss in the WM or GM may be more informative to explain impairment in specific cognitive domains.

WM Atrophy

Only a few studies have focused solely on WM loss; these showed that, in contrast to brain parenchymal fraction, ventricular width correlated negatively (*r* of approximately –0.3) with verbal learning and memory (CVLT; Hildebrandt et al., 2006). Other studies replicated this negative correlation between ventricular width and the performance on tests assessing verbal learning and memory (Benedict et al., 2006) but also found a negative association with information processing speed (SDMT) and sustained attention and working memory (PASAT; Benedict et al., 2006). A study that more accurately estimated WM volume by using (automated) software also found that lower WM volume could be related to worse verbal learning and memory (Selective Reminding Test [SRT]; $r = .5$; Sacco et al., 2015).

A longitudinal study that predicted cognitive functioning over a period of 7 years, using MRI data from baseline and Year 2, found that a decrease in memory function (as measured with the SRT and Spatial Recall Test) was related to an increase in ventricular width in the first 2 years (Deloire et al., 2011). Additionally, reductions in information processing speed (SDMT) were predicted by an increase in ventricular width and a decrease in brain parenchymal fraction (Deloire et al., 2011). A specific WM bundle important for information transfer between both hemispheres is the corpus callosum. Damage to this bundle has been related to cognitive problems in MS (Lin, Tench, Morgan, & Constantinescu, 2008). Atrophy of the corpus callosum over a period of 9 years (Bergendal et al., 2013) and 17 years (Granberg et al., 2015) has been investigated in relationship with information processing speed (SDMT) performance. Baseline corpus callosum volume was strongly correlated with information processing speed at Year 17 ($r = 0.8$; Granberg et al., 2015), whereas in the other study, no such correlation analysis was performed (i.e., correlating baseline volume with performance at Year 9). The WM can be seen as the structural connection between remote GM regions that enables information flow through the brain, and thus WM abnormalities are often related to MS-related problems with information processing speed.

GM Atrophy

In past decades, it became clear that MS is not solely an inflammatory WM disease but also includes a major neurodegenerative component that plays an important role in the disease course (Stys, Zamponi, van Minnen, & Geurts, 2012). When the disease progresses, it seems that especially GM atrophy rate increases relative to that of the WM and also relates more strongly to physical disability (Fisniku et al., 2008). Hence, the main focus shifted from WM pathology toward GM damage with regard to physical and cognitive disability. GM can refer to the *cortex* as well as the *subcortical* or *deep* GM structures. As one can imagine, damage to cortical and subcortical GM can severely affect neuronal signaling and might therefore be closely related to cognitive symptoms in MS (Geurts, Calabrese, Fisher, & Rudick, 2012; van Munster, Jonkman, Weinstein, Uitdehaag, & Geurts, 2015).

Cortical Atrophy

Several studies have shown that cognitively impaired MS patients have lower total GM volume (cortical and subcortical) compared with cognitively preserved patients (Roosendaal et al., 2011), whereas other studies only found differences in cortical volume (Calabrese et al., 2009; Riccitelli et al., 2011). Regional changes in cortical volume usually relate to specific cognitive problems. For example, atrophy of frontal regions correlates negatively with information processing speed (SDMT; Nocentini et al., 2014; Tekok-Kilic et al., 2007), sustained attention and working memory (PASAT; Steenwijk et al., 2016; Tekok-Kilic et al., 2007), verbal learning and memory (CVLT; Nocentini et al., 2014; Tekok-Kilic et al., 2007) and visual episodic memory (Brief Visuospatial Memory Test [BVMT]; Tekok-Kilic et al., 2007). Interestingly, one study observed a pattern of frontotemporal thinning in cognitively preserved patients versus healthy control subjects, which might suggest that cortical thinning starts in these regions, whereas cognitively impaired patients showed thinning of the entire cortex (Calabrese et al., 2010). Additionally, atrophy of the parietal cortex can be related to slower information processing speed (PASAT; Morgen et al., 2006) and temporal cortex atrophy is negatively correlated with performance on information processing speed (SDMT) and a test for verbal memory (CVLT; Nocentini et al., 2014). Although in general the pattern of cortical atrophy in MS seems to be random, it has been suggested that, at least for long-standing MS, various cortical atrophy patterns can be observed on top of global cortical thinning (Steenwijk et al., 2016). In turn, these atrophy patterns, including the frontal, temporal, and cingulate cortex, were related to worse performance on tests assessing information processing speed (SDMT), attention (Stroop), executive functioning (Concept Shifting Task and Word List Generation), and visuospatial memory (Spatial Recall Test; Steenwijk et al., 2016). It remains to be investigated whether cortical atrophy indeed follows a certain pattern over time, by using longitudinal studies.

Subcortical Atrophy—The Thalamus and Hippocampus Highlighted

Deep GM structures that have often been studied in the context of cognitive dysfunction in MS include, among others, the thalamus and hippocampus. Although the hippocampus is officially part of the cortex, we categorized it as deep GM in this chapter for the sake of clarity. The main reason for particular focus on the thalamus and hippocampus is twofold. First, the thalamus and hippocampus play an important role in global integration of (cognitive) information and memory function, respectively. Second, histopathological studies have found pronounced pathology in these structures, such as lesions and neuronal loss (Geurts et al., 2007), which, in case of the hippocampus, has been linked to cognitive decline (Geurts et al., 2007). Other deep GM structures (e.g., caudate nucleus and amygdala) are also involved in MS (Popescu et al., 2016). However, their link with (specific) cognitive problems seems to be less strong compared with that of the thalamus and hippocampus and is therefore not discussed in this section.

Thalamus. The thalamus is an old structure located at the most medial part of the brain and acts as a relay station for incoming information. That is, incoming information projects to the thalamus, which in turn conveys information to remote cortical brain regions for further processing, making it one of the key players in terms of cognitive functioning. Damage to this structure is thought to influence the function of other brain regions and efficiency of information transfer, thereby having a large effect on clinical disability in MS, including cognitive functioning (Minagar et al., 2013).

Only in the past decade have studies selectively focused on specific brain structures to explain cognitive functioning in MS. The thalamus was found to be highly important in understanding cognitive deficits in MS, showing moderate to strong correlations ($r = .5–.7$) between thalamic atrophy and impaired performance on all cognitive tests of the Minimal Assessment of Cognitive Function in Multiple Sclerosis (MACFIMS; Houtchens et al., 2007). Various studies have replicated the relationship between thalamus atrophy and cognitive problems, including performance on tests of verbal memory (CVLT; Benedict et al., 2013), visuospatial memory (BVMT, Rey Complex Figure Test; Benedict et al., 2013; Debernard et al., 2015), information processing speed (SDMT; Batista et al., 2012; R. H. Benedict et al., 2013; Debernard et al., 2015), sustained attention and working memory (PASAT; Batista et al., 2012; Debernard et al., 2015), executive functioning (Delis–Kaplan Executive Function System Sorting Test and Wisconsin Card Sorting Test; Benedict et al., 2013; Debernard et al., 2015), and average cognitive performance (Schoonheim, Popescu, et al., 2012).

Hippocampus. The hippocampus is located in the medial temporal lobe and plays a central role in verbal and visuospatial memory. In MS tissue, lesions and extensive demyelination of the hippocampus can be observed, especially in the CA1 subregion of the hippocampus (Geurts et al., 2007). In vivo, with the availability of DIR, hippocampal lesions can be detected in MS, and the number of hippocampal lesions has been related to problems with visuospatial memory (LLT) performance (Roosendaal et al., 2009). Atrophy of the hippocampus can already be observed in patients with a short disease duration and intact visuospatial memory function (LLT; Roosendaal, Hulst, et al., 2010). As the disease progresses, hippocampal atrophy becomes more pronounced. That is, in SPMS the hippocampus is smaller than in relapsing–remitting MS (RRMS; Sicotte et al., 2008). Furthermore, hippocampal atrophy can be linked to worse performance on verbal memory (SRT, word-pair learning task, CVLT; Koenig et al., 2014; Sacco et al., 2015; Sicotte et al., 2008), visuospatial memory (BVMT; Koenig et al., 2014) and information processing speed (SDMT; Koenig et al., 2014).

To summarize, correlation coefficients between atrophy and cognitive functioning (ranging between 0.3 and 0.8) seem to be higher than those between WM lesion load and cognitive functioning (r ranging between .1 and .4). This is particularly evident for (regional) cortical and subcortical GM atrophy, with a focus on the thalamus and hippocampus, because atrophy of those structures is closely related to impaired cognitive functioning on various cognitive domains. However, not all variation in cognitive dysfunction can be explained by atrophy alone or in combination with lesion load. Hence, more sophisticated MRI techniques might provide additional information on the underlying brain mechanisms involved in cognitive dysfunction.

ADVANCED STRUCTURAL IMAGING TECHNIQUES

Advanced imaging techniques offer unique opportunities to further quantify specific (pathological) processes that might help to better understand cognitive problems in MS. For example, *diffusion tensor imaging* (DTI) and *magnetic resonance spectroscopy* (MRS) have been applied in the field of MS and cognition (for more information on these techniques, see Exhibit 2.1).

Diffusion Tensor Imaging

A more subtle measure of MS pathology, compared with lesions and atrophy, is the integrity of the tissue, which can be measured using DTI. With regard to cognitive performance, it has been demonstrated that cognitively impaired patients display more extensive and severe WM damage in cognitively relevant WM tracts compared with cognitively preserved MS patients (Hulst et al., 2013; Meijer et al., 2016; Schoonheim et al., 2014). These WM tracts include the corpus callosum, thalamic radiation, uncinate fasciculus, superior longitudinal fasciculus, and forceps minor. Additionally, slower information processing speed (SDMT; Yu et al., 2012) and poor sustained attention and working memory (PASAT; Dineen et al., 2009) have been related to lower WM integrity of various tracts, including the corpus callosum, whereas verbal memory (CVLT) and visuospatial memory (BVMT) can be related to damage in, among other tracts, the cingulum, forceps major, and inferior longitudinal fasciculus (Dineen et al., 2009). DTI also offers the opportunity to focus on specific WM tracts. For example, damage to specific corticothalamic tracts, including the occipitothalamic tract, has been found to affect global cognitive functioning, whereas spatial memory problems were related to motor-thalamic and temporothalamic tracts (connecting thalamic subregions with frontal and temporal areas; Bisecco et al., 2015). Taken together, these results suggest that regional WM damage, in terms of decreased integrity, can be related to specific cognitive problems.

Magnetic Resonance Spectroscopy

Using MRS, molecular changes in vivo can be measured and linked to cognitive performance. For example, it was found that MS patients with impaired auditory selective attention (dichotic listening test) have axonal damage in the locus coeruleus, a structure important for attention, memory, and arousal, reflected by an increased N-acetylaspartate/creatine ratio (Gadea et al., 2004). Also, higher levels of glutamate in the hippocampus and cingulate cortex were related to better visuospatial memory function in patients (r between 0.5 and 0.6) but not in healthy control participants (Muhlert et al., 2014). To summarize, it seems that molecular changes can be related to cognitive functioning.

Where conventional MRI techniques (WM and GM lesions) show weak to moderate correlations with cognitive functioning in MS, more advanced imaging techniques provide stronger correlations with cognition. At the same time, using more advanced neuroimaging measures will provide additional, or sometimes complementary, information about pathological processes related to cognitive dysfunction. Next to the structural brain changes, it is important to focus on the relationship between cognitive deficits and functional brain changes. The next section discusses the functional changes that are associated with cognitive decline in MS.

Functional Brain Imaging

Besides the previously described structural MRI measures, functional MRI (fMRI) measures could also help us to better understand the underlying mechanisms of cognitive decline in MS. Functional neuroimaging techniques can be used to examine the impact of disease-related tissue damage on brain function. In this section, the relationship between cognitive deficits in MS and findings from functional neuroimaging studies is described. The interpretation of these findings is discussed more extensively in Chapter 3 of this volume. Only conclusions drawn by the authors of the described studies are shortly mentioned in this chapter.

INTRODUCTION TO FUNCTIONAL BRAIN
IMAGING METHODS

In our brain, the activity of neurons constantly fluctuates as one engages in different activities, from simple tasks, such as controlling your hand, to complex cognitive activities, such as memorizing a grocery list.

The knowledge that MRI could be made sensitive to brain activity is only about 25 years old. Seiji Ogawa and colleagues (1992) provided proof-of-concept in 1992, after an experiment demonstrated that an increase in neural activity was accompanied with a small increase in MR signal. Today it is known that fMRI maps the change in the level of blood oxygenation via the blood oxygen level–dependent contrast (Exhibit 2.2).

Within the functional neuroimaging field, a distinction can be made between task-related fMRI and resting-state fMRI. In other words, brain function can be investigated either during the performance of certain cognitive tasks (i.e., task-related fMRI) or in a so-called rest condition (i.e., resting-state fMRI). The most commonly used task-related fMRI experiment is a paradigm that alternates between periods of performing a particular task and a control state, such as looking at a visual stimulus. The images acquired during the task are then subtracted from those acquired when not performing the task (i.e., control condition) to determine which brain regions show signal changes that may indicate neuronal activity. Resting-state fMRI experiments measure the brain activity during the so-called resting-state and are therefore not influenced by task performance, which may differ from that of healthy subjects or other patient groups. Subjects are usually instructed to lie in the scanner with their eyes closed and not to think of anything in particular. Whether to use resting-state fMRI or task-based fMRI to investigate brain function depends highly on the research question.

Next to mapping activity of brain regions, it is possible to measure how well brain regions are connected to each other. Functional connectivity is defined as the temporal dependence of activity patterns of anatomically separated brain regions (Sporns, Chialvo, Kaiser, & Hilgetag, 2004) and can be analyzed in various ways (see Exhibit 2.2). These patterns of correlated activity (i.e., functional connectivity) in the human brain reflect functional communication between neuronal populations (Shmuel & Leopold, 2008).

Task-Related Functional Brain Activation

Shortly after the observation of expanded brain activation during a simple motor task (e.g., a finger-tapping paradigm) in MS patients with normal motor function compared with healthy subjects (Reddy et al., 2000),

EXHIBIT 2.2.
Functional MRI Methods

Functional magnetic resonance imaging (fMRI) is based on the assumption that cerebral blood flow is indirectly linked to neuronal activity (it is important to note that it does not directly measure neuronal activity). When a brain area is more active, it needs more oxygen, and therefore, the blood flow increases to this area (Friston, Jezzard, & Turner, 1994). Oxygen is delivered to neurons by hemoglobin in capillary red blood cells. Hemoglobin has different magnetic properties in its oxygenated and deoxygenated forms. Hemoglobin without bound oxygen molecules (i.e., deoxy-hemoglobin) is paramagnetic, whereas oxygen-bound hemoglobin (i.e., oxyhemoglobin) is diamagnetic. The various magnetic properties of hemoglobin lead to magnetic signal variation that can be detected using a MRI scanner.

Several fMRI analysis techniques are based on this hemodynamic response. The level of activity of brain regions is most commonly assessed by task-based fMRI paradigms. The functional communication between regions is measured by computing the degree of functional connectivity between regions. The most commonly applied methods to do so are the analysis of (a) so-called resting-state networks and (b) specific regions of interest (i.e., seed-based analysis). Independent component analysis (ICA) is a data-driven, whole-brain approach that can separate the brain into several resting-state networks. This is based on the assumption that the statistical independence of the blood oxygen level–dependent contrast (BOLD) signal is decomposed into temporally and spatially distinct maps. These maps represent resting-state networks that share similar BOLD fluctuations over time. The best-known resting-state networks are the default mode, frontoparietal, sensorimotor, and visual and executive resting-state networks (Smith et al., 2009). Seed-based analyses explore the changes in connectivity from a prespecified region of interest with other regions in the brain (van den Heuvel & Hulshoff Pol, 2010). The level of functional connectivity is defined independently of whether the connectivity was changed from Region A to Region B or the other way around. To explore whether the communication from Region A to Region B is disturbed, so-called effective connectivity can be computed that refers explicitly to the influence that one neural system exerts over another. Functional connectivity and effective connectivity require different procedural and statistical implications for data analysis (Stephan & Friston, 2010).

The brain can be also analyzed as one large complex network. Complex networks can be examined by using "graph theory" (Color Plate 3). A graph (or network) is a basic representation of a network consisting of a collection of nodes (or vertices) and links (or edges or connections) interconnecting the nodes of the graph (Stam & Reijneveld, 2007). This mathematical method can be used to gain a better understanding of the topological organization of the brain. In functional brain networks, the nodes will be defined according to the anatomical location of brain regions, whereas the functional connectivity among these regions represents the links. The cluster coefficient and the path length are describing factors of a graph. The cluster coefficient reflects the local interconnectedness of the graph, whereas the path length is an indicator of its overall connectedness (Stam & Reijneveld, 2007).

---

the question arose as to whether such changes in activity patterns could also be observed when MS patients are performing cognitive tasks. The first task-related fMRI studies used the PASAT to measure cognitive function in MS patients. Including the PASAT was advantageous because the PASAT has been included in the Multiple Sclerosis Functional Composite score (i.e., composite score for clinical disability) and has long been recommended as an outcome measure in clinical trials for cognitive evaluation of MS patients (Cutter et al., 1999). This cognitive task requires working memory, sustained attention and information processing speed—processes that are frequently impaired in MS (Chiaravalloti & DeLuca, 2008). In MS patients, during the performance of the PASAT, two phenomena were observed: (a) increased activation of regions also activated in healthy subjects in response to the task and (b) recruitment of additional areas that were not attributed to the task in healthy subjects. Despite these differences in activation patterns, patients did not differ on task performance compared with healthy subjects (Staffen et al., 2002). These findings were replicated in other studies, although next to the patterns of increased activation, some studies also reported recruitment of additional regions during PASAT performance in early MS patients (Audoin et al., 2005) and RRMS patients (Mainero et al., 2004) with no or only mild cognitive impairment. In general, it seems that in early MS patients with no or minimal cognitive impairment, PASAT performance was consistently associated with increased activation of frontoparietal brain areas, which was expected on the basis of the origin of the task. When the patients were categorized according to their PASAT performance during fMRI, the level of activation was higher in the patients, whose performance was similar or even higher than that of healthy subjects, than the patients with PASAT scores lower than the healthy subjects (Mainero et al., 2004). These findings argue in favor of the existence of adaptive compensatory activations that contribute to maintenance of cognitive functions in early MS patients. The study design of comparing task-related activation patterns of cognitively preserved patients to cognitively impaired patients is commonly used and also applied to study the brain activation patterns during other cognitive paradigms.

During an episodic memory task, patients with preserved cognitive functioning showed increased brain activation in parahippocampal areas, whereas patients with impaired cognitive functioning showed decreased brain activation in parahippocampal areas relative to healthy subjects (Hulst et al., 2012). The increase in brain activation was interpreted as a compensatory mechanism to preserve cognitive function (see Color Plate 2). Comparable findings were observed in cognitively preserved versus cognitively impaired patients during the performance of a recall task (Mainero et al., 2004) and working memory task (N-back task; Rocca, Valsasina, Hulst, et al., 2014). These MRI studies also showed decreased activity in patients with worse cognitive function, whereas increased activity was observed in cognitively preserved patients. Other functional studies during the performance of a working memory task (N-back task) reported stronger activation in the dorsolateral prefrontal cortex compared with healthy subjects, whereas reaction time and accuracy on the task were similar (Sweet, Rao, Primeau, Durgerian, & Cohen, 2006; Sweet, Rao, Primeau, Mayer, & Cohen, 2004). On the basis of these studies, it seems that patients who had preserved cognitive functioning showed a greater extent of brain activation.

Moderately impaired patients, whose performance was significantly worse than those of healthy subject but not fulfilling the definition of cognitive impairment, did not show significant differences in brain activation during the performance of a planning task (Tower of London) compared with healthy subjects (Lazeron, Rombouts, Scheltens, Polman, & Barkhof, 2004). The lack of increased activity in this mildly cognitively impaired patient group was interpreted as evidence of the exhaustion of the adaptive mechanisms. Although the general tendency seems to be that higher brain activation during a task is associated with better performance, contradicting results are described in the literature. Increased brain activation in cognitively impaired compared with cognitively preserved patients during the performance of tasks requiring working memory (PASAT and N-back) were also observed (Forn et al., 2012; Koini et al., 2016). This is often interpreted as a reorganization mechanism capable of mitigating, at least to a certain extent, the cognitive impairment.

From a meta-analysis, it was learned that brain activation during an attention and working memory task was decreased in the inferior parietal lobule and the dorsolateral prefrontal cortex, but increased in the left ventrolateral prefrontal cortex and the right premotor area in patients with MS relative to healthy control subjects (Kollndorfer et al., 2013). To gain a better understanding of the meaning of these changes in brain activation, several studies linked brain activation patterns to measures of disease burden. Some studies have found a correlation between the extent of task-fMRI activations and measures of structural damage in terms of lesion load (Mainero et al., 2004; Rocca, Valsasina, Hulst, et al., 2014) and the integrity of the WM (Audoin et al., 2005; Bonzano, Pardini, Mancardi, Pizzorno, & Roccatagliata, 2009). Further exploration of the influence of WM integrity on functional brain activation pattern revealed that RRMS patients with loss of WM integrity (i.e., low FA) in the superior longitudinal fasciculus showed more bilateral cortical activation during PASAT performance than both healthy subjects and patients without WM impairment (i.e., high FA) in this tract (Bonzano et al., 2009). It is noteworthy that the behavioral performance was not significantly different between patients with and without WM impairment.

At present, the role of altered activation patterns during the performance of a behavioral task is largely debated because available studies in MS demonstrate varied and sometimes conflicting results. The involvement of heterogeneous methodological paradigms and study populations, such as early and late patients or patients with and without cognitive impairment, most likely contribute to these diverse findings. Nevertheless, fMRI changes in brain activation patterns by using different cognitive paradigms have been disclosed in all MS phenotypes (Audoin et al., 2005; Mainero et al., 2004; Mesaros et al., 2009). In general, the deviation from the activation pattern observed in healthy subjects tends to increase with disease progression (Loitfelder et al., 2011; for more information on this topic, see Chapter 3, this volume).

Task-Related Functional Connectivity

Findings regarding changes in brain activation patterns during the performance of a cognitive task were described in the previous section. To investigate the communication between brain regions, functional connectivity can be measured. Functional connectivity is conceptually quite different from task-related brain activation and reflects the degree of communication between brain regions (see Exhibit 2.2). Mapping the level of functional connectivity between brain regions could help us to understand whether the communication between regions is changed in MS patients and how this relates to cognitive performance.

The first task-related fMRI connectivity study appeared a few years later than the task-fMRI activation studies and measured brain connectivity during PASAT performance, allowing investigation of whether functional connectivity changes were associated with PASAT performance and with clinical and structural MRI abnormalities (e.g., lesion load, WM integrity, and atrophy). The ventrolateral prefrontal cortex became functionally active during the performance of the PASAT in healthy subjects (Audoin et al., 2003), and so this region was selected as a seed region for further connectivity analyses (see Exhibit 2.2). It was of particular interest to investigate whether this region showed, next to the observed increased activity during the performance of the PASAT, changes in connectivity as well. Very early MS patients (i.e., patients with clinically isolated syndrome) with impaired task performance, showed increased levels of activity in the ventrolateral prefrontal cortex during the performance of the PASAT relative to healthy control subjects (Audoin et al., 2005). Additionally, in the same cohort of patients, a decrease in functional connectivity from the seed region with several other regions of the brain, including the left dorsolateral prefrontal cortex, right primary somatosensory cortex, and anterior cingulate cortex, was observed during the PASAT

(Au Duong, Audoin, et al., 2005). Already during the very early stages of MS, impaired task performance was observed and, on top of differences in the level of activity during the performance of the PASAT, changes in the communication between brain regions were observed as well. The functional connectivity changes were related to WM lesion load and WM integrity (Au Duong, Audoin, et al., 2005). In very early MS patients with impaired task performance, attention and working memory deficits were predicted according to structural and functional measures, including WM integrity, functional activation, and functional connectivity between the ventrolateral prefrontal cortex (i.e., seed region) and the thalamus, left supramarginal gyrus, left anterior cingulate gyrus (Ranjeva et al., 2006). A closer look at connectivity changes of the ventrolateral prefrontal cortex during the performance of the PASAT revealed decreased effective connectivity (see Exhibit 2.2) from the right to left ventrolateral prefrontal cortex and the left anterior cingulate cortex to the ipsilateral ventrolateral prefrontal cortex in patients with MS compared with healthy subjects. Moreover, increased effective connectivity in both directions between the right anterior cingulate cortex and right ventrolateral prefrontal cortex and from right to left anterior cingulate cortex was observed in patients with MS compared with healthy subjects. These findings are interpreted as an adaptive mechanism of the working memory network that may limit cognitive dysfunction. However, these very early MS patients scored worse on the PASAT compared with healthy subjects (Au Duong, Boulanouar, et al., 2005). A few years later, a PASAT paradigm was again used to investigate connectivity changes in very early MS patients. This time the middle frontal gyrus, inferior frontal gyrus, anterior cingulate cortex, and inferior parietal lobe, known to be related to working memory, were chosen as seed regions. Compared with both cognitively preserved patients and healthy subjects, cognitively impaired patients had significantly increased connectivity from the right inferior frontal gyrus to the right inferior parietal lobe, from left to right inferior parietal lobe, and right inferior parietal lobe to right inferior frontal gyrus (Forn et al., 2012). In contrast to the previously described effective connectivity study in very early MS patients (Au Duong, Boulanouar, et al., 2005), no decreased connectivity was observed in cognitively impaired or cognitively preserved patients compared with healthy subjects. These results suggest that impaired PASAT performance was mainly driven by increased connectivity between several regions and might be maladaptive.

Functional connectivity was also investigated during the performance of the symbol digit modalities task (SDMT). It was hypothesized that an increased number of functional connections must be recruited in MS patients to maintain a similar performance level as healthy subjects. In line with the hypothesis, more connections in the posterior and dorsal prefrontal cortex were observed in MS patients than healthy subjects (Leavitt, Wylie, Genova,

Chiaravalloti, & DeLuca, 2012). Additionally, another study revealed increased functional connectivity in MS patients with impaired information processing performance relative to those with a preserved information processing performance (Dobryakova et al., 2016).

In short, task-related functional connectivity changes are present in MS patients, even during the early stages of the disease and are related to specific cognitive functions. Increased connectivity was observed, as well as decreased connectivity and loss of the number of connections. It is difficult to pinpoint why these contradicting results are observed and further research is necessary. For a more thoroughly interpretation of these findings, see Chapter 3 of this volume.

Resting-State Connectivity Studies

In addition to fMRI studies that have addressed activity and connectivity changes during the performance of cognitive tasks, it is also possible to explore regional interactions during the so-called resting-state of the brain, that is, when a subject is not performing an explicit task. For these studies, different methodological approaches were used, including independent-components analysis to explore certain resting-state networks and regions of interest analysis (see Exhibit 2.2).

The first resting-state connectivity studies in MS explored the so-called default mode network (DMN). Regions belonging to this network, including the posterior cingulate, medial frontal areas, inferior parietal cortex, and the precuneus, are highly correlated with each other and are coherently active during resting-state. In the DMN, increased connectivity in clinically isolated syndrome patients who were suggestive of MS (Roosendaal, Schoonheim, et al., 2010) and decreased connectivity in progressive MS (Rocca et al., 2010) have been reported relative to RRMS patients and healthy subjects, respectively. In progressive patients, reduced connectivity of the DMN was more pronounced in cognitively impaired patients than patients without cognitive deficits. The functional connectivity of the DMN decreased gradually with increasing structural damage (Roosendaal, Schoonheim, et al., 2010). These findings led to the hypothesis that during the early phases of the disease, increased connectivity reflected a compensatory mechanism to preserve cognitive functions, whereas decreased connectivity observed in the progressive phase was explained as a result of accumulating structural damage (Schoonheim, Geurts, & Barkhof, 2010). However, many contradictory findings in relation to cognitive function are reported. For example, when looking to the DMN, increased (Basile et al., 2014; Hawellek, Hipp, Lewis, Corbetta, & Engel, 2011), decreased (Cruz-Gómez, Ventura-Campos, Belenguer, Ávila, & Forn, 2014; Leavitt, Paxton, & Sumowski, 2014) and both increased and decreased connectivity (Bonavita et al., 2011) have been associated with cognitive deficits in MS. Unlike the first findings regarding the DMN, these findings are partially consistent with the previously stated hypothesis (Schoonheim et al., 2010).

Next to the commonly investigated DMN, seed-based resting-state fMRI studies have shown widespread functional connectivity changes in both deep GM structures and cortical brain regions, including the anterior cingulate cortex (Loitfelder et al., 2012), posterior cingulate cortex (Hawellek et al., 2011), dorsolateral prefrontal cortex (Bonnet et al., 2010), thalamus (Schoonheim, Hulst, et al., 2015; Tona et al., 2014), and hippocampus (Hulst et al., 2015) in MS. Although some of the studies related increased functional connectivity with better cognitive performance (Loitfelder et al., 2012), increased connectivity was most often related to worse cognitive function (Hawellek et al., 2011; Hulst et al., 2015; Schoonheim, Hulst, et al., 2015; Tona et al., 2014). In addition, increased connectivity of the thalamus (Schoonheim, Hulst, et al., 2015) and hippocampus (Hulst et al., 2015) appeared to be independent predictors of cognitive function. The influence of atrophy on functional connectivity measures was shown by findings demonstrating that in MS patients with hippocampal atrophy, decreased functional connectivity of the hippocampus was observed, whereas only subtle connectivity changes were observed between patients with normal hippocampal volumes and healthy subjects (Roosendaal, Hulst, et al., 2010).

Resting-state fMRI studies have taught us that the communication between brain regions is disturbed in MS patients. These abnormalities are mostly associated with cognitive dysfunction. However, the exact relation between resting-state functional connectivity changes and cognitive deficits needs to be further elucidated. The current hypothesis and interpretation of these resting-state studies in relation with cognitive function are further described in Chapter 3 of this volume.

Brain Network Efficiency

As described earlier, local changes in brain activation or connectivity can be observed in patients with MS. Although it can be assumed that these local changes influence the efficiency and balance of the entire brain network, studies that directly investigated the changes in the brain network topology were needed to support the long-distance effects. Using graph analysis, different parameters such as clustering coefficient and path length can be calculated to describe the efficiency of the brain's network (see Exhibit 2.2; Color Plate 3). This relatively novel method has so far been applied a small number of times in MS. Nevertheless, graph analytical studies in MS have shown that cognitive function is related to reduced network efficiency, as seen by changes in clustering coefficient and increases in path length (Schoonheim, Hulst, et al., 2012; Van Schependom et al., 2014) as well as impaired integration of information (Rocca, Valsasina, Meani, et al., 2016). However, in early MS patients, loss of network efficiency was especially observed in male MS patients. This gender effect was related to the worse performance on cognitive tests of male MS patients relative to female patients with similar disease duration (Schoonheim, Hulst, et al., 2012). It was suggested that the functional network topology of female patients provides more possibilities to reorganize on structural damage, therefore resulting in less severe cognitive deficits relative to male patients.

Investigating changes in brain function by using a holistic model of the entire brain helps us to understand more global changes in the efficiency of communication within the brain. Although this technique is seldom applied in MS, the current available graph-analytical studies in MS show that cognitive dysfunction is related to an inefficient brain network.

CONCLUSIONS AND FUTURE DIRECTIONS

On MRI, both structural and functional changes can be linked to specific cognitive deficits that patients with MS suffer from. To date, MRI is the main method to study the underlying neurobiological mechanisms of cognitive impairment in MS. Measures of neurodegeneration (i.e., cortical and subcortical atrophy) and subtle changes in WM integrity seem more informative than the classical WM (or GM) lesions. Functional measures (i.e., task-related fMRI, resting-state fMRI, connectivity) allow us to study the function of the brain under pathological conditions. A standardized MRI protocol for detecting cognitive deficits in MS currently does not exist. Therefore, we propose the following (Table 2.2): For measuring GM abnormalities and neurodegeneration, include a DIR or PSIR sequence (or both), as well as a three-dimensional T1 sequence in your scanning protocol. To be even more sophisticated and state of the art, one might include DTI and task-related and resting-state fMRI measures in the protocol, although these are more difficult to use in the postprocessing phase.

To move beyond the relatively poorly understood local increases and decreases in brain activation and connectivity, it is now time to look at these functional measures slightly differently by using a more holistic approach (Schoonheim, Meijer, & Geurts, 2015). We need to understand what happens to the global status of the entire brain network in MS patients with cognitive impairment. How is the efficiency of the brain network changed? Does the importance of certain brain regions in relation to the overall network change in the presence of pathology, and how does that explain cognitive

TABLE 2.2
Recommendation for MRI Protocol to Image the Pathological Changes
Related to Cognitive Decline in Multiple Sclerosis

Technique	Used for	Applicability in clinical practice
Phase-sensitive inversion recovery and/or Double Inversion Recovery	Detection of GM lesions	++++
Three-dimensional T1-weighted MRI	Whole brain and regional (subcortical) atrophy	+++
Diffusion tensor imaging	Quantification of WM integrity	++
Task-related functional MRI	Brain activation and connectivity during a specific cognitive task	+
Resting-state functional MRI	Brain activation and connectivity during a rest (i.e., network dynamics)	+

Note. GM = gray matter; MRI = magnetic resonance imaging; WM = white matter. ++++ = easy to apply in clinical practice; images will be available without pre-processing; +++ = moderately easy to apply in clinical practice; some straightforward computer calculations will be necessary; ++ = more difficult to apply in clinical practice; more advanced computer processing will be necessary; + difficult to apply in clinical practice; high-end computer computation will be necessary.

functioning? Understanding these changes in network characteristics might, for example, help us to understand individual differences among patients, such as cognitive reserve (see Chapters 3 and 15, this volume) and how this might limit the influence of pathology on cognitive functioning.

In the end, the brain should be regarded as a complex network, with both local and global characteristics influencing patients' cognitive functioning. Understanding the changing aspects of the entire brain network is the future if we wish to unravel the pathological mechanisms leading to, or explaining, cognitive decline in MS.

REFERENCES

Arnett, P. A., Rao, S. M., Bernardin, L., Grafman, J., Yetkin, F. Z., & Lobeck, L. (1994). Relationship between frontal lobe lesions and Wisconsin Card Sorting Test performance in patients with multiple sclerosis. *Neurology, 44,* 420–425. http://dx.doi.org/10.1212/WNL.44.3_Part_1.420

Au Duong, M. V., Audoin, B., Boulanouar, K., Ibarrola, D., Malikova, I., Confort-Gouny, S., . . . Ranjeva, J. P. (2005). Altered functional connectivity related to white matter changes inside the working memory network at the very early stage of MS. *Journal of Cerebral Blood Flow and Metabolism, 25,* 1245–1253. http://dx.doi.org/10.1038/sj.jcbfm.9600122

Au Duong, M. V., Boulanouar, K., Audoin, B., Treseras, S., Ibarrola, D., Malikova, I., . . . Ranjeva, J. P. (2005). Modulation of effective connectivity inside the working memory network in patients at the earliest stage of multiple sclerosis. *NeuroImage, 24*, 533–538. http://dx.doi.org/10.1016/j.neuroimage.2004.08.038

Audoin, B., Au Duong, M. V., Ranjeva, J. P., Ibarrola, D., Malikova, I., Confort-Gouny, S., . . . Cozzone, P. J. (2005). Magnetic resonance study of the influence of tissue damage and cortical reorganization on PASAT performance at the earliest stage of multiple sclerosis. *Human Brain Mapping, 24*, 216–228. http://dx.doi.org/10.1002/hbm.20083

Audoin, B., Ibarrola, D., Ranjeva, J. P., Confort-Gouny, S., Malikova, I., Ali-Chérif, A., . . . Cozzone, P. (2003). Compensatory cortical activation observed by fMRI during a cognitive task at the earliest stage of multiple sclerosis. *Human Brain Mapping, 20*, 51–58. http://dx.doi.org/10.1002/hbm.10128

Basile, B., Castelli, M., Monteleone, F., Nocentini, U., Caltagirone, C., Centonze, D., . . . Bozzali, M. (2014). Functional connectivity changes within specific networks parallel the clinical evolution of multiple sclerosis. *Multiple Sclerosis Journal, 20*, 1050–1057. http://dx.doi.org/10.1177/1352458513515082

Batista, S., Zivadinov, R., Hoogs, M., Bergsland, N., Heininen-Brown, M., Dwyer, M. G., . . . Benedict, R. H. B. (2012). Basal ganglia, thalamus and neocortical atrophy predicting slowed cognitive processing in multiple sclerosis. *Journal of Neurology, 259*, 139–146. http://dx.doi.org/10.1007/s00415-011-6147-1

Benedict, R. H. B., Bruce, J. M., Dwyer, M. G., Abdelrahman, N., Hussein, S., Weinstock-Guttman, B., . . . Zivadinov, R. (2006). Neocortical atrophy, third ventricular width, and cognitive dysfunction in multiple sclerosis. *Archives of Neurology, 63*, 1301–1306. http://dx.doi.org/10.1001/archneur.63.9.1301

Benedict, R. H. B., Hulst, H. E., Bergsland, N., Schoonheim, M. M., Dwyer, M. G., Weinstock-Guttman, B., . . . Zivadinov, R. (2013). Clinical significance of atrophy and white matter mean diffusivity within the thalamus of multiple sclerosis patients. *Multiple Sclerosis Journal, 19*, 1478–1484. http://dx.doi.org/10.1177/1352458513478675

Bergendal, G., Martola, J., Stawiarz, L., Kristoffersen-Wiberg, M., Fredrikson, S., & Almkvist, O. (2013). Callosal atrophy in multiple sclerosis is related to cognitive speed. *Acta Neurologica Scandinavica, 127*, 281–289. http://dx.doi.org/10.1111/ane.12006

Bisecco, A., Rocca, M. A., Pagani, E., Mancini, L., Enzinger, C., Gallo, A., . . . the MAGNIMS Network. (2015). Connectivity-based parcellation of the thalamus in multiple sclerosis and its implications for cognitive impairment: A multi-center study. *Human Brain Mapping, 36*, 2809–2825. http://dx.doi.org/10.1002/hbm.22809

Bonavita, S., Gallo, A., Sacco, R., Corte, M. D., Bisecco, A., Docimo, R., . . . Tedeschi, G. (2011). Distributed changes in default-mode resting-state connectivity in multiple sclerosis. *Multiple Sclerosis Journal, 17*, 411–422. http://dx.doi.org/10.1177/1352458510394609

Bonnet, M. C., Allard, M., Dilharreguy, B., Deloire, M., Petry, K. G., & Brochet, B. (2010). Cognitive compensation failure in multiple sclerosis. *Neurology, 75,* 1241–1248. http://dx.doi.org/10.1212/WNL.0b013e3181f612e3

Bonzano, L., Pardini, M., Mancardi, G. L., Pizzorno, M., & Roccatagliata, L. (2009). Structural connectivity influences brain activation during PVSAT in multiple sclerosis. *NeuroImage, 44,* 9–15. http://dx.doi.org/10.1016/j.neuroimage.2008.08.015

Brex, P. A., Jenkins, R., Fox, N. C., Crum, W. R., O'Riordan, J. I., Plant, G. T., & Miller, D. H. (2000). Detection of ventricular enlargement in patients at the earliest clinical stage of MS. *Neurology, 54,* 1689–1691. http://dx.doi.org/10.1212/WNL.54.8.1689

Cala, L. A., Mastaglia, F. L., & Black, J. L. (1978). Computerized tomography of brain and optic nerve in multiple sclerosis. Observations in 100 patients, including serial studies in 16. *Journal of the Neurological Sciences, 36,* 411–426. http://dx.doi.org/10.1016/0022-510X(78)90048-5

Calabrese, M., Agosta, F., Rinaldi, F., Mattisi, I., Grossi, P., Favaretto, A., . . . Filippi, M. (2009). Cortical lesions and atrophy associated with cognitive impairment in relapsing-remitting multiple sclerosis. *Archives of Neurology, 66,* 1144–1150. http://dx.doi.org/10.1001/archneurol.2009.174

Calabrese, M., Rinaldi, F., Mattisi, I., Grossi, P., Favaretto, A., Atzori, M., . . . Gallo, P. (2010). Widespread cortical thinning characterizes patients with MS with mild cognitive impairment. *Neurology, 74,* 321–328. http://dx.doi.org/10.1212/WNL.0b013e3181cbcd03

Chiaravalloti, N. D., & DeLuca, J. (2008). Cognitive impairment in multiple sclerosis. *The Lancet Neurology, 7,* 1139–1151. http://dx.doi.org/10.1016/S1474-4422(08)70259-X

Chu, R., Tauhid, S., Glanz, B. I., Healy, B. C., Kim, G., Oommen, V. V., . . . Bakshi, R. (2016). Whole brain volume measured from 1.5T versus 3T MRI in healthy subjects and patients with multiple sclerosis. *Journal of Neuroimaging, 26,* 62–67. http://dx.doi.org/10.1111/jon.12271

Cruz-Gómez, Á. J., Ventura-Campos, N., Belenguer, A., Ávila, C., & Forn, C. (2014). The link between resting-state functional connectivity and cognition in MS patients. *Multiple Sclerosis Journal, 20,* 338–348. http://dx.doi.org/10.1177/1352458513495584

Cutter, G. R., Baier, M. L., Rudick, R. A., Cookfair, D. L., Fischer, J. S., Petkau, J., . . . Willoughby, E. (1999). Development of a multiple sclerosis functional composite as a clinical trial outcome measure. *Brain: A Journal of Neurology, 122,* 871–882. http://dx.doi.org/10.1093/brain/122.5.871

Dalton, C. M., Chard, D. T., Davies, G. R., Miszkiel, K. A., Altmann, D. R., Fernando, K., . . . Miller, D. H. (2004). Early development of multiple sclerosis is associated with progressive grey matter atrophy in patients presenting with clinically isolated syndromes. *Brain: A Journal of Neurology, 127,* 1101–1107. http://dx.doi.org/10.1093/brain/awh126

Debernard, L., Melzer, T. R., Alla, S., Eagle, J., Van Stockum, S., Graham, C., . . . Mason, D. F. (2015). Deep grey matter MRI abnormalities and cognitive function in relapsing-remitting multiple sclerosis. *Psychiatry Research: Neuroimaging, 234*, 352–361. http://dx.doi.org/10.1016/j.pscychresns.2015.10.004

Deloire, M. S. A., Ruet, A., Hamel, D., Bonnet, M., Dousset, V., & Brochet, B. (2011). MRI predictors of cognitive outcome in early multiple sclerosis. *Neurology, 76*, 1161–1167. http://dx.doi.org/10.1212/WNL.0b013e318212a8be

Dineen, R. A., Vilisaar, J., Hlinka, J., Bradshaw, C. M., Morgan, P. S., Constantinescu, C. S., & Auer, D. P. (2009). Disconnection as a mechanism for cognitive dysfunction in multiple sclerosis. *Brain: A Journal of Neurology, 132*, 239–249. http://dx.doi.org/10.1093/brain/awn275

Dobryakova, E., Costa, S. L., Wylie, G. R., DeLuca, J., & Genova, H. M. (2016). Altered effective connectivity during a processing speed task in individuals with multiple sclerosis. *Journal of the International Neuropsychological Society, 22*, 216–224.

Filippi, M., Rocca, M. A., Ciccarelli, O., De Stefano, N., Evangelou, N., Kappos, L., . . . the MAGNIMS Study Group. (2016). MRI criteria for the diagnosis of multiple sclerosis: MAGNIMS consensus guidelines. *The Lancet Neurology, 15*, 292–303. http://dx.doi.org/10.1016/S1474-4422(15)00393-2

Fisniku, L. K., Chard, D. T., Jackson, J. S., Anderson, V. M., Altmann, D. R., Miszkiel, K. A., . . . Miller, D. H. (2008). Gray matter atrophy is related to long-term disability in multiple sclerosis. *Annals of Neurology, 64*, 247–254. http://dx.doi.org/10.1002/ana.21423

Forn, C., Rocca, M. A., Valsasina, P., Boscá, I., Casanova, B., Sanjuan, A., . . . Filippi, M. (2012). Functional magnetic resonance imaging correlates of cognitive performance in patients with a clinically isolated syndrome suggestive of multiple sclerosis at presentation: An activation and connectivity study. *Multiple Sclerosis Journal, 18*, 153–163. http://dx.doi.org/10.1177/1352458511417744

Friston, K. J., Jezzard, P., & Turner, R. (1994). Analysis of functional MRI time-series. *Human Brain Mapping, 1*, 153–171. http://dx.doi.org/10.1002/hbm.460010207

Gadea, M., Martínez-Bisbal, M. C., Marti-Bonmatí, L., Espert, R., Casanova, B., Coret, F., & Celda, B. (2004). Spectroscopic axonal damage of the right locus coeruleus relates to selective attention impairment in early stage relapsing-remitting multiple sclerosis. *Brain: A Journal of Neurology, 127*, 89–98. http://dx.doi.org/10.1093/brain/awh002

Geurts, J. J. G., Bö, L., Roosendaal, S. D., Hazes, T., Daniëls, R., Barkhof, F., . . . van der Valk, P. (2007). Extensive hippocampal demyelination in multiple sclerosis. *Journal of Neuropathology and Experimental Neurology, 66*, 819–827. http://dx.doi.org/10.1097/nen.0b013e3181461f54

Geurts, J. J. G., Calabrese, M., Fisher, E., & Rudick, R. A. (2012). Measurement and clinical effect of grey matter pathology in multiple sclerosis. *The Lancet Neurology, 11*, 1082–1092. http://dx.doi.org/10.1016/S1474-4422(12)70230-2

Geurts, J. J. G., Pouwels, P. J. W., Uitdehaag, B. M. J., Polman, C. H., Barkhof, F., & Castelijns, J. A. (2005). Intracortical lesions in multiple sclerosis: Improved detection with 3D double inversion-recovery MR imaging. *Radiology, 236,* 254–260. http://dx.doi.org/10.1148/radiol.2361040450

Granberg, T., Martola, J., Bergendal, G., Shams, S., Damangir, S., Aspelin, P., . . . Kristoffersen-Wiberg, M. (2015). Corpus callosum atrophy is strongly associated with cognitive impairment in multiple sclerosis: Results of a 17-year longitudinal study. *Multiple Sclerosis Journal, 21,* 1151–1158. http://dx.doi.org/10.1177/1352458514560928

Harel, A., Ceccarelli, A., Farrell, C., Fabian, M., Howard, J., Riley, C., . . . Inglese, M. (2016). Phase-sensitive inversion-recovery MRI improves longitudinal cortical lesion detection in progressive MS. *PLoS One, 11,* e0152180. http://dx.doi.org/10.1371/journal.pone.0152180

Harrison, D. M., Roy, S., Oh, J., Izbudak, I., Pham, D., Courtney, S., . . . Calabresi, P. A. (2015). Association of cortical lesion burden on 7-T magnetic resonance imaging with cognition and disability in multiple sclerosis. *JAMA Neurology, 72,* 1004–1012. http://dx.doi.org/10.1001/jamaneurol.2015.1241

Hawellek, D. J., Hipp, J. F., Lewis, C. M., Corbetta, M., & Engel, A. K. (2011). Increased functional connectivity indicates the severity of cognitive impairment in multiple sclerosis. *Proceedings of the National Academy of Sciences of the United States of America, 108,* 19066–19071. http://dx.doi.org/10.1073/pnas.1110024108

Hildebrandt, H., Hahn, H. K., Kraus, J. A., Schulte-Herbrüggen, A., Schwarze, B., & Schwendemann, G. (2006). Memory performance in multiple sclerosis patients correlates with central brain atrophy. *Multiple Sclerosis Journal, 12,* 428–436. http://dx.doi.org/10.1191/1352458506ms1286oa

Hou, P., Hasan, K. M., Sitton, C. W., Wolinsky, J. S., & Narayana, P. A. (2005). Phase-sensitive T1 inversion recovery imaging: A time-efficient interleaved technique for improved tissue contrast in neuroimaging. *American Journal of Neuroradiology, 26,* 1432–1438.

Houtchens, M. K., Benedict, R. H. B., Killiany, R., Sharma, J., Jaisani, Z., Singh, B., . . . Bakshi, R. (2007). Thalamic atrophy and cognition in multiple sclerosis. *Neurology, 69,* 1213–1223. http://dx.doi.org/10.1212/01.wnl.0000276992.17011.b5

Hulst, H. E., Schoonheim, M. M., Roosendaal, S. D., Popescu, V., Schweren, L. J. S., van der Werf, Y. D., . . . Geurts, J. J. G. (2012). Functional adaptive changes within the hippocampal memory system of patients with multiple sclerosis. *Human Brain Mapping, 33,* 2268–2280. http://dx.doi.org/10.1002/hbm.21359

Hulst, H. E., Schoonheim, M. M., Van Geest, Q., Uitdehaag, B. M. J., Barkhof, F., & Geurts, J. J. G. (2015). Memory impairment in multiple sclerosis: Relevance of hippocampal activation and hippocampal connectivity. *Multiple Sclerosis Journal, 21,* 1705–1712. http://dx.doi.org/10.1177/1352458514567727

Hulst, H. E., Steenwijk, M. D., Versteeg, A., Pouwels, P. J. W., Vrenken, H., Uitdehaag, B. M. J., . . . Barkhof, F. (2013). Cognitive impairment in MS: Impact of white matter integrity, gray matter volume, and lesions. *Neurology, 80,* 1025–1032. http://dx.doi.org/10.1212/WNL.0b013e31828726cc

Koenig, K. A., Sakaie, K. E., Lowe, M. J., Lin, J., Stone, L., Bermel, R. A., . . . Phillips, M. D. (2014). Hippocampal volume is related to cognitive decline and fornicial diffusion measures in multiple sclerosis. *Magnetic Resonance Imaging, 32,* 354–358. http://dx.doi.org/10.1016/j.mri.2013.12.012

Koini, M., Filippi, M., Rocca, M. A., Yousry, T., Ciccarelli, O., Tedeschi, G., . . . the MAGNIMS fMRI Study Group. (2016). Correlates of executive functions in multiple sclerosis based on structural and functional MR imaging: Insights from a multicenter study. *Radiology, 280,* 869–879. http://dx.doi.org/10.1148/radiol.2016151809

Kollndorfer, K., Krajnik, J., Woitek, R., Freiherr, J., Prayer, D., & Schöpf, V. (2013). Altered likelihood of brain activation in attention and working memory networks in patients with multiple sclerosis: An ALE meta-analysis. *Neuroscience and Biobehavioral Reviews, 37,* 2699–2708. http://dx.doi.org/10.1016/j.neubiorev.2013.09.005

Lazeron, R. H. C., Rombouts, S. A., Scheltens, P., Polman, C. H., & Barkhof, F. (2004). An fMRI study of planning-related brain activity in patients with moderately advanced multiple sclerosis. *Multiple Sclerosis Journal, 10,* 549–555. http://dx.doi.org/10.1191/1352458504ms1072oa

Leavitt, V. M., Paxton, J., & Sumowski, J. F. (2014). Default network connectivity is linked to memory status in multiple sclerosis. *Journal of the International Neuropsychological Society, 20,* 937–944.

Leavitt, V. M., Wylie, G., Genova, H. M., Chiaravalloti, N. D., & DeLuca, J. (2012). Altered effective connectivity during performance of an information processing speed task in multiple sclerosis. *Multiple Sclerosis Journal, 18,* 409–417. http://dx.doi.org/10.1177/1352458511423651

Lin, X., Tench, C. R., Morgan, P. S., & Constantinescu, C. S. (2008). Use of combined conventional and quantitative MRI to quantify pathology related to cognitive impairment in multiple sclerosis. *Journal of Neurology, Neurosurgery, and Psychiatry, 79,* 437–441.

Locatelli, L., Zivadinov, R., Grop, A., & Zorzon, M. (2004). Frontal parenchymal atrophy measures in multiple sclerosis. *Multiple Sclerosis Journal, 10,* 562–568. http://dx.doi.org/10.1191/1352458504ms1093oa

Loitfelder, M., Fazekas, F., Petrovic, K., Fuchs, S., Ropele, S., Wallner-Blazek, M., . . . Enzinger, C. (2011). Reorganization in cognitive networks with progression of multiple sclerosis: Insights from fMRI. *Neurology, 76,* 526–533. http://dx.doi.org/10.1212/WNL.0b013e31820b75cf

Loitfelder, M., Filippi, M., Rocca, M., Valsasina, P., Ropele, S., Jehna, M., . . . Enzinger, C. (2012). Abnormalities of resting state functional connectivity are related to sustained attention deficits in MS. *PLoS One, 7,* e42862. http://dx.doi.org/10.1371/journal.pone.0042862

Mainero, C., Caramia, F., Pozzilli, C., Pisani, A., Pestalozza, I., Borriello, G., . . . Pantano, P. (2004). fMRI evidence of brain reorganization during attention and memory tasks in multiple sclerosis. *NeuroImage, 21*, 858–867. http://dx.doi.org/10.1016/j.neuroimage.2003.10.004

Medaer, R., Nelissen, E., Appel, B., Swerts, M., Geutjens, J., & Callaert, H. (1987). Magnetic resonance imaging and cognitive functioning in multiple sclerosis. *Journal of Neurology, 235*, 86–89. http://dx.doi.org/10.1007/BF00718015

Meijer, K. A., Muhlert, N., Cercignani, M., Sethi, V., Ron, M. A., Thompson, A. J., . . . Ciccarelli, O. (2016). White matter tract abnormalities are associated with cognitive dysfunction in secondary progressive multiple sclerosis. *Multiple Sclerosis Journal, 22*, 1429–1437. http://dx.doi.org/10.1177/1352458515622694

Mesaros, S., Rocca, M. A., Riccitelli, G., Pagani, E., Rovaris, M., Caputo, D., . . . Filippi, M. (2009). Corpus callosum damage and cognitive dysfunction in benign MS. *Human Brain Mapping, 30*, 2656–2666. http://dx.doi.org/10.1002/hbm.20692

Mike, A., Glanz, B. I., Hildenbrand, P., Meier, D., Bolden, K., Liguori, M., . . . Guttmann, C. R. G. (2011). Identification and clinical impact of multiple sclerosis cortical lesions as assessed by routine 3T MR imaging. *American Journal of Neuroradiology, 32*, 515–521. http://dx.doi.org/10.3174/ajnr.A2340

Minagar, A., Barnett, M. H., Benedict, R. H. B., Pelletier, D., Pirko, I., Sahraian, M. A., . . . Zivadinov, R. (2013). The thalamus and multiple sclerosis: Modern views on pathologic, imaging, and clinical aspects. *Neurology, 80*, 210–219. http://dx.doi.org/10.1212/WNL.0b013e31827b910b

Morgen, K., Sammer, G., Courtney, S. M., Wolters, T., Melchior, H., Blecker, C. R., . . . Vaitl, D. (2006). Evidence for a direct association between cortical atrophy and cognitive impairment in relapsing-remitting MS. *NeuroImage, 30*, 891–898. http://dx.doi.org/10.1016/j.neuroimage.2005.10.032

Muhlert, N., Atzori, M., De Vita, E., Thomas, D. L., Samson, R. S., Wheeler-Kingshott, C. A., . . . Ciccarelli, O. (2014). Memory in multiple sclerosis is linked to glutamate concentration in grey matter regions. *Journal of Neurology, Neurosurgery and Psychiatry, 85*, 833–839. http://dx.doi.org/10.1136/jnnp-2013-306662

Nelson, F., Poonawalla, A. H., Hou, P., Huang, F., Wolinsky, J. S., & Narayana, P. A. (2007). Improved identification of intracortical lesions in multiple sclerosis with phase-sensitive inversion recovery in combination with fast double inversion recovery MR imaging. *American Journal of Neuroradiology, 28*, 1645–1649. http://dx.doi.org/10.3174/ajnr.A0645

Nocentini, U., Bozzali, M., Spanò, B., Cercignani, M., Serra, L., Basile, B., . . . DeLuca, J. (2014). Exploration of the relationships between regional grey matter atrophy and cognition in multiple sclerosis. *Brain Imaging and Behavior, 8*, 378–386. http://dx.doi.org/10.1007/s11682-012-9170-7

Ogawa, S., Tank, D. W., Menon, R., Ellermann, J. M., Kim, S. G., Merkle, H., & Ugurbil, K. (1992). Intrinsic signal changes accompanying sensory stimulation:

Functional brain mapping with magnetic resonance imaging. *Proceedings of the National Academy of Sciences of the United States of America, 89,* 5951–5955. http://dx.doi.org/10.1073/pnas.89.13.5951

Popescu, V., Schoonheim, M. M., Versteeg, A., Chaturvedi, N., Jonker, M., Xavier de Menezes, R., . . . Vrenken, H. (2016). Grey matter atrophy in multiple sclerosis: Clinical interpretation depends on choice of analysis method. *PLoS One, 11,* e0143942. http://dx.doi.org/10.1371/journal.pone.0143942

Ranjeva, J. P., Audoin, B., Au Duong, M. V., Confort-Gouny, S., Malikova, I., Viout, P., . . . Cozzone, P. J. (2006). Structural and functional surrogates of cognitive impairment at the very early stage of multiple sclerosis. *Journal of the Neurological Sciences, 245,* 161–167. http://dx.doi.org/10.1016/j.jns.2005.09.019

Rao, S. M., Glatt, S., Hammeke, T. A., McQuillen, M. P., Khatri, B. O., Rhodes, A. M., & Pollard, S. (1985). Chronic progressive multiple sclerosis. Relationship between cerebral ventricular size and neuropsychological impairment. *Archives of Neurology, 42,* 678–682. http://dx.doi.org/10.1001/archneur.1985.04060070068018

Rao, S. M., Martin, A. L., Huelin, R., Wissinger, E., Khankhel, Z., Kim, E., & Fahrbach, K. (2014). Correlations between MRI and information processing speed in MS: A meta-analysis. *Multiple Sclerosis International, 2014,* 975803. http://dx.doi.org/10.1155/2014/975803

Reddy, H., Narayanan, S., Arnoutelis, R., Jenkinson, M., Antel, J., Matthews, P. M., & Arnold, D. L. (2000). Evidence for adaptive functional changes in the cerebral cortex with axonal injury from multiple sclerosis. *Brain: A Journal of Neurology, 123,* 2314–2320. http://dx.doi.org/10.1093/brain/123.11.2314

Riccitelli, G., Rocca, M. A., Pagani, E., Rodegher, M. E., Rossi, P., Falini, A., . . . Filippi, M. (2011). Cognitive impairment in multiple sclerosis is associated to different patterns of gray matter atrophy according to clinical phenotype. *Human Brain Mapping, 32,* 1535–1543. http://dx.doi.org/10.1002/hbm.21125

Rocca, M. A., Valsasina, P., Absinta, M., Riccitelli, G., Rodegher, M. E., Misci, P., . . . Filippi, M. (2010). Default-mode network dysfunction and cognitive impairment in progressive MS [see correction at http://dx.doi.org/10.1212/WNL.0b013e3182817f5f]. *Neurology, 74,* 1252–1259. http://dx.doi.org/10.1212/WNL.0b013e3181d9ed91

Rocca, M. A., Valsasina, P., Hulst, H. E., Abdel-Aziz, K., Enzinger, C., Gallo, A., . . . the MAGNIMS fMRI Study Group. (2014). Functional correlates of cognitive dysfunction in multiple sclerosis: A multicenter fMRI Study. *Human Brain Mapping, 35,* 5799–5814. http://dx.doi.org/10.1002/hbm.22586

Rocca, M. A., Valsasina, P., Meani, A., Falini, A., Comi, G., & Filippi, M. (2016). Impaired functional integration in multiple sclerosis: A graph theory study. *Brain Structure & Function, 221,* 115–131. http://dx.doi.org/10.1007/s00429-014-0896-4

Roosendaal, S. D., Bendfeldt, K., Vrenken, H., Polman, C. H., Borgwardt, S., Radue, E. W., . . . Geurts, J. J. G. (2011). Grey matter volume in a large cohort of MS patients: Relation to MRI parameters and disability. *Multiple Sclerosis Journal*, *17*, 1098–1106. http://dx.doi.org/10.1177/1352458511404916

Roosendaal, S. D., Hulst, H. E., Vrenken, H., Feenstra, H. E. M., Castelijns, J. A., Pouwels, P. J., ... Geurts, J. J. G. (2010). Structural and functional hippocampal changes in multiple sclerosis patients with intact memory function. *Radiology*, *255*, 595–604. http://dx.doi.org/10.1148/radiol.10091433

Roosendaal, S. D., Moraal, B., Pouwels, P. J., Vrenken, H., Castelijns, J. A., Barkhof, F., & Geurts, J. J. G. (2009). Accumulation of cortical lesions in MS: Relation with cognitive impairment. *Multiple Sclerosis Journal*, *15*, 708–714. http://dx.doi.org/10.1177/1352458509102907

Roosendaal, S. D., Schoonheim, M. M., Hulst, H. E., Sanz-Arigita, E. J., Smith, S. M., Geurts, J. J. G., & Barkhof, F. (2010). Resting state networks change in clinically isolated syndrome. *Brain: A Journal of Neurology*, *133*, 1612–1621. http://dx.doi.org/10.1093/brain/awq058

Rovaris, M., Comi, G., & Filippi, M. (2006). MRI markers of destructive pathology in multiple sclerosis-related cognitive dysfunction. *Journal of the Neurological Sciences*, *245*, 111–116. http://dx.doi.org/10.1016/j.jns.2005.07.014

Runge, V. M., Aoki, S., Bradley, W. G., Jr., Chang, K. H., Essig, M., Ma, L., ... Valavanis, A. (2015). Magnetic resonance imaging and computed tomography of the brain—50 years of innovation, with a focus on the future. *Investigative Radiology*, *50*, 551–556. http://dx.doi.org/10.1097/RLI.0000000000000170

Sacco, R., Bisecco, A., Corbo, D., Della Corte, M., d'Ambrosio, A., Docimo, R., ... Bonavita, S. (2015). Cognitive impairment and memory disorders in relapsing-remitting multiple sclerosis: The role of white matter, gray matter and hippocampus. *Journal of Neurology*, *262*, 1691–1697. http://dx.doi.org/10.1007/s00415-015-7763-y

Schoonheim, M. M., Geurts, J. J. G., & Barkhof, F. (2010). The limits of functional reorganization in multiple sclerosis. *Neurology*, *74*, 1246–1247. http://dx.doi.org/10.1212/WNL.0b013e3181db9957

Schoonheim, M. M., Hulst, H. E., Brandt, R. B., Strik, M., Wink, A. M., Uitdehaag, B. M., ... Geurts, J. J. G. (2015). Thalamus structure and function determine severity of cognitive impairment in multiple sclerosis. *Neurology*, *84*, 776–783. http://dx.doi.org/10.1212/WNL.0000000000001285

Schoonheim, M. M., Hulst, H. E., Landi, D., Ciccarelli, O., Roosendaal, S. D., Sanz-Arigita, E. J., ... Geurts, J. J. G. (2012). Gender-related differences in functional connectivity in multiple sclerosis. *Multiple Sclerosis Journal*, *18*, 164–173. http://dx.doi.org/10.1177/1352458511422245

Schoonheim, M. M., Meijer, K. A., & Geurts, J. J. G. (2015, April). Network collapse and cognitive impairment in multiple sclerosis. *Frontiers in Neurology*, *6*, 1–5. Retrieved from https://www.frontiersin.org/articles/10.3389/fneur.2015.00082/full

Schoonheim, M. M., Popescu, V., Rueda Lopes, F. C., Wiebenga, O. T., Vrenken, H., Douw, L., . . . Barkhof, F. (2012). Subcortical atrophy and cognition: Sex effects in multiple sclerosis. *Neurology, 79*, 1754–1761. http://dx.doi.org/10.1212/WNL.0b013e3182703f46

Schoonheim, M. M., Vigeveno, R. M., Rueda Lopes, F. C., Pouwels, P. J. W., Polman, C. H., Barkhof, F., & Geurts, J. J. G. (2014). Sex-specific extent and severity of white matter damage in multiple sclerosis: Implications for cognitive decline. *Human Brain Mapping, 35*, 2348–2358. http://dx.doi.org/10.1002/hbm.22332

Seewann, A., Kooi, E. J., Roosendaal, S. D., Pouwels, P. J. W., Wattjes, M. P., van der Valk, P., . . . Geurts, J. J. G. (2012). Postmortem verification of MS cortical lesion detection with 3D DIR. *Neurology, 78*, 302–308. http://dx.doi.org/10.1212/WNL.0b013e31824528a0

Shmuel, A., & Leopold, D. A. (2008). Neuronal correlates of spontaneous fluctuations in fMRI signals in monkey visual cortex: Implications for functional connectivity at rest. *Human Brain Mapping, 29*, 751–761. http://dx.doi.org/10.1002/hbm.20580

Sicotte, N. L., Kern, K. C., Giesser, B. S., Arshanapalli, A., Schultz, A., Montag, M., . . . Bookheimer, S. Y. (2008). Regional hippocampal atrophy in multiple sclerosis. *Brain: A Journal of Neurology, 131*, 1134–1141. http://dx.doi.org/10.1093/brain/awn030

Smith, S. M., Fox, P. T., Miller, K. L., Glahn, D. C., Fox, P. M., Mackay, C. E., . . . Beckmann, C. F. (2009). Correspondence of the brain's functional architecture during activation and rest. *Proceedings of the National Academy of Sciences of the United States of America, 106*, 13040–5.

Sporns, O., Chialvo, D. R., Kaiser, M., & Hilgetag, C. C. (2004). Organization, development and function of complex brain networks. *Trends in Cognitive Sciences, 8*, 418–425. http://dx.doi.org/10.1016/j.tics.2004.07.008

Staffen, W., Mair, A., Zauner, H., Unterrainer, J., Niederhofer, H., Kutzelnigg, A., . . . Ladurner, G. (2002). Cognitive function and fMRI in patients with multiple sclerosis: Evidence for compensatory cortical activation during an attention task. *Brain: A Journal of Neurology, 125*, 1275–1282. http://dx.doi.org/10.1093/brain/awf125

Stam, C. J., & Reijneveld, J. C. (2007). Graph theoretical analysis of complex networks in the brain. *Nonlinear Biomedical Physics, 1*, 3. http://dx.doi.org/10.1186/1753-4631-1-3

Steenwijk, M. D., Geurts, J. J. G., Daams, M., Tijms, B. M., Wink, A. M., Balk, L. J., . . . Pouwels, P. J. W. (2016). Cortical atrophy patterns in multiple sclerosis are non-random and clinically relevant. *Brain: A Journal of Neurology, 139*, 115–126. http://dx.doi.org/10.1093/brain/awv337

Stephan, K. E., & Friston, K. J. (2010). Analyzing effective connectivity with functional magnetic resonance imaging. *Wiley Interdisciplinary Reviews: Cognitive Science, 1*, 446–459. http://dx.doi.org/10.1002/wcs.58

Stys, P. K., Zamponi, G. W., van Minnen, J., & Geurts, J. J. G. (2012). Will the real multiple sclerosis please stand up? *Nature Reviews Neuroscience, 13,* 507–514. http://dx.doi.org/10.1038/nrn3275

Sweet, L. H., Rao, S. M., Primeau, M., Durgerian, S., & Cohen, R. A. (2006). Functional magnetic resonance imaging response to increased verbal working memory demands among patients with multiple sclerosis. *Human Brain Mapping, 27,* 28–36. http://dx.doi.org/10.1002/hbm.20163

Sweet, L. H., Rao, S. M., Primeau, M., Mayer, A. R., & Cohen, R. A. (2004). Functional magnetic resonance imaging of working memory among multiple sclerosis patients. *Journal of Neuroimaging, 14,* 150–157. http://dx.doi.org/10.1111/j.1552-6569.2004.tb00232.x

Tekok-Kilic, A., Benedict, R. H. B., Weinstock-Guttman, B., Dwyer, M. G., Carone, D., Srinivasaraghavan, B., . . . Zivadinov, R. (2007). Independent contributions of cortical gray matter atrophy and ventricle enlargement for predicting neuropsychological impairment in multiple sclerosis. *NeuroImage, 36,* 1294–1300. http://dx.doi.org/10.1016/j.neuroimage.2007.04.017

Tona, F., Petsas, N., Sbardella, E., Prosperini, L., Carmellini, M., Pozzilli, C., & Pantano, P. (2014). Multiple sclerosis: Altered thalamic resting-state functional connectivity and its effect on cognitive function. *Radiology, 271,* 814–821. http://dx.doi.org/10.1148/radiol.14131688

van den Heuvel, M. P., & Hulshoff Pol, H. E. (2010). Exploring the brain network: A review on resting-state fMRI functional connectivity. *European Neuropsychopharmacology, 20,* 519–534. http://dx.doi.org/10.1016/j.euroneuro.2010.03.008

van Munster, C. E. P., Jonkman, L. E., Weinstein, H. C., Uitdehaag, B. M. J., & Geurts, J. J. G. (2015). Gray matter damage in multiple sclerosis: Impact on clinical symptoms. *Neuroscience, 303,* 446–461. http://dx.doi.org/10.1016/j.neuroscience.2015.07.006

Van Schependom, J., Gielen, J., Laton, J., D'hooghe, M. B., De Keyser, J., & Nagels, G. (2014). Graph theoretical analysis indicates cognitive impairment in MS stems from neural disconnection. *NeuroImage. Clinical, 4,* 403–410. http://dx.doi.org/10.1016/j.nicl.2014.01.012

Vollmer, T., Huynh, L., Kelley, C., Galebach, P., Signorovitch, J., DiBernardo, A., & Sasane, R. (2016). Relationship between brain volume loss and cognitive outcomes among patients with multiple sclerosis: A systematic literature review. *Neurological Sciences, 37,* 165–179. http://dx.doi.org/10.1007/s10072-015-2400-1

Vollmer, T., Signorovitch, J., Huynh, L., Galebach, P., Kelley, C., DiBernardo, A., & Sasane, R. (2015). The natural history of brain volume loss among patients with multiple sclerosis: A systematic literature review and meta-analysis. *Journal of the Neurological Sciences, 357*(1-2), 8–18. http://dx.doi.org/10.1016/j.jns.2015.07.014

Yu, H. J., Christodoulou, C., Bhise, V., Greenblatt, D., Patel, Y., Serafin, D., . . . Wagshul, M. E. (2012). Multiple white matter tract abnormalities underlie cognitive impairment in RRMS. *NeuroImage, 59*, 3713–3722. http://dx.doi.org/10.1016/j.neuroimage.2011.10.053

Zivadinov, R., Sepcic, J., Nasuelli, D., De Masi, R., Bragadin, L. M., Tommasi, M. A., . . . Zorzon, M. (2001). A longitudinal study of brain atrophy and cognitive disturbances in the early phase of relapsing-remitting multiple sclerosis. *Journal of Neurology, Neurosurgery and Psychiatry, 70*, 773–780. http://dx.doi.org/10.1136/jnnp.70.6.773

3

CEREBRAL REORGANIZATION AND COGNITION IN MULTIPLE SCLEROSIS

EKATERINA DOBRYAKOVA, MARIA ASSUNTA ROCCA,
AND MASSIMO FILIPPI

Among one of the first things one learns about the brain is that it is an incredibly plastic organ. It has the ability to reorganize and change during the course of development in response to either its environment or injury. Our brains go through developmental changes from the day we are born until about age 22 years. During this developmental period, the brain goes through a process called *synaptic pruning* in which it actively eliminates certain connections to increase the efficiency of others. In healthy individuals, these neural changes lead to the acquisition of necessary skills, such as language, memories, motor function, and balance (Johnson, 2001). However, what happens when these acquired skills and abilities are affected by multiple sclerosis (MS)? Does cerebral reorganization have to be maladaptive, causing negative consequences on cognition, or can it also be adaptive?

Great technological advances in brain imaging and analysis have emerged in recent decades, paving the way for a more accurate investigation

http://dx.doi.org/10.1037/0000097-004
Cognition and Behavior in Multiple Sclerosis, J. DeLuca and B. M. Sandroff (Editors)

of MS-related cerebral reorganization. Examination of cerebral reorganization in MS has been especially fruitful using magnetic resonance imaging (MRI). A simple keyword search of *multiple sclerosis* and *MRI* on PubMed produces an astonishing 12,457 peer-reviewed articles in English (as of January 2018), covering a wide range of studies concerning the brains of individuals with MS. These studies use an array of different acquisition and analysis methods, such as diffusion tensor imaging (DTI), atrophy analysis, and functional MRI (fMRI). They also investigate the role of damaging and reparative mechanisms at different stages of the disease as well as the effects of treatment. The current chapter provides a review of recent developments in the field of MS, particularly focusing on cerebral reorganization and cognition. The topics covered primarily involve findings from fMRI, including activation and connectivity, and structural MRI abnormalities in patients at different stages of the disease. The burgeoning field of research on cognitive rehabilitation in MS is also mentioned (see Chapter 13 of this volume by Chiaravalloti and DeLuca for a more detailed review). Meanwhile, we begin with a description of the basic mechanisms involved in cerebral reorganization.

LEVELS OF CEREBRAL REORGANIZATION

In general, cerebral reorganization can occur at different neurobiological levels, including both microstructural and macrostructural changes (Kolb, Muhammad, & Gibb, 2011). In addition, it can occur throughout the various stages of life, with a great deal of cerebral reorganization occurring during development. For years, it was thought that once an organism reaches maturity, cerebral reorganization stops. This idea led to the conclusion that our brain, which is organized into different networks, would not be able to adapt to a changing environment or compensate for injury if a region within a network was damaged. Several investigations have shown that this is not the case. Training and experience allows the brain to adapt to its environment after damage, with cerebral plasticity being evident at both the microstructural and macrostructural levels (Duffau, 2006; Will, Dalrymple-Alford, Wolff, & Cassel, 2008a).

Microstructural Level

At the microstructural level, cerebral reorganization manifests as neurogenesis (the process of new neural cell development), synaptogenesis (the development of new neuronal connections), and the amplification of synaptic transmission. It was previously believed that neurogenesis occurs only early on in life: New dendrites and axons are created during the early stages of development but not during adulthood. Recent evidence shows that neuro-genesis continues to influence cognition in the mature healthy brain (Duffau, 2006; Ksiazek-Winiarek, Szpakowski, & Glabinski, 2015). However, axonal regression and neural cell elimination also occur, allowing a neural network to specialize and thus remove unnecessary connections that prevent network efficiency (i.e., the processes of pruning).

Hebbian learning or Hebb's rule is another especially pertinent concept in cerebral reorganization at the microstructural level. Hebbian learning can be characterized as an increase of synaptic strength between neurons that fire together during a recurring event. Cells that are not engaged in particular processes are pruned out and are not included in future neural networks. Donald Hebb was a proponent of use-dependent plasticity, as described in his 1949 book, *The Organization of Behavior. A Neuropsychological Theory*. A decade later, empirical findings indeed confirmed the occurrence of neuro-chemical changes induced by training and experience.

Pathological Evidence

Historically, MS has been considered a demyelinating disease. However, histological studies have revealed that axonal damage also occurs (Bjartmar, Battistuta, Terada, Dupree, & Trapp, 2002; Trapp et al., 1998). For example, Trapp et al. (1998) examined brain tissue from 11 MS patients and showed the presence of axonal transection in MS lesions. Early studies also showed that lesions in the white matter (WM) occur around inflamed veins, whereas gray matter (GM) lesions occur in the tissue that surrounds veins. More recently, Haider et al. (2016) showed that demyelination and neurodegen-eration in the MS brain have a certain topography. Specifically, demyelin-ation was characterized by the presence of inflammatory infiltrates in the meninges and demyelinated lesions in the WM at sites with high venous density. Neurodegeneration was due to oxidative injury of cortical neurons and retrograde neurodegeneration secondary to axonal injury in the WM.

Neuroimaging Evidence

Demyelination and axonal loss are the primary factors that contrib-ute to both cognitive and motor decline (Tomassini et al., 2012). Proton magnetic resonance spectroscopy (1H-MRS) is a noninvasive method that allows one to capture changes reflective of axonal damage in normal-appearing WM (Cifelli & Matthews, 2002). The majority of 1H-MRS studies examine brain concentration of N-acetylaspartate (NAA), a marker of neu-ronal integrity. Reduced levels of NAA have been shown to be associated with longer disease duration and increased disability (Bjartmar et al., 2002). Several 1H-MRS studies also linked decreased levels of NAA with impaired cognitive functioning in MS (Giorgio & De Stefano, 2010). Further, Genova et al. (2014) showed that higher NAA levels were associated with increased functional brain activity during a processing speed task in which MS patients performed slower than healthy control subjects (HCs; discussed later in the chapter). Given that MS participants performed the task as well as HC participants, these results suggest a complex interplay between metabolic abnormalities and blood oxygen level–dependent (BOLD) activation. Thus, microstructural changes do not occur in isolation and can be linked to cerebral reorganization on the macrostructural level.

Macrostructural Level

MRI provides several techniques for examining cerebral reorganization on the macrostructural level, allowing dynamic examination of cerebral reorganization specifically associated with cognition, either by observing brain function during a cognitive task (fMRI) or by examining the association between structural parameters and performance on standardized cognitive tests (e.g., DTI).

Task fMRI

Task fMRI is an approach that allows for the observation of brain changes during task performance. Several fMRI studies demonstrated cerebral reorganization in MS patients by showing that these patients exhibited an altered activation of brain regions compared with HCs (Color Plate 4) during performance of cognitive tasks testing selected cognitive domains.

One of the domains frequently affected in individuals with MS is working memory, that is, the ability to manipulate and hold information for a short period after it is no longer present in the environment (e.g., N. Chiaravalloti et al., 2005). By administering the Paced Auditory Addition Test (PASAT) during fMRI, a series of studies by Audoin et al. (2003, 2005) revealed significant cerebral reorganization within the working memory network in MS patients who were at the earliest stage of the disease. Specifically, patients with intact task performance had greater activation in areas shown to be involved in working memory and attention compared with HCs. Similar findings were presented by Staffen et al. (2002), supporting the claim that cerebral reorganization during working memory functioning can be compensatory and adaptive in MS patients without cognitive impairment.

Another cognitive domain that is affected by MS is information processing speed, defined as "the amount of information that can be processed in a certain unit of time" (N. D. Chiaravalloti, Stojanovic-Radic, & DeLuca, 2013, p. 181). Several studies have examined the functionality of brain networks involved in processing speed in individuals with MS compared with

HCs. The study by Genova, Hillary, Wylie, Rypma, and DeLuca (2009) adapted the Symbol Digit Modalities Test (SDMT) for use during MRI. Instead of having a page with digits and symbols (as during the pencil-and-paper test), participants were presented with a panel containing nine number–symbol combinations during each trial and had to indicate whether the probe, presented below the number–symbol panel, matched any of the number–symbol pairs in the panel (Figure 3.1). Although performance accuracy was similar between groups, MS participants' response time was significantly slower than that of HCs. Importantly, MS participants showed reduced activation compared with HCs in the frontoparietal network. The results of this study suggest that MS participants use different neural mechanisms than HCs when processing speed is taxed. Although this adaptive cerebral reorganization might have supported adequate performance for MS patients (i.e., accuracy), it came at a cost of slowed responding.

Functional Connectivity Studies

Now that we looked at how task-based fMRI can inform us about the regions that are engaged during task performance, we can go a step further and examine the interaction between brain regions. Focusing on brain network interaction, rather than on individual areas, is important because MS affects the central nervous system so diffusely. In general, researchers use one of two advanced statistical analyses to examine such interactions: functional or effective connectivity analysis. Evidence from both approaches points to the association between cerebral reorganization and cognition in MS.

Functional connectivity analysis provides correlational information about the BOLD signal from brain regions. This approach can be applied to both task fMRI and resting-state fMRI (to analyze the interaction between brain regions while the brain is not engaged in any task). Au Duong et al.

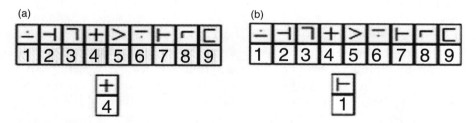

Figure 3.1. A representation of a number–symbol panel from the modified Symbol Digit Modalities Test. (a) Match trial. (b) Nonmatch trial. From "Examination of Processing Speed Deficits in Multiple Sclerosis Using Functional Magnetic Resonance Imaging," by H. M. Genova, F. G. Hillary, G. Wylie, B. Rypma, and J. DeLuca, 2009, *Journal of the International Neuropsychological Society, 15*, p. 385. Copyright 2009 by Cambridge University Press. Reprinted with permission.

(2005) conducted a functional connectivity analysis on the regions identified in their previous studies (Audoin et al., 2003, 2005) to examine the interplay between working memory regions. Although there were no differences in PASAT performance between the two groups, the working memory regions showed decreased functional connectivity in the patient sample, with HCs exhibiting greater connectivity between these areas. Thus, these findings suggest that the observed altered functional connectivity in working memory regions is compensatory and adaptive.

One of the main issues when comparing brain changes between healthy individuals and a clinical population is that results from studies on patients performing active tasks can be influenced by the patients' ability to match task performance with HCs. Analyzing brain connectivity at rest (or resting state functional connectivity [RSFC]) potentially solves this problem. Roosendaal et al. (2010) examined RSFC in subjects with clinically isolated syndrome (CIS), with relapsing–remitting MS (RRMS), and HCs. Compared with HCs, CIS patients showed increased RSFC in the majority of functional brain networks, including the default-mode network (DMN) and the sensorimotor network, possibly reflecting the recruitment of reserve capacity to compensate for structural damage. Consistent with the hypothesis of an early-occurring, but limited, reorganization process, RSFC modifications were not found in cognitively impaired (CI) RRMS patients (Roosendaal et al., 2010).

Better cognitive performance in MS patients has been associated with increased functional connectivity among several regions of the attention network, thus supporting the adaptive role of these functional modifications (Loitfelder et al., 2012). Conversely, in CI patients, a reduced RSFC of frontal regions (Bonavita et al., 2011; Rocca, Valsasina, et al., 2010, 2014) has been observed, which was related not only to the severity of cognitive impairment but also to the structural disruption of connecting cognitive-related WM tracts (Rocca, Valsasina, et al., 2010). This is contrary to the hypothesis that cerebral reorganization is always adaptive. To that end, a handful of studies (Hawellek, Hipp, Lewis, Corbetta, & Engel, 2011; Schoonheim et al., 2015) have reported correlations between increased RSFC and worsened cognitive performance based on neuropsychological testing. Recent studies suggest a distributed and complex pattern of RSFC abnormalities that correlate with T2 lesion volume and disability status (Rocca, Bonnet, et al., 2012; Rocca, Valsasina, et al., 2010). These data suggest that the increased RSFC associated with cognitive impairment can also be maladaptive.

Graph analysis represents the state-of-the-art methodology to assess functional connectivity in the brain, contributing to the characterization of functional disconnection and efficiency loss in neurological conditions (Filippi et al., 2013). This method schematizes the brain as a set of nodes connected by edges and identifies the so-called hubs, defined as nodes with a high number of connections and central position in the topological organization of a network. A recent study applying graph theory in 246 MS patients and 55 matched control subjects found that regional redistribution and impaired functional integration of network properties in MS patients contributed to cognitive status and MS clinical course (Rocca et al., 2016). These findings suggested that the loss of "critical" hubs and the functional incompetence of alternative hubs might contribute to a progressive disease course. Further, the capacity to maintain the functional integrity and specialization of specific brain regions over time might be among the main factors responsible for the preservation of clinical and cognitive functions (Bonnet et al., 2010; Rocca, Riccitelli, et al., 2010; Staffen et al., 2002).

Despite the clear advantages of RS fMRI for comparing MS patients to HCs, it is important to note that there might be some mechanisms related to cognitive network function that are unlikely to be captured properly using a resting paradigm. Specifically, it has been suggested that MS patients might have a limited ability to optimize cognitive network recruitment with increasing cognitive load (i.e., the ability to match brain activity to increasing cognitive demand), reflecting an impaired cognitive functional reserve (Loitfelder et al., 2011; Tortorella et al., 2013). Such an impaired functional reserve is likely to be a maladaptive mechanism contributing to MS clinical manifestations. This mechanism is usually present from the beginning of the disease, including in CIS patients (Tortorella et al., 2013), but is more pronounced in patients with progressive MS (Loitfelder et al., 2011) and in those with CI (Rocca, Parisi, et al., 2014).

Effective Connectivity Studies

Whereas functional connectivity examines correlational information about the BOLD signal from brain regions, effective connectivity allows examination of the influence of one brain region on another brain region (Friston, 1994). Several statistical algorithms exist that are able to reflect changes in effective connectivity, and thus possibly a higher degree of cerebral reorganization.

Additional studies support this idea of compensatory or adaptive changes in functional connectivity within MS by using the Stroop task, a cognitively demanding interference task that taxes the regions of the executive brain network. Work by Rocca et al. (2009) shows that patients with benign MS (BMS) exhibit increased effective connectivity among several cortical areas of the sensorimotor network, as well as decreased effective connectivity between the ACC and the left secondary sensorimotor cortex, right cerebellum, and prefrontal regions. These results suggest an altered interhemispheric balance in favor of the right hemisphere recruitment in BMS patients. Another Stroop fMRI study (Rocca, Bonnet, et al., 2012) explored modifications of effective connectivity between cerebellar and prefrontal areas in patients with relapse-onset MS at different stages of the disease and their association with cognitive failure. Abnormalities in activation and effective connectivity between the right cerebellum and frontoparietal areas were detected between MS and HC, and these contribute to inefficient cortical reorganization with increasing cognitive load.

Throughout this chapter, we have described research that compares individuals with MS to HCs. Studies that approach the analysis of patients with and without cognitive deficits are sparse. However, recently, Dobryakova, Costa, et al. (2016) examined differences in processing speed and the associated effective connectivity patterns in a sample of 18 HC and 21 MS patients, eight of whom had processing speed deficits, defined by performance on the SDMT (Parmenter, Testa, Schretlen, Weinstock-Guttman, & Benedict, 2010). All participants performed the modified SDMT during MRI scanning. The authors first determined brain regions engaged in modified SDMT in HCs and then applied a novel effective connectivity analysis method based on causal Bayes networks (Ramsey, Hanson, & Glymour, 2011) to examine whether the neurotypical connectivity pattern is altered in the two groups of MS patients (i.e., those with and without processing speed deficits). As expected, the connectivity pattern of MS patients with processing speed impairment was significantly different from the connectivity pattern of MS patients without processing speed impairment and that of HCs. Interestingly, the connectivity pattern of MS patients without processing speed impairment shared certain connections with the HC connectivity pattern, whereas other connections were shared with the connectivity pattern observed in MS patients with processing speed impairment (Figure 3.2). The study by Dobryakova et al. is the first to date that examined MS patients based on processing speed impairment, thus approaching the analysis of cerebral reorganization dimensionally. The results of this study suggest that the cerebral reorganization in MS patients with processing speed impairment is qualitatively and quantitatively different from HCs and thus might be maladaptive.

Although it is evident from the preceding work that individuals with MS have alterations in effective connectivity reflective of cerebral reorganization, a few studies compared more than a single group of MS patients to HCs. Dobryakova, Rocca, et al. (2016) examined brain interaction patterns in three MS phenotypes during the Stroop task, providing a detailed description of alterations in effective connectivity. Connectivity patterns of 33 patients with RRMS, 18 patients with BMS, and 33 patients with secondary progressive MS (SPMS) were compared with 37 HCs. Behavioral results

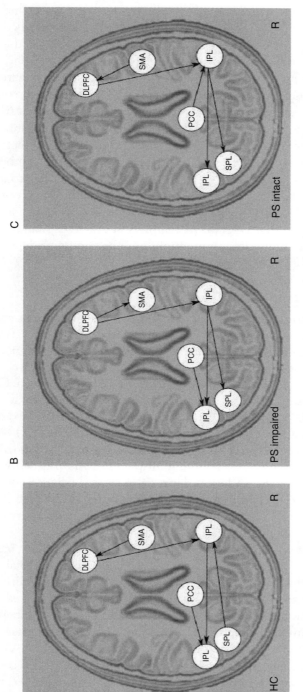

Figure 3.2. Graphs that represent connectivity patterns of the three groups of subjects. Note the similarities and differences in information flow between multiple sclerosis patients with and without processing speed impairment (PS impaired vs. PS intact). From "Altered Effective Connectivity During a Processing Speed Task in Individuals With Multiple Sclerosis," by E. Dobryakova, S. L. Costa, G. R. Wylie, J. DeLuca, and H. M. Genova, 2016, *Journal of the International Neuropsychological Society, 22*, p. 221. Copyright 2016 by Cambridge University Press. Reprinted with permission.

showed that compared with HCs, all MS phenotypes were slower and exhibited lower performance accuracy during trials requiring increased cognitive control (i.e., when participants were required to name the color of the font of a color word, e.g., the word *red* presented in green ink). All MS phenotypes also exhibited connectivity abnormalities, reflected as weaker shared connections (i.e., connections that were present in all four groups), the presence of extra connections (i.e., connections that were absent in the connectivity pattern of HCs), connection reversal (i.e., a switch from the HC connectivity pattern in causal influence of one region on another), and connection loss (i.e., the absence of connections that were present in the HC connectivity pattern; Color Plate 5). Importantly, in the SPMS and BMS groups (the phenotypes with longer disease duration) but not in the RRMS group, extra connections were associated with deficits in Stroop performance accuracy. These results suggest that cerebral reorganization differs depending on the MS phenotype and that extra connections may become maladaptive with disease and disability progression.

Structural MRI

In addition to an abnormal pattern of functional activations and connectivity, the majority of existing studies describe variable relationships among cognition, functional brain activation, and tissue damage derived from structural imaging techniques (Au Duong et al., 2005; Filippi, Rocca, Falini, et al., 2002; Mainero et al., 2004; Rocca, Falini, et al., 2002; Rocca, Gavazzi, et al., 2003; Rocca, Matthews, et al., 2002; Rocca, Mezzapesa, et al., 2003), thus also reflecting cerebral reorganization. For example, increased recruitment of several brain areas with increasing T2 lesion volume (LV) has been shown in RRMS (Au Duong et al., 2005; Bobholz et al., 2006; Mainero et al., 2004) and primary progressive multiple sclerosis (PPMS) patients. The severity of intrinsic T2 lesion damage, measured using T1-weighted images (Pantano et al., 2002), magnetization transfer (MT), and diffusion tensor imaging (DTI) (Rocca, Falini, et al., 2002), has been found to modulate the activity of some brain areas.

The severity of normal-appearing brain tissue (NABT) injury, measured using (Rocca, Mezzapesa, et al., 2003) MT MRI (Au Duong et al., 2005; Filippi, Rocca, Falini, et al., 2002) and DTI (Filippi, Rocca, Falini, et al., 2002; Rocca, Mezzapesa, et al., 2003), is another important factor associated with increased recruitment of motor- and cognitive-related brain regions. A seminal study by Audoin et al. (2005) found significant correlations between functional activation in the lateral prefrontal cortices during PASAT execution in CIS patients and the severity of NABT damage, quantified using MT MRI. By combining fMRI and DTI measures, Bonzano et al. (2009) found a relationship between structural damage to strategic WM tracts.

Although MS is thought to primarily affect WM, recent evidence suggests that there is also cerebral reorganization within GM, with GM pathology being a significant contributor to cognitive impairment (e.g., Hulst & Geurts, 2011). For example, Batista et al. (2012) assessed basal ganglia and thalamic volume, as well as information processing speed in 86 MS patients and 25 HCs (Color Plate 6). Controlling for neocortex volume, the results showed that atrophy of these GM structures independently contributes to slowed processing speed in MS. Similarly, Sanfilipo, Benedict, Weinstock-Guttman, and Bakshi (2006) showed that not only WM but also GM volume explains deficits in memory and processing speed in individuals with MS.

Amato et al. (2004) examined GM pathology in 41 RRMS patients, further characterizing them as CI and CP based on performance using the Brief Repeatable Battery (BRB). CI patients had significantly more GM atrophy compared with CP patients. More detailed findings were provided recently by Nocentini et al. (2014) who used voxel-based morphometry to show a significant association between SDMT performance and GM volume reduction.

Longitudinal Studies and Cognitive Rehabilitation

Only a few studies have used fMRI techniques to explore the longitudinal modifications of cognitive network recruitment and their impact on patients' cognitive status (Enzinger et al., 2016). A 1-year longitudinal study in patients with early MS found an association between increased activation of the right dorsolateral prefrontal cortex during a cognitive task and improved working memory and processing speed performance (Audoin et al., 2008). A 20-month longitudinal study (Loitfelder et al., 2014) showed that worsening of SDMT performance in RRMS patients was correlated with increased activity of the left inferior parietal lobule over time, probably reflecting a maladaptive mechanism.

Rehabilitation can be described as "the action of restoring someone to health or normal life through training and therapy after imprisonment, addiction, or illness" (Oxford Dictionary; https://en.oxforddictionaries.com) for the purpose of facilitating brain plasticity, leading to increased usage of a skill (Duffau, 2006). Several investigations examined neural changes after rehabilitation in various cognitive domains. A study that applied 3-month computer-assisted cognitive rehabilitation in RRMS patients with selective attention and executive function deficits detected an enhanced recruitment of brain networks subserving the trained functions in the rehabilitation group (Filippi et al., 2012). Interestingly enough, changes in RSFC of cognitive-related networks helped explain the persistence of the cognitive rehabilitation effects several months after treatment termination. In addition, the observed changes helped explain patients' improvement on depression and quality-of-life scales, suggesting that cognitive rehabilitation exerts a positive effect not limited to the trained function, but extending to several additional domains (Parisi et al., 2014). Another study also supported a cerebral reorganization effect in CI MS patients as assessed by fMRI during PASAT. The cognitive rehabilitation program targeted processing speed, attention, executive functions, memory, and high-level language function and lasted for 5 weeks (Sastre-Garriga et al., 2011).

It is no exaggeration to say that longitudinal MRI and cognitive rehabilitation studies are uniquely suited to reflect cerebral reorganization associated with cognition in individuals with MS. Regardless of the paucity of such studies, there are promising findings showing cognitive rehabilitation leading to changes in brain activity in association with working memory (Huiskamp, Dobryakova, Wylie, DeLuca, & Chiaravalloti, 2016), long-term memory acquisition and encoding (N. D. Chiaravalloti, Wylie, Leavitt, & DeLuca, 2012), as well as persistence of effects from cognitive rehabilitation (Dobryakova, Wylie, DeLuca, & Chiaravalloti, 2014; Parisi et al., 2014). Moving forward, innovative treatments for cognitive dysfunction may be developed from current research using fMRI to guide the combined use of computer-based cognitive rehabilitation and noninvasive brain stimulation (Mattioli, Bellomi, Stampatori, Capra, & Miniussi, 2016). Chapter 13 of this volume goes beyond neuroimaging findings and provides a more detailed look at cognitive rehabilitation in MS.

ADAPTIVE VERSUS MALADAPTIVE CHANGES

As previously discussed, studies that found altered brain recruitment or connectivity in cognitively preserved MS patients, often related to the severity of structural MRI damage, have argued for a possible adaptive role of fMRI modifications to counteract the progressive accumulation of irreversible, disease-related tissue damage. However, there are also studies suggesting that, occasionally, what is being measured by fMRI is not beneficial for the patients, reflecting maladaptive mechanisms associated with the presence of cognitive deficits or specific symptoms, such as fatigue. Penner, Rausch, Kappos, Opwis, and Radü (2003) examined mildly impaired and severely impaired MS patients, as well as HCs, while they were performing three cognitive tasks. Although performance of mildly impaired MS patients did not differ from HCs on any task, they exhibited adaptive reorganization, showing higher and more bilateral recruitment of prefrontal and parietal regions compared with HCs. Severely impaired MS patients, whose performance was significantly different from both mildly impaired MS subjects and HCs, had a weakened pattern of brain recruitment compared with HCs, suggestive of maladaptive cerebral reorganization.

Similarly, Rocca, Bonnet, et al. (2012) showed likely maladaptive activation differences between CI and CP PPMS patients as they were related to CI severity and measures of brain tissue damage. These studies thus suggest that the extent of cerebral reorganization might be exhausted when cognitive impairment is severe.

Although not in the category of cognition, fatigue is another common symptom of MS (see Chapter 6) associated with altered patterns of cerebral reorganization. Several recent studies implicate the frontostriatal network, which is heavily innervated by the neurotransmitter dopamine in fatigue (Dobryakova, Genova, DeLuca, & Wylie, 2015; Filippi, Rocca, Colombo, et al., 2002; Rocca et al., 2007). Additional functional connectivity studies show alterations within this network in individuals with MS compared with HCs. Importantly, this brain network is also engaged in cognitive processes such as working memory and attention (Cools, 2011). Thus, this evidence potentially points to a dysregulation of the dopamine within the MS-affected brain, bringing about fatigue, deficits in the cognition, and thus maladaptive patterns of brain activation. Fatigue has also been shown to be associated with disease type, duration, and disability (Ghajarzadeh et al., 2013). Thus, early in the disease, cerebral reorganization might be adaptive and aid in maintaining cognitive function. However, as the disease progresses, cerebral reorganization becomes maladaptive resulting in cognitive deficits and fatigue.

FROM THEORIES TO DATA

Throughout this chapter, cerebral reorganization, or neural plasticity, has been generally defined as the brain's ability to go through functional or structural changes. Regardless of such a seemingly straightforward definition, there is some debate about what cerebral reorganization really is and what processes it specifically encompasses. According to Paillard, a French neuroscientist who has done extensive work on the topic of long-term potentiation, "The term *plasticity* is only appropriate in terms of the ability of a system to achieve novel functions, either by transforming its internal connectivity or by changing the elements of which it is made" (Will, Dalrymple-Alford, Wolff, & Cassel, 2008a, p. 2). In other words, *cerebral reorganization*, or *neural plasticity*, is an appropriate term only when it leads to a development of a new function and to a structural change (Will, Dalrymple-Alford, Wolff, & Cassel, 2008b). A majority of literature on cognition in MS interprets increased activation, in conjunction with the absence of behavioral deficits compared with HCs, as compensatory cerebral reorganization (as discussed earlier). However, that would contradict Paillard's definition because the activation changes observed through fMRI produce neural changes but occur in the absence of behavioral changes. More recently, it has also been proposed that the observed increase in functional brain activity is not a result of adaptive cerebral reorganization or neural compensation but rather is due to increased cognitive control, a native support mechanism (Hillary, 2008). Thus, only maladaptive cerebral reorganization would constitute true neural plasticity according to Paillard's definition.

Regardless of the preceding theories and their extent, the MRI evidence in support of cerebral reorganization, be it adaptive or maladaptive, is only as strong as the data analysis method. The majority of MRI studies on cerebral reorganization usually have a low number of participants, with only two comparison groups. Furthermore, unlike other imaging modalities that can be easily used in a clinical setting, such as computed tomography (CT) for assessing traumatic brain injury severity, MRI analysis usually involves cumbersome data processing. These multistep data processing pipelines rely on statistical algorithms that are updated and improved constantly, even as you read this chapter. Thus, MRI results must be interpreted with caution and are pending replication. That being said, so far, MRI has shown to be the best noninvasive method for observing cerebral reorganization on the macrostructural level, despite the method's practical and methodological limitations. As technology and research advance, it is doubtless these limitations, too, will subsequently be surmounted.

CONCLUSIONS AND FUTURE DIRECTIONS

Although a topic of debate in the 20th century, it is now generally accepted that the adult brain goes through cerebral reorganization. Cerebral reorganization occurs during the course of development or through changes to the environment. However, it can also occur as a result of injury or disease. The current chapter provided ample evidence for both adaptive and maladaptive cerebral reorganization as a result of MS from investigations using MRI and various approaches to data analyses.

Current studies provide valuable evidence about cerebral reorganization, but there is a need for longitudinal and randomized controlled rehabilitation studies that would reflect the influence of disease course and rehabilitation strategies on brain plasticity, respectively. As data acquisition and analysis methods improve, researchers will be able to garner evidence that is more robust and thus better address the theories of cerebral reorganization.

REFERENCES

Amato, M. P., Bartolozzi, M. L., Zipoli, V., Portaccio, E., Mortilla, M., Guidi, L., . . . De Stefano, N. (2004). Neocortical volume decrease in relapsing-remitting MS patients with mild cognitive impairment. *Neurology, 63,* 89–93. http://dx.doi.org/10.1212/01.WNL.0000129544.79539.D5

Au Duong, M. V., Audoin, B., Boulanouar, K., Ibarrola, D., Malikova, I., Confort-Gouny, S., . . . Ranjeva, J.-P. (2005). Altered functional connectivity related to white matter changes inside the working memory network at the very early stage of MS. *Journal of Cerebral Blood Flow and Metabolism, 25,* 1245–1253. http://dx.doi.org/10.1038/sj.jcbfm.9600122

Audoin, B., Au Duong, M. V., Ranjeva, J. P., Ibarrola, D., Malikova, I., Confort-Gouny, S., . . . Cozzone, P. J. (2005). Magnetic resonance study of the influence of tissue damage and cortical reorganization on PASAT performance at the earliest stage of multiple sclerosis. *Human Brain Mapping, 24,* 216–228.

Audoin, B., Ibarrola, D., Ranjeva, J.-P., Confort-Gouny, S., Malikova, I., Ali-Chérif, A., . . . Cozzone, P. (2003). Compensatory cortical activation observed by fMRI during a cognitive task at the earliest stage of multiple sclerosis. *Human Brain Mapping, 20,* 51–58. http://dx.doi.org/10.1002/hbm.10128

Audoin, B., Reuter, F., Duong, M. V. A., Malikova, I., Confort-Gouny, S., Cherif, A. A., . . . Ranjeva, J. P. (2008). Efficiency of cognitive control recruitment in the very early stage of multiple sclerosis: A one-year fMRI follow-up study. *Multiple Sclerosis Journal, 14,* 786–792. http://dx.doi.org/10.1177/1352458508089360

Batista, S., Zivadinov, R., Hoogs, M., Bergsland, N., Heininen-Brown, M., Dwyer, M. G., . . . Benedict, R. H. B. (2012). Basal ganglia, thalamus and neocortical atrophy predicting slowed cognitive processing in multiple sclerosis. *Journal of Neurology, 259,* 139–146. http://dx.doi.org/10.1007/s00415-011-6147-1

Bjartmar, C., Battistuta, J., Terada, N., Dupree, E., & Trapp, B. D. (2002). N-acetylaspartate is an axon-specific marker of mature white matter in vivo: A biochemical and immunohistochemical study on the rat optic nerve. *Annals of Neurology, 51,* 51–58. http://dx.doi.org/10.1002/ana.10052

Bobholz, J. A., Rao, S. M., Lobeck, L., Elsinger, C., Gleason, A., Kanz, J., . . . Maas, E. (2006). fMRI study of episodic memory in relapsing-remitting MS: Correlation with T2 lesion volume. *Neurology, 67,* 1640–1645.

Bonavita, S., Gallo, A., Sacco, R., Corte, M. D., Bisecco, A., Docimo, R., . . . Tedeschi, G. (2011). Distributed changes in default-mode resting-state connectivity in multiple sclerosis. *Multiple Sclerosis Journal, 17,* 411–422. http://dx.doi.org/10.1177/1352458510394609

Bonnet, M. C., Allard, M., Dilharreguy, B., Deloire, M., Petry, K. G., & Brochet, B. (2010). Cognitive compensation failure in multiple sclerosis. *Neurology, 75,* 1241–1248. http://dx.doi.org/10.1212/WNL.0b013e3181f612e3

Bonzano, L., Pardini, M., Mancardi, G. L., Pizzorno, M., & Roccatagliata, L. (2009). Structural connectivity influences brain activation during PVSAT in multiple sclerosis. *NeuroImage, 44,* 9–15. http://dx.doi.org/10.1016/j.neuroimage.2008.08.015

Chiaravalloti, N., Hillary, F., Ricker, J., Christodoulou, C., Kalnin, A., Liu, W.-C., . . . DeLuca, J. (2005). Cerebral activation patterns during working memory performance in multiple sclerosis using FMRI. *Journal of Clinical and Experimental Neuropsychology, 27,* 33–54. http://dx.doi.org/10.1080/138033990513609

Chiaravalloti, N. D., Stojanovic-Radic, J., & DeLuca, J. (2013). The role of speed versus working memory in predicting learning new information in multiple sclerosis. *Journal of Clinical and Experimental Neuropsychology, 35,* 180–191. http://dx.doi.org/10.1080/13803395.2012.760537

Chiaravalloti, N. D., Wylie, G., Leavitt, V., & DeLuca, J. (2012). Increased cerebral activation after behavioral treatment for memory deficits in MS. *Journal of Neurology, 259,* 1337–1346. http://dx.doi.org/10.1007/s00415-011-6353-x

Cifelli, A., & Matthews, P. M. (2002). Cerebral plasticity in multiple sclerosis: Insights from fMRI. *Multiple Sclerosis Journal, 8,* 193–199. http://dx.doi.org/10.1191/1352458502ms820oa

Cools, R. (2011). Dopaminergic control of the striatum for high-level cognition. *Current Opinion in Neurobiology, 21,* 402–407. http://dx.doi.org/10.1016/j.conb.2011.04.002

Dobryakova, E., Costa, S. L., Wylie, G. R., DeLuca, J., & Genova, H. M. (2016). Altered effective connectivity during a processing speed task in individuals with multiple sclerosis. *Journal of the International Neuropsychological Society, 22,* 216–224. http://dx.doi.org/10.1017/S1355617715001034

Dobryakova, E., Genova, H. M., DeLuca, J., & Wylie, G. R. (2015). The dopamine imbalance hypothesis of fatigue in multiple sclerosis and other neurological disorders. *Frontiers in Neurology, 6,* 52. http://dx.doi.org/10.3389/fneur.2015.00052

Dobryakova, E., Rocca, M. A., Valsasina, P., Ghezzi, A., Colombo, B., Martinelli, V., . . . Filippi, M. (2016). Abnormalities of the executive control network in multiple sclerosis phenotypes: An fMRI effective connectivity study. *Human Brain Mapping, 37,* 2293–2304.

Dobryakova, E., Wylie, G. R., DeLuca, J., & Chiaravalloti, N. D. (2014). A pilot study examining functional brain activity 6 months after memory retraining in MS: The MEMREHAB trial. *Brain Imaging and Behavior, 8,* 403–406. http://dx.doi.org/10.1007/s11682-014-9309-9

Duffau, H. (2006). Brain plasticity: From pathophysiological mechanisms to therapeutic applications. *Journal of Clinical Neuroscience, 13,* 885–897. http://dx.doi.org/10.1016/j.jocn.2005.11.045

Enzinger, C., Pinter, D., Rocca, M. A., DeLuca, J., Sastre-Garriga, J., Audoin, B., & Filippi, M. (2016). Longitudinal fMRI studies: Exploring brain plasticity and repair in MS. *Multiple Sclerosis Journal, 22,* 269–278. http://dx.doi.org/10.1177/1352458515619781

Filippi, M., Riccitelli, G., Mattioli, F., Capra, R., Stampatori, C., Pagani, E., . . . Rocca, M. A. (2012). Multiple sclerosis: Effects of cognitive rehabilitation on structural and functional MR imaging measures—An explorative study. *Radiology*, *262*, 932–940. http://dx.doi.org/10.1148/radiol.11111299

Filippi, M., Rocca, M. A., Colombo, B., Falini, A., Codella, M., Scotti, G., & Comi, G. (2002). Functional magnetic resonance imaging correlates of fatigue in multiple sclerosis. *NeuroImage*, *15*, 559–567. http://dx.doi.org/10.1006/nimg.2001.1011

Filippi, M., Rocca, M. A., Falini, A., Caputo, D., Ghezzi, A., Colombo, B., . . . Comi, G. (2002). Correlations between structural CNS damage and functional MRI changes in primary progressive MS. *NeuroImage*, *15*, 537–546. http://dx.doi.org/10.1006/nimg.2001.1023

Filippi, M., van den Heuvel, M. P., Fornito, A., He, Y., Hulshoff Pol, H. E., Agosta, F., . . . Rocca, M. A. (2013). Assessment of system dysfunction in the brain through MRI-based connectomics. *The Lancet Neurology*, *12*, 1189–1199. http://dx.doi.org/10.1016/S1474-4422(13)70144-3

Friston, K. J. (1994). Functional and effective connectivity in neuroimaging: A synthesis. *Human Brain Mapping*, *2*, 56–78. http://dx.doi.org/10.1002/hbm.460020107

Genova, H. M., Dobryakova, E., Gonen, O., Hillary, F., Wylie, G., Wu, W. E., . . . DeLuca, J. (2014). Examination of functional reorganization in multiple sclerosis using fMRI-guided magnetic resonance spectroscopy: A pilot study. *Journal of Multiple Sclerosis*, *2*, 1–6.

Genova, H. M., Hillary, F. G., Wylie, G., Rypma, B., & DeLuca, J. (2009). Examination of processing speed deficits in multiple sclerosis using functional magnetic resonance imaging. *Journal of the International Neuropsychological Society*, *15*, 383–393. http://dx.doi.org/10.1017/S1355617709090535

Ghajarzadeh, M., Jalilian, R., Eskandari, G., Sahraian, M. A., Azimi, A., & Mohammadifar, M. (2013). Fatigue in multiple sclerosis: Relationship with disease duration, physical disability, disease pattern, age and sex. *Acta Neurologica Belgica*, *113*, 411–414. http://dx.doi.org/10.1007/s13760-013-0198-2

Giorgio, A., & De Stefano, N. (2010). Cognition in multiple sclerosis: Relevance of lesions, brain atrophy and proton MR spectroscopy. *Neurological Sciences*, *31*(Suppl. 2), S245–S248. http://dx.doi.org/10.1007/s10072-010-0370-x

Haider, L., Zrzavy, T., Hametner, S., Höftberger, R., Bagnato, F., Grabner, G., . . . Lassmann, H. (2016). The topography of demyelination and neurodegeneration in the multiple sclerosis brain. *Brain: A Journal of Neurology*, *139*, 807–815. http://dx.doi.org/10.1093/brain/awv398

Hawellek, D. J., Hipp, J. F., Lewis, C. M., Corbetta, M., & Engel, A. K. (2011). Increased functional connectivity indicates the severity of cognitive impairment in multiple sclerosis. *Proceedings of the National Academy of Sciences of the United States of America*, *108*, 19066–19071. http://dx.doi.org/10.1073/pnas.1110024108

Hillary, F. G. (2008). Neuroimaging of working memory dysfunction and the dilemma with brain reorganization hypotheses. *Journal of the International Neuropsychological Society*, *14*, 526–534. http://dx.doi.org/10.1017/S1355617708080788

Huiskamp, M., Dobryakova, E., Wylie, G. D., DeLuca, J., & Chiaravalloti, N. D. (2016). A pilot study of changes in functional brain activity during a working memory task after mSMT treatment: The MEMREHAB trial. *Multiple Sclerosis and Related Disorders, 7*, 76–82. http://dx.doi.org/10.1016/j.msard.2016.03.012

Hulst, H. E. H., & Geurts, J. G. (2011). Gray matter imaging in multiple sclerosis: What have we learned? *BMC Neurology, 11*, 153. http://dx.doi.org/10.1186/1471-2377-11-153

Johnson, M. H. (2001). Functional brain development in humans. *Nature Reviews Neuroscience, 2*, 475–483. http://dx.doi.org/10.1038/35081509

Kolb, B., Muhammad, A., & Gibb, R. (2011). Searching for factors underlying cerebral plasticity in the normal and injured brain. *Journal of Communication Disorders, 44*, 503–514. http://dx.doi.org/10.1016/j.jcomdis.2011.04.007

Ksiazek-Winiarek, D. J., Szpakowski, P., & Glabinski, A. (2015). Neural plasticity in multiple sclerosis: The functional and molecular background. *Neural Plasticity, 2015*, 307175. http://dx.doi.org/10.1155/2015/307175

Loitfelder, M., Fazekas, F., Koschutnig, K., Fuchs, S., Petrovic, K., Ropele, S., . . . Enzinger, C. (2014). Brain activity changes in cognitive networks in relapsing-remitting multiple sclerosis—Insights from a longitudinal FMRI study. *PLoS One, 9*, e93715. http://dx.doi.org/10.1371/journal.pone.0093715

Loitfelder, M., Fazekas, F., Petrovic, K., Fuchs, S., Ropele, S., Wallner-Blazek, M., . . . Enzinger, C. (2011). Reorganization in cognitive networks with progression of multiple sclerosis: Insights from fMRI. *Neurology, 76*, 526–533. http://dx.doi.org/10.1212/WNL.0b013e31820b75cf

Loitfelder, M., Filippi, M., Rocca, M., Valsasina, P., Ropele, S., Jehna, M., . . . Enzinger, C. (2012). Abnormalities of resting state functional connectivity are related to sustained attention deficits in MS. *PLoS One, 7*, e42862. http://dx.doi.org/10.1371/journal.pone.0042862

Mainero, C., Caramia, F., Pozzilli, C., Pisani, A., Pestalozza, I., Borriello, G., . . . Pantano, P. (2004). fMRI evidence of brain reorganization during attention and memory tasks in multiple sclerosis. *NeuroImage, 21*, 858–867. http://dx.doi.org/10.1016/j.neuroimage.2003.10.004

Mattioli, F., Bellomi, F., Stampatori, C., Capra, R., & Miniussi, C. (2016). Neuro-enhancement through cognitive training and anodal tDCS in multiple sclerosis. *Multiple Sclerosis Journal, 22*, 222–230. http://dx.doi.org/10.1177/1352458515587597

Nocentini, U., Bozzali, M., Spanò, B., Cercignani, M., Serra, L., Basile, B., . . . DeLuca, J. (2014). Exploration of the relationships between regional grey matter atrophy and cognition in multiple sclerosis. *Brain Imaging and Behavior, 8*, 378–386. http://dx.doi.org/10.1007/s11682-012-9170-7

Pantano, P., Mainero, C., Iannetti, G. D., Caramia, F., Di Legge, S., Piattella, M. C., . . . Lenzi, G. L. (2002). Cortical motor reorganization after a single clinical attack of multiple sclerosis. *Brain, 125*, 1607–1615. http://dx.doi.org/10.1093/brain/awf164

Parisi, L., Rocca, M. A., Mattioli, F., Copetti, M., Capra, R., Valsasina, P., . . . Filippi, M. (2014). Changes of brain resting state functional connectivity predict the persistence of cognitive rehabilitation effects in patients with multiple sclerosis. *Multiple Sclerosis Journal, 20,* 686–694. http://dx.doi.org/10.1177/1352458513505692

Parmenter, B. A., Testa, S. M., Schretlen, D. J., Weinstock-Guttman, B., & Benedict, R. H. B. (2010). The utility of regression-based norms in interpreting the minimal assessment of cognitive function in multiple sclerosis (MACFIMS). *Journal of the International Neuropsychological Society, 16,* 6–16. http://dx.doi.org/10.1017/S1355617709990750

Penner, I.-K., Rausch, M., Kappos, L., Opwis, K., & Radü, E. W. (2003). Analysis of impairment related functional architecture in MS patients during performance of different attention tasks. *Journal of Neurology, 250,* 461–472. http://dx.doi.org/10.1007/s00415-003-1025-0

Ramsey, J. D., Hanson, S. J., & Glymour, C. (2011). Multi-subject search correctly identifies causal connections and most causal directions in the DCM models of the Smith et al. simulation study. *NeuroImage, 58,* 838–848. http://dx.doi.org/10.1016/j.neuroimage.2011.06.068

Rocca, M. A., Agosta, F., Colombo, B., Mezzapesa, D. M., Falini, A., Comi, G., & Filippi, M. (2007). fMRI changes in relapsing-remitting multiple sclerosis patients complaining of fatigue after IFNbeta-1a injection. *Human Brain Mapping, 28,* 373–382. http://dx.doi.org/10.1002/hbm.20279

Rocca, M. A., Bonnet, M. C., Meani, A., Valsasina, P., Colombo, B., Comi, G., & Filippi, M. (2012). Differential cerebellar functional interactions during an interference task across multiple sclerosis phenotypes. *Radiology, 265,* 864–873. http://dx.doi.org/10.1148/radiol.12120216

Rocca, M. A., Falini, A., Colombo, B., Scotti, G., Comi, G., & Filippi, M. (2002). Adaptive functional changes in the cerebral cortex of patients with nondisabling multiple sclerosis correlate with the extent of brain structural damage. *Annals of Neurology, 51,* 330–339. http://dx.doi.org/10.1002/ana.10120

Rocca, M. A., Gavazzi, C., Mezzapesa, D. M., Falini, A., Colombo, B., Mascalchi, M., . . . Filippi, M. (2003). A functional magnetic resonance imaging study of patients with secondary progressive multiple sclerosis. *NeuroImage, 19,* 1770–1777. http://dx.doi.org/10.1016/S1053-8119(03)00242-8

Rocca, M. A., Matthews, P. M., Caputo, D., Ghezzi, A., Falini, A., Scotti, G., . . . Filippi, M. (2002). Evidence for widespread movement-associated functional MRI changes in patients with PPMS. *Neurology, 58,* 866–872. http://dx.doi.org/10.1212/WNL.58.6.866

Rocca, M. A., Mezzapesa, D. M., Falini, A., Ghezzi, A., Martinelli, V., Scotti, G., . . . Filippi, M. (2003). Evidence for axonal pathology and adaptive cortical reorganization in patients at presentation with clinically isolated syndromes suggestive of multiple sclerosis. *NeuroImage, 18,* 847–855. http://dx.doi.org/10.1016/S1053-8119(03)00043-0

Rocca, M. A., Parisi, L., Pagani, E., Copetti, M., Rodegher, M., Colombo, B., . . . Filippi, M. (2014). Regional but not global brain damage contributes to fatigue in multiple sclerosis. *Radiology*, *273*, 511–520. http://dx.doi.org/10.1148/radiol.14140417

Rocca, M. A., Riccitelli, G., Rodegher, M., Ceccarelli, A., Falini, A., Falautano, M., . . . Filippi, M. (2010). Functional MR imaging correlates of neuropsychological impairment in primary-progressive multiple sclerosis. *American Journal of Neuroradiology*, *31*, 1240–1246. http://dx.doi.org/10.3174/ajnr.A2071

Rocca, M. A., Valsasina, P., Absinta, M., Riccitelli, G., Rodegher, M. E., Misci, P., . . . Filippi, M. (2010). Default-mode network dysfunction and cognitive impairment in progressive MS [see correction at http://dx.doi.org/10.1212/WNL.0b013e3182817f5f]. *Neurology*, *74*, 1252–1259. http://dx.doi.org/10.1212/WNL.0b013e3181d9ed91

Rocca, M. A., Valsasina, P., Ceccarelli, A., Absinta, M., Ghezzi, A., Riccitelli, G., . . . Filippi, M. (2009). Structural and functional MRI correlates of Stroop control in benign MS. *Human Brain Mapping*, *30*, 276–290. http://dx.doi.org/10.1002/hbm.20504

Rocca, M. A., Valsasina, P., Hulst, H. E., Abdel-Aziz, K., Enzinger, C., Gallo, A., . . . the MAGNIMS fMRI Study Group. (2014). Functional correlates of cognitive dysfunction in multiple sclerosis: A multicenter fMRI Study. *Human Brain Mapping*, *35*, 5799–5814. http://dx.doi.org/10.1002/hbm.22586

Rocca, M. A., Valsasina, P., Meani, A., Falini, A., Comi, G., & Filippi, M. (2016). Impaired functional integration in multiple sclerosis: A graph theory study. *Brain Structure & Function*, *221*, 115–131. http://dx.doi.org/10.1007/s00429-014-0896-4

Roosendaal, S. D., Schoonheim, M. M., Hulst, H. E., Sanz-Arigita, E. J., Smith, S. M., Geurts, J. J. G., & Barkhof, F. (2010). Resting state networks change in clinically isolated syndrome. *Brain: A Journal of Neurology*, *133*, 1612–1621. http://dx.doi.org/10.1093/brain/awq058

Sanfilipo, M. P., Benedict, R. H. B., Weinstock-Guttman, B., & Bakshi, R. (2006). Gray and white matter brain atrophy and neuropsychological impairment in multiple sclerosis. *Neurology*, *66*, 685–692. http://dx.doi.org/10.1212/01.wnl.0000201238.93586.d9

Sastre-Garriga, J., Alonso, J., Renom, M., Arévalo, M. J., González, I., Galán, I., . . . Rovira, A. (2011). A functional magnetic resonance proof of concept pilot trial of cognitive rehabilitation in multiple sclerosis. *Multiple Sclerosis Journal*, *17*, 457–467. http://dx.doi.org/10.1177/1352458510389219

Schoonheim, M. M., Hulst, H. E., Brandt, R. B., Strik, M., Wink, A. M., Uitdehaag, B. M. J., . . . Geurts, J. J. G. (2015). Thalamus structure and function determine severity of cognitive impairment in multiple sclerosis. *Neurology*, *84*, 776–783. http://dx.doi.org/10.1212/WNL.0000000000001285

Staffen, W., Mair, A., Zauner, H., Unterrainer, J., Niederhofer, H., Kutzelnigg, A., . . . Ladurner, G. (2002). Cognitive function and fMRI in patients with multiple sclerosis: Evidence for compensatory cortical activation during an attention task. *Brain: A Journal of Neurology, 125,* 1275–1282. http://dx.doi.org/10.1093/brain/awf125

Tomassini, V., Matthews, P. M., Thompson, A. J., Fuglø, D., Geurts, J. J., Johansen-Berg, H., . . . Palace, J. (2012). Neuroplasticity and functional recovery in multiple sclerosis. *Nature Reviews. Neurology, 8,* 635–646. http://dx.doi.org/10.1038/nrneurol.2012.179

Tortorella, C., Romano, R., Direnzo, V., Taurisano, P., Zoccolella, S., Iaffaldano, P., . . . Trojano, M. (2013). Load-dependent dysfunction of the putamen during attentional processing in patients with clinically isolated syndrome suggestive of multiple sclerosis. *Multiple Sclerosis Journal, 19,* 1153–1160. http://dx.doi.org/10.1177/1352458512473671

Trapp, B. D., Peterson, J., Ransohoff, R. M., Rudick, R., Mörk, S., & Bö, L. (1998). Axonal transection in the lesions of multiple sclerosis. *The New England Journal of Medicine, 338,* 278–285. http://dx.doi.org/10.1056/NEJM199801293380502

Will, B., Dalrymple-Alford, J., Wolff, M., & Cassel, J.-C. (2008a). The concept of brain plasticity—Paillard's systemic analysis and emphasis on structure and function (followed by the translation of a seminal paper by Paillard on plasticity). *Behavioural Brain Research, 192,* 2–7. http://dx.doi.org/10.1016/j.bbr.2007.11.030

Will, B., Dalrymple-Alford, J., Wolff, M., & Cassel, J.-C. (2008b). Reflections on the use of the concept of plasticity in neurobiology. Translation and adaptation by Bruno Will, John Dalrymple-Alford, Mathieu Wolff and Jean-Christophe Cassel from J. Paillard, *J Psychol 1976, 1,* 33–47. *Behavioural Brain Research, 192,* 7–11. http://dx.doi.org/10.1016/j.bbr.2007.11.031

4

COGNITION AND DEPRESSION IN MULTIPLE SCLEROSIS

PETER A. ARNETT, MARGARET CADDEN,
CRISTINA ROMAN, AND ERIN GUTY

DEPRESSION IN MULTIPLE SCLEROSIS

The challenges of dealing with a severely debilitating illness, such as multiple sclerosis (MS), could understandably induce depressive moods or episodes. The prevalence of depression is high in patients with MS (Arnett, Barwick, & Beeney, 2008; Fischer et al., 1994; Goldman Consensus Group, 2005), with the lifetime risk approximately 50% (Patten & Metz, 1997; Sadovnick et al., 1996), compared with a lifetime risk in the general population of approximately 16% (Kessler et al., 2003). Point prevalence rates in MS are also high, with the most rigorous community-based study showing 26%, with a confidence interval ranging from about 19% to 33% (Viner et al., 2014), a finding consistent with a recent study using a variety of self-report depression measures (Strober & Arnett, 2015). Notably, this rate of depression in MS populations is also 2 times higher than in other chronic illnesses

http://dx.doi.org/10.1037/0000097-005
Cognition and Behavior in Multiple Sclerosis, J. DeLuca and B. M. Sandroff (Editors)

89

and even some other neurological disorders (Byatt, Rothschild, Riskind, Ionete, & Hunt, 2011). These discrepancies highlight the unique nature of depression in MS as well as the need for greater understanding of the diagnosis and etiology of depression in this disorder.

Due to its high prevalence and association with well-being (Kenealy, Beaumont, Lintern, & Murrell, 2000), disease course (Mohr et al., 2000), medication adherence (Bruce, Hancock, Arnett, & Lynch, 2010), and cognitive dysfunction (Arnett, Higginson, Voss, Wright, et al., 1999; Grech et al., 2015; Niino et al., 2014), among other factors, depression has been intensively studied in MS.

COGNITIVE IMPAIRMENTS IN MS

Cognitive dysfunction is also common in MS. Since Rao and colleagues' (Rao, Leo, Bernardin, & Unverzagt, 1991) seminal study on the prevalence of cognitive deficits in MS, other investigators have supported their finding of a close to 45% prevalence in community-based samples (Amato, Zipoli, & Portaccio, 2006; Jonsson et al., 2006). More than half of patients in clinically based samples (approximately 55%–65%) have typically been shown to have significant cognitive problems (Amato et al., 2006; Feinstein et al., 2004). There is also evidence of impairments in social cognition. One study found that individuals with MS show impairments in detecting lies and sarcasm compared with healthy control subjects (Genova et al., 2016), and other work has shown impairments in emotional processing (e.g., Kraemer et al., 2013) and theory of mind (e.g., Mike et al., 2013). Overall, it appears that both cognitive and social cognitive function can be impaired individuals with MS.

DEPRESSION AND COGNITIVE
IMPAIRMENTS IN MS

Despite the high prevalence of depression and cognitive dysfunction in MS, early studies surprisingly did not typically find a relationship between these two common sequelae of the disease. In fact, a consensus paper published about 25 years ago in the mid-1990s indicated that depression and cognitive dysfunction in MS were not related (Fischer et al., 1994). Subsequent research, however, has produced numerous studies demonstrating that depression and cognitive dysfunction in MS are in fact often correlated (Arnett et al., 2008; Grech et al., 2015; Niino et al., 2014), although it is important to note that this finding has not been universal, and some studies still do not report a significant relationship (Glanz et al., 2010).

Prevalence of Comorbid Depression
and Cognitive Impairment

In some of our initial work, we reasoned that past studies may not have found a relationship between depression and cognitive dysfunction because the overlap between neurovegetative depression symptoms and MS symptoms may have confounded the diagnosis of depression and thus made it more difficult to actually examine a direct depression–cognitive dysfunction relationship (Arnett, Higginson, Voss, Bender, et al., 1999; Arnett, Higginson, Voss, Wright, et al., 1999). Some of the clinical features of depression, as defined by the fifth edition of the *Diagnostic and Statistical Manual of Mental Disorders* (American Psychiatric Association, 2013), include somatic symptoms such as fatigue, disturbed sleep, altered appetite, concentration difficulties, and memory impairments (Feinstein, Magalhaes, Richard, Audet, & Moore, 2014). Because of this overlap, specific measures of depression can be used, such as the Hospital Anxiety and Depression Scale or the Beck Depression Inventory—Fast Screen (BDI–FS), which assess nonsomatic symptoms of depression. The Chicago Multiscale Depression Inventory is also useful because it has separate scales for mood, negative evaluative, and neurovegetative symptoms of depression. The use of such depression measures that have been validated for this population allows for a more precise exploration into the specific association of depression and functional ability in individuals with MS (Feinstein et al., 2014). In relapsing–remitting MS patients, there is evidence that after a relapse occurs, depression scores correlate with disability scores, but in the months after the relapse, as physical improvement occurs, depression scores decrease. However, despite this apparent remission of physical MS symptoms, depression scores are still elevated 6 months after a relapse, indicating that in a subset of patients, depression does not abate (Feinstein et al., 2014). These findings support the notion that, in addition to the physical challenges that likely contribute to depression, there are also other underlying mechanisms of depression in MS.

With consideration of these overlapping depression and MS disease symptoms in mind, we used the Chicago Multiscale Depression Inventory and found that mood and negative evaluative symptoms of depression were associated with cognitive dysfunction but not neurovegetative symptoms (Arnett, Higginson, Voss, Wright, et al., 1999). In other studies, we found that people with MS (PWMS) who used more adaptive coping strategies did not report depression even when they were cognitively impaired. In contrast, those PWMS who used maladaptive coping strategies and had cognitive impairments tended to be depressed (Arnett, Higginson, Voss, Randolph, & Grandey, 2002; Rabinowitz & Arnett, 2009; see Figure 4.1).

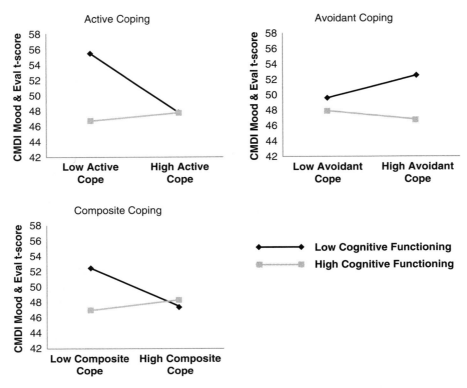

Figure 4.1. Active coping moderation model: Simple slopes for low and high cognitive functioning. For the active, avoidant, and composite coping models, respectively, the unstandardized simple slopes for participants scoring high on the cognitive index are 0.78, –1.02, and 0.73; the unstandardized simple slopes for participants scoring low on the cognitive index are –5.67, 2.37, and –2.68. From "A Longitudinal Analysis of Cognitive Dysfunction, Coping, and Depression in Multiple Sclerosis," by A. R. Rabinowitz & P. A. Arnett, 2009, *Neuropsychology, 23*, p. 587. Copyright 2009 by American Psychological Association.

Impact of Depression on Cognitive Functioning

In depression populations more generally, depression has been associated with various aspects of functioning, including cognition. Specifically, individuals with depression consistently demonstrate difficulties in the cognitive domains of memory and attention (e.g., Mathews & MacLeod, 2005), as well as cognitively effortful tasks more generally (Ellis & Ashbrook, 1988). A meta-analysis revealed that in the general population, depression severity is associated with performance on measures of episodic memory, executive functioning, and processing speed (McDermott & Ebmeier, 2009).

Research exploring cognition and depression in the general population has revealed a few potential underlying mechanisms. Depressed individuals often ruminate on negative thoughts, and this repetitive thinking may interfere with the formation of other memories. Research suggests that when depressed individuals perform tasks in structured situations that remove opportunities for rumination, they are able to perform at the same level as individuals who are not depressed (Hertel, 2004). These results imply that perhaps memory deficits in depressed individuals are a reflection of an inability to filter out irrelevant information and negative thoughts. Another proposed mechanism behind the cognitive deficits among individuals with depression is a lack of motivation (Egeland et al., 2003). Reduced performance on working memory tasks has mainly been found to be due to slower processing speed and lower vigilance that is often consistent with reduced effort. When depressed participants are given "goal-setting" instructions before their neuropsychological evaluations to increase motivation, their performance is superior to depressed individuals who are given the standard instructions (Scheurich et al., 2008). Targeting the mechanisms of rumination and diminished motivation may thus be a way to improve cognitive functioning in depressed PWMS.

Other Variables Associated With Depression and Cognitive Impairment in MS

One study found that cognitively impaired PWMS had higher levels of depression and fatigue compared with those patients without cognitive impairments (Heesen et al., 2010). Furthermore, fatigue had a greater association with attention measures, whereas depression was more strongly related to tests of memory. Another study by Niino and colleagues (2014) found that PWMS performed significantly worse than control subjects on a battery of neurocognitive tests, and patients also had higher scores on a measure of apathy and the Beck Depression Inventory—II (BDI–II). In PWMS, scores on information processing speed and attention tasks from the Brief Repeatable Neuropsychological Battery were also correlated with apathy and depression scores. Contrary to the finding from the aforementioned study by Heesen and colleagues (2010), Niino and colleagues did not find a strong association between fatigue scores and neuropsychological performance. Another study on patients with relapsing–remitting MS found that cognitive performance was predicted by the nonphysical symptoms of depression (Sundgren, Maurex, Wahlin, Piehl, & Brismar, 2013), similar to the findings of our initial study reported earlier (Arnett, Higginson, Voss, Wright, et al., 1999).

Given the relationship between depression and cognition in many individuals with MS, targeting depression in MS could alleviate some cognitive problems in addition to depressive symptoms. A study examining the effects of telephone-administered cognitive behavior therapy and emotion-focused therapy for depressed PWMS found that changes in depression and fatigue after therapy predicted changes in subjective assessments of cognitive performance (Kinsinger, Lattie, & Mohr, 2010). Patients were more accurate in their judgments of their cognitive performance after the depression treatments; however, objective measures of cognitive performance did not improve with treatment. This study is one of the few of its kind, and more research clearly needs to be conducted exploring the effects of therapy on depression and cognition. With all this said, it is important to note that depression is unlikely to account for all cognitive problems in MS. In Niino et al.'s study (2014), for example, even though depression was correlated with cognitive dysfunction in PWMS, MS patients were still impaired cognitively relative to control subjects even when depression was controlled for statistically.

COGNITIVE RESERVE AND DEPRESSION

Examining the construct of cognitive reserve is another way to consider the relationship between cognitive functioning and depression in MS. Like coping, as discussed earlier, cognitive reserve has the potential to moderate this relationship. First, we discuss the construct of cognitive reserve. Then we summarize what is known about cognitive reserve in MS. Last, we put forth the concept that cognitive reserve may moderate the relationship between brain pathology and depression symptoms in MS.

What Is Cognitive Reserve?

The construct of cognitive reserve (CR) developed from the repeated clinical observation that there is no consistent one-to-one relationship between degree of brain pathology and its functional manifestations (Stern, 2002). For example, two individuals with identical brain damage may functionally look very different in their mobility, cognitive abilities, and day-to-day functioning depending on their level of cognitive reserve. The construct was made popular by Yaakov Stern through his work on individuals with Alzheimer's disease (AD). Support for the validity of the CR construct has been found in other neurodegenerative populations including Parkinson's disease and MS (Hindle, Martyr, & Clare, 2014; Sumowski, Chiaravalloti, & DeLuca, 2009). CR, unlike the related concept of brain reserve capacity (BRC), is hypothesized as an active process in which the brain can adapt to damage more efficiently and thus limit functional impairment (Stern, 2002). For example, consider the metaphor of the brain as the engine of a car. In the

BRC conceptualization, Engine 1 has more gasoline at baseline than Engine 2. Therefore, when both Engine 1 and 2 lose a liter of gasoline, Engine 1 has enough gas in reserve to keep functioning, while Engine 2 does not. In the CR conceptualization, both engines have the same amount of gas at baseline, and each loses 1 liter of gasoline. Engine 1 has the capacity to become more fuel-efficient and thus can continue to function on this amount of gas. However, Engine 2 does not have this capacity (i.e., is less fuel efficient) and becomes nonfunctional despite having the same amount gas initially as Engine 1. In other words, BRC is about how much is in the tank, whereas CR is about the efficiency of the engine. Although parsimonious in metaphor, it is more difficult to parse these constructs in real life. BRC and CR are likely related and correlated with factors such as growing up in an enriched environment, although it has been argued that BRB is primarily genetically determined. Also, proxies used to measure these constructs likely confound them during their approximations.

How is Cognitive Reserve Measured?

Typically, damage is assessed through either structural images of the brain or passage of time (the assumption being that damage occurs in neurodegenerative diseases over time; Stern, 2002). Measures of functional outcome vary as well. In the AD literature, the traditional functional outcome is whether diagnostic criteria for dementia are met (Stern, 2002). Recently, neuropsychological measures that capture more nuanced aspects of functioning, such as processing speed or memory, have become popular as well (Amato et al., 2013; Benedict, Morrow, Weinstock-Guttman, Cookfair, & Schretlen, 2010).

There is no standard way of measuring CR, but measures of intelligence, education level, level of occupation, and time spent in enriching leisure-time activities are common (Amato et al., 2013; Stern, 2002; Sumowski & Leavitt, 2013). When measuring CR, it is crucial to consider whether the operationalization of reserve is confounded with the chosen measure of functional outcome. For example, using education as the proxy for CR and then a reading test as the functional outcome measure could be problematic because reading test performance is confounded by educational attainment. All and all, careful thought must be given to choosing measurements of both CR and functional outcome if the CR hypothesis is to be appropriately tested.

What Do We Know About Cognitive Reserve in MS?

MS causes myriad symptoms including pain, muscle weakness, loss of sensation, mental and physical fatigue, visual impairment, sexual dysfunction, depression, and cognitive impairment (Arnett, Ukueberuwa, & Cadden, 2015). Literature examining CR in MS has focused almost exclusively on cognitive functioning as the functional outcome. Several studies have demonstrated that proxies of CR moderate the relationship between disease burden and cognitive performance in MS. For a more detailed review of studies demonstrating an effect of cognitive reserve in MS, see Chapter 15 of this volume. A recent study (Sumowski & Leavitt, 2013) examined unique moderating contributions of both BRC and CR (measured by intellectually enriching leisure activities) while simultaneously considering education. This study found that BRC moderated the relationship between lesion load and cognitive performance. It also demonstrated that education level predicts cognitive performance after controlling for brain reserve. In addition, CR moderated the relationship between lesion load and cognitive performance even after controlling for education level, brain reserve, and the interaction of lesion load and brain reserve. These results suggest a unique and protective role of brain reserve, education, and cognitively enriching daily activities. Overall, it is clear that the construct of CR has some validity for the MS population.

Depression as the Functional Outcome Measure

As noted earlier, depression in MS is about as common as cognitive symptoms. More important, depression affects individuals' daily functional ability, is often associated with poorer cognitive functioning, and can worsen disease progression through increased fatigue and decreased adherence to potentially disease modifying behaviors (e.g., medication adherence and exercise; Arnett, Higginson, & Randolph, 2001; Bruce, Hancock, Arnett, & Lynch, 2010). Thus far, the CR literature in MS has largely ignored the potential importance of depression. Depression level in the more general CR literature discussed earlier has been used as an exclusionary criterion, statistically controlled for, or simply not considered. Instead of ignoring or statistically controlling for depression, depression could be considered as a functional outcome variable. This logic closely mirrors initial studies examining the relationship between depression and cognitive functioning more generally in MS. The risk for depression increases at the onset of MS, and there is typically a medium to large effect size of disease burden (Expanded Disability Status Scale [EDSS]) and measures of brain integrity (including lesions, atrophy, white matter tract integrity, etc.) on depression status in MS (Arnett et al., 2008; Bakshi et al., 2000). However, the relationship between disease burden/brain pathology and depression is not one to one, suggesting a potential role for a construct such as CR.

Recent work from our lab suggests that CR can moderate the effect of disease burden on depression status. Cadden and Arnett (2016) found that an index of CR (Shipley Vocabulary subtest) and years of education, moderated the relationship between disease burden (EDSS) and depression status (BDI–FS) in PWMS. Specifically, only individuals with high disease burden and low levels of CR met criteria for clinical depression (i.e., BDI–FS score ≥ 4; see Figure 4.2).

Potential Problems With Examining Depression as a Functional Outcome in MS

A couple of unique problems manifest when conceptualizing depression status as the functional outcome measure in a CR model. First and foremost, some of the available constructs for CR likely have a direct effect on depression symptoms. For example, there is a rich literature on the protective effects of educational attainment on depression symptoms, particularly in aging populations (Miech & Shanahan, 2000). Although this relationship is not inherently problematic, future models need to demonstrate that CR is interacting with damage to predict depression and thus show that it is working in a reserve fashion and is not simply a direct effect of education status on depression symptoms. Additionally, careful attention should be given to understanding whether depression symptoms affect measurements of CR. For example, MS studies have reported significantly lower fluid intelligence in

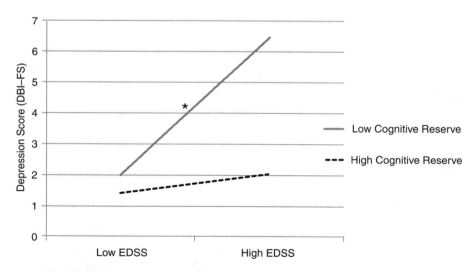

Figure 4.2. Cognitive reserve moderates the effect of disease burden (Expanded Disability Status Scale [EDSS]) on depression status (Beck Depression Inventory—Fast Screen [BDI–FS]). Only individuals with high disease burden and low cognitive reserve met clinical criteria for depression (BDI–FS ≥4).

depressed compared with non-depressed patients (Barwick & Arnett, 2011). Therefore, fluid intelligence measures might not be good candidates for CR in a model examining depression as the functional outcome. It is also possible that individuals suffering from especially chronic depression are less likely to engage in cognitively enriching leisure-time activity due to symptoms of anhedonia; therefore, using enriched leisure time as a measure of CR independent of depression may also be problematic. Lastly, there is no equivalent "rapid decline" in depression (such as from diagnosis of dementia to death in AD literature), meaning that CR in this conceptualization may never "run out" and thus, in some ways, is inherently different from the CR developed from AD literature. In other words, we would not expect someone with advanced brain pathology due to MS to become severely and permanently depressed. The relationship between brain pathology and depression appears to be more complex than brain pathology and cognitive functioning. For example, loss of brain tissue will result in cognitive impairment and emotional dysfunction, but emotional dysfunction does not necessarily mean depressed mood.

NEURAL UNDERPINNINGS OF COGNITIVE IMPAIRMENT AND DEPRESSION IN MS

MS is characterized by significant neuropathological damage brought on by recurrent inflammatory "attacks" within the central nervous system, resulting in sclerotic lesions, demyelination, axonal loss and damage, and whole-brain and regional atrophy (Paty & Ebers, 1998; Raine, McFarland, & Hohlfeld, 2008). Conventional (e.g., T1-weighted imaging, functional magnetic resonance imaging) and nonconventional (e.g., diffusion tensor imaging, or DTI) neuroimaging have become integral to exploring these structural and functional neural underpinnings of the disease and linking them to cognitive impairment and depression in MS. In this section, we first explore neural correlates of cognitive impairment and then depression; we then explore possible common neural underpinnings that may help explain why depression and cognitive dysfunction are often comorbid in MS.

Neural Correlates of Cognitive Impairment

Rao, Leo, Haughton, St. Aubin-Faubert, and Bernardin (1989) were among the first to explore the relationship between structural brain damage and cognitive functioning in MS. In their study, they showed that total lesion area was the best predictor of cognitive impairment, predicting poorer performance in more than 50% of the administered tests (i.e., 18 of 34 tests), and after dividing the MS group into cognitively impaired and cognitively intact groups, the authors found that the impaired group had significantly greater TLA than the cognitively intact group. Subsequent studies examining overall lesion load found similar associations between lesion volume and cognitive functioning (Calabrese et al., 2009; Deloire et al., 2005; Hohol et al., 1997; Papadopoulou et al., 2013). Additionally, these associations persist even when examining specific brain regions. A study by Arnett and colleagues (1994), for example, showed that patients with a higher ratio of frontal white matter lesions performed worse on the Wisconsin Card Sorting Test compared with a low ratio of frontal white matter lesions or minimal lesions overall. Lesion load in the frontal, parietal, and temporal brain areas have also been shown to individually predict cognitive functioning (Lazeron et al., 2005)

Whole-brain and regional atrophy have also been shown to contribute to cognitive dysfunction in MS, sometimes even surpassing the predictive power of sclerotic lesions. Benedict and colleagues (2004) examined lesion burden and third ventricle width in a sample of 37 PWMS. After controlling for age and premorbid intelligence, they found that third ventricle width accounted for the greatest amount of variance in learning, recall, attention, and processing speed scores. When third ventricle width was removed from their regression analyses, a second measure of brain atrophy, brain parenchymal fraction (BPF), served as the best predictor of performance on recall, attention, and processing speed scores. Subsequent work highlighted the influence of atrophy on cognitive functioning in MS, with measures of brain atrophy associated with greater overall cognitive dysfunction, impairment status, and cognitive deterioration over a 2.5-year period (Amato et al., 2007; Calabrese et al., 2009; Lazeron et al., 2005).

Regional analyses of atrophy, as measured by BPF and thalamic and basal ganglia volumes, have also been shown to be linked to cognitive impairment in MS. Houtchens et al. (2007) investigated the effect of thalamic atrophy on cognitive functioning in a subgroup of 31 PWMS. Overall, total normalized thalamic volume in the MS patient group was 16.8% smaller than that of healthy control participants, and thalamic fraction was shown to be the single best predictor of performance on the Controlled Oral Word Association Test, California Verbal Learning Test—II (CVLT–II) total and delayed recall, Brief Visuospatial Memory Test—Revised (BVMT–R) total and delayed recall, Paced Auditory Addition Test (PASAT), and Symbol Digit Modalities Test (SDMT). Atrophy in other deep gray matter structures, namely the putamen, has also been linked to poorer performance on the PASAT and SDMT (Batista et al., 2012).

Conventional MRI allows for the quantification of lesion load and various measures of brain atrophy but does not provide information about the microstructure of white matter tracts. Diffusion-weighted imaging, particularly DTI, has emerged in recent years as an instrumental tool for quantifying microstructural damage in sclerotic lesions and normal appearing white matter and linking them to cognitive impairment. In a study of PWMS and healthy control subjects, tract-based spatial statistics (TBSS) were used to investigate white matter disconnection as a mechanism for cognitive impairment in MS (Dineen et al., 2009). Results from voxelwise comparisons found positive correlations between tract fractional anisotropy (FA; in various tracts) and performance on the PASAT, BVMT–R, and CVLT–II, suggesting that cognitive dysfunction in MS may be driven by damage-induced white matter disconnection. Hecke et al. (2010) further explored the impact of microstructural white matter damage by examining diffusivity measures (axial diffusivity, radial diffusivity [RD], mean diffusivity [MD]) in conjunction with FA. Significant correlations were found between PASAT performance and FA, RD, and MD in various tracts. Group differences between cognitively impaired and cognitively preserved PWMS have also been found across DTI metrics, with cognitively impaired patients having worse measures of FA, MD, and RD in the corpus callosum, superior and inferior longitudinal fasciculus, corticospinal tracts, forceps minor, cingulum, and fornices and more extensive white matter damage in the thalamus, uncinate fasciculus, juxtacortical areas, brainstem, and cerebellum compared to cognitively intact patients (Hulst et al., 2013).

As these studies show, a strong link exists between structural brain damage and cognitive impairment in MS, but brain structure is not the sole determinant of cognitive functioning; functional components and networks underlie cognitive functioning and are therefore important to investigate in MS. Genova, Hillary, Wylie, Rypma, and DeLuca (2009) examined processing speed and functional activation in a group of PWMS and healthy control subjects using an in-scanner modified SDMT task and found that slower reaction times in PWMS were positively associated with activation in left and right insula, left anterior cingulate gyrus, and right thalamus. Increased activation has also been observed during a sustained attention task (i.e., Paced Visual Serial Addition Task–PVSAT), such that PWMS showed significant activation in more brain areas than healthy control subjects (Staffen et al., 2002). The authors suggest that this increased activation pattern in the MS group may represent a compensatory process brought on by increased cerebral efforts.

Further evidence for compensatory brain activation can be seen in studies examining functional connectivity. PWMS have been shown to have decreased functional reserve and altered and increased connectivity, something thought to reflect a compensatory mechanism by way of recruitment of homologous regions (Cader, Cifelli, Abu-Omar, Palace, and Matthews, 2006). Studies exploring nontask connectivity (i.e., resting state connectivity), on the other hand, have had mixed results, with some studies linking increased resting state connectivity to poorer cognitive functioning (Faivre et al., 2012), others linking reduced resting state connectivity to cognitive functioning (Louapre et al., 2014), and still others pointing to variable connectivity–cognitive functioning patterns depending on the exhibited MS phenotype (Dobryakova et al., 2016). Overall, fMRI studies in PWMS show that atypical activation patterns are associated with aberrant cognitive functioning; however, additional studies are needed so that more unequivocal inferences about the functional neural underpinnings of cognition in MS.

Neural Correlates of Depression

Given the high prevalence of depression in MS, it is important to understand the neuropathological sequelae that underlie depressive symptoms. The limbic system has long been known to contribute to emotional functioning in both healthy individuals and individuals suffering from psychiatric disorders. As such, it has often been the focus of MS depression research. One of the first studies to examine the relationship between the limbic system and depression in MS was conducted by Sabatini et al. (1996). They used single-photon emission computed tomography to evaluate regional cerebral blood flow (rCBF) in 10 depressed and 10 nondepressed PWMS. Significant correlations were found between perfusion asymmetry in the limbic cortex and BDI and Hamilton Depression Rating Scale scores. Furthermore, the depressed group had greater rCBF in the left limbic cortex, whereas the nondepressed group had greater rCBF in the right limbic cortex. The authors posited that this asymmetry in rCBF reflected impaired limbic system activity brought on by a cortex–limbic system disconnection, which contributed to either hyperactivity in the left limbic cortex or hypoactivity in the right limbic cortex.

A more recent study examined connectivity during an emotion processing task by using two limbic areas shown to be involved in the psychophysiology of depression—the amygdala and hippocampus—as seed regions (Riccelli et al., 2015). Altered connectivity was found between the left amygdala and ventral and dorsal prefrontal cortices in PWMS but not in healthy control subjects. In addition, depression scores were negatively correlated with left hippocampus–orbitofrontal cortex and left hippocampus–dorsal lateral prefrontal cortex connectivity. Structural "connectomic" examinations of the limbic system, which use graph-theoretical indices to characterize structural brain networks, have also illuminated the neurobiological substrates of depression. Nigro and colleagues (2014), for example, used deterministic tractography and graph theoretical analysis to assess white matter connectivity in 20 depressed and 22 nondepressed PWMS and 16 healthy control subjects. Global and local network measures were analyzed, and results indicated that depressed PWMS had increased "shortest distance" between the right hippocampus–right amygdala and frontal and prefrontal cortices compared with nondepressed MS patients and healthy control subjects. Additionally, a trend correlation was found between BDI–II scores and local path length in the right hippocampus and inferior frontal gyrus pars orbitalis.

Whole-brain and regional structural analyses outside of the limbic system have also pointed to a relationship between MS-induced damage and depression. Feinstein et al. (2004) found that depressed PWMS were found to have more extensive hyperintense and hypointense lesions in the left medial inferior frontal area and greater CSF volume in the left anterior temporal region. Regression analyses further showed that these affected regions accounted for 42% of the variance in explaining depression. Severity of depression has also been linked to superior frontal, superior parietal, and temporal T1 holes, lateral ventricle enlargement, superior frontal and inferior frontal sulcal enlargement, third ventricle enlargement, overall lesion load, and brain parenchymal volume (Bakshi et al., 2000; Zorzon et al., 2002). Furthermore, DTI analyses have shown that regional white matter damage, as measured by MD and FA, can differentiate depressed and nondepressed MS groups, add to the overall variance accounted for by conventional structural brain indices, and significantly predict depression severity scores (Feinstein et al., 2009; Shen et al., 2014).

The aforementioned studies provide insight into the neural correlates of depression in MS, pointing to aberrations in limbic system activity and regional structural damage as drivers for depressive symptoms and status. Given the high prevalence of depression in MS, it will be important to continue to explore these relationships using conventional, nonconventional, and multimodal neuroimaging approaches.

Commonalities in Brain Indices Underlying Cognitive Impairment and Depression

Few studies have been published examining the specific overlap in brain pathology between cognitive impairment and depression in MS. From the studies described in the preceding text, it can be deduced that certain brain abnormalities (e.g., lesion load, microstructural white matter damage, altered connectivity) appear to contribute to both outcomes. Yet the difficulty arises when trying to identify brain areas that carry comparable associations with depression and cognitive functioning when both are analyzed together. Regionally speaking, various studies have shown that the limbic system has been strongly, albeit independently, implicated in depression and cognitive functioning (e.g., Batista et al., 2012; Benedict et al., 2013; Houtchens et al., 2007; Sabatini et al., 1996). However, Kiy and colleagues (2011) are, to the authors' knowledge, one of the few groups to examine the overlap in limbic system pathology in relation to both depression and cognitive functioning in the same MS sample. These investigators measured lateral ventricle temporal horn volumetry (a proxy for hippocampal volume), depression (BDI), Multiple Sclerosis Functional Composite performance, and CVLT–II memory encoding, retrieval, and consolidation in 72 PWMS and 16 healthy control subjects. MS patients were divided into three groups based on their consolidation performance: (a) a loss of information during consolidation, (b) equal short- and long-delay free recall performance, and (c) a gain during the consolidation period. Overall, patients experiencing a high loss of information during the consolidation period had larger right lateral ventricle temporal horn volumes (i.e., greater atrophy) compared with the equal performance and healthy control groups. Similar results were found for the left temporal horn of the lateral ventricle, with significant differences between the high-loss group and healthy control subjects. Left temporal horn lateral ventricle volume positively correlated with psychic items of the BDI (e.g., sadness, failure, disappointment) but not fatigue or somatic items. In the end, there is evidence for overlap of neuropathological correlates of both depression and cognitive functioning, but clearly more studies will need to be conducted to better solidify the variance that these variables share.

CONCLUSIONS AND FUTURE DIRECTIONS

With the benefit of more than 20 years of additional research since Fischer et al.'s (1994) consensus paper, the weight of the evidence clearly shows that there is an association between depression and cognitive impairment in many PWMS. However, this is not a universal finding. Additionally, some studies show that only nonsomatic depression symptoms are associated with cognitive dysfunction in MS. Also, there appear to be moderators at work in this relationship, with coping being especially important; cognitive dysfunction in the context of maladaptive coping is most likely to show a relationship with depression.

CR is a concept that has only been examined relatively recently in MS, having initially been developed as a construct in the context of AD research. Cognitive functional outcomes have primarily been examined in MS, and studies have shown that CR moderates cognitive outcomes from disease burden. Far less attention has been given to other important functional outcomes, such as depression. Our recent research has begun to explore this, and we have found that individuals with a high disease burden combined with lower CR are more likely to report clinically significant depression. Thus, in addition to depression being associated with traditional cognitive outcome measures in MS, it also appears to be related to cognitive reserve in the context of varying disease burdens. However, this conclusion is only based on one limited study, so clearly this is an area with great potential for future exploration.

Finally, although there is considerable evidence for both structural and functional brain underpinnings of cognitive dysfunction and depression in MS, limited research has explored common neural underpinnings. In considering these separate literatures, dysfunction and damage in a number of limbic structures seems be common to both depression and cognitive dysfunction in MS. Where the neural underpinnings of depression and cognitive dysfunction are both the primary focus of examination in the same study, it appears that damage and dysfunction in subcortical structures, such as the hippocampus (in this case measured indirectly), may underlie both. However, this conclusion is based on only one study, so this is another area in the exploration of depression and cognitive links in MS where much future work needs to be done. Given that many studies examining cognition in MS use depression as an exclusionary criterion, it will be important to find ways to include these individuals in future studies to account for the depressive symptoms that so often co-occur with cognitive impairment in PWMS.

In the final analysis, there is a rich literature examining the connection between depression and cognitive functioning in MS. However, much additional work needs to be done, especially in the realm of exploring depression as an outcome in CR models and in clarifying the common neural underpinnings to these extremely shared and debilitating sequelae of MS. Through such work, treatment outcomes of depression may be improved and subsequently result in a mitigation of cognitive difficulties in MS.

REFERENCES

Amato, M. P., Portaccio, E., Goretti, B., Zipoli, V., Battaglini, M., Bartolozzi, M. L., . . . De Stefano, N. (2007). Association of neocortical volume changes with cognitive deterioration in relapsing-remitting multiple sclerosis. *Archives of Neurology*, 64, 1157–1161. http://dx.doi.org/10.1001/archneur.64.8.1157

Amato, M. P., Razzolini, L., Goretti, B., Stromillo, M. L., Rossi, F., Giorgio, A., . . . De Stefano, N. (2013). Cognitive reserve and cortical atrophy in multiple sclerosis: A longitudinal study. *Neurology*, 80, 1728–1733. http://dx.doi.org/10.1212/WNL.0b013e3182918c6f

Amato, M. P., Zipoli, V., & Portaccio, E. (2006). Multiple sclerosis-related cognitive changes: A review of cross-sectional and longitudinal studies. *Journal of the Neurological Sciences*, 245, 41–46.

American Psychiatric Association. (2013). *Diagnostic and statistical manual of mental disorders* (5th ed.). Washington, DC: Author.

Arnett, P. A., Barwick, F. H., & Beeney, J. E. (2008). Depression in multiple sclerosis: Review and theoretical proposal. *Journal of the International Neuropsychological Society, 14*, 691–724. http://dx.doi.org/10.1017/S1355617708081174

Arnett, P. A., Higginson, C. I., & Randolph, J. J. (2001). Depression in multiple sclerosis: Relationship to planning ability. *Journal of the International Neuropsychological Society, 7*, 665–674. http://dx.doi.org/10.1017/S1355617701766027

Arnett, P. A., Higginson, C. I., Voss, W. D., Bender, W. I., Wurst, J. M., & Tippin, J. M. (1999). Depression in multiple sclerosis: Relationship to working memory capacity. *Neuropsychology, 13*, 546–556. http://dx.doi.org/10.1037/0894-4105.13.4.546

Arnett, P. A., Higginson, C. I., Voss, W. D., Randolph, J. J., & Grandey, A. A. (2002). Relationship between coping, depression, and cognitive dysfunction in multiple sclerosis. *The Clinical Neuropsychologist, 16*, 341–355. http://dx.doi.org/10.1076/clin.16.3.341.13852

Arnett, P. A., Higginson, C. I., Voss, W. D., Wright, B., Bender, W. I., Wurst, J. M., & Tippin, J. M. (1999). Depressed mood in multiple sclerosis: Relationship to capacity-demanding memory and attentional functioning. *Neuropsychology, 13*, 434–446. http://dx.doi.org/10.1037/0894-4105.13.3.434

Arnett, P. A., Rao, S. M., Bernardin, L., Grafman, J., Yetkin, F. Z., & Lobeck, L. (1994). Relationship between frontal lobe lesions and Wisconsin Card Sorting Test performance in patients with multiple sclerosis. *Neurology, 44*, 420–425. http://dx.doi.org/10.1212/WNL.44.3_Part_1.420

Arnett, P. A., Ukueberuwa, D., & Cadden, M. (2015). Psychological and behavioral therapies in MS. In B. Brochet (Ed.), *Neuropsychiatric Symptoms of Inflammatory Demyelinating Diseases* (pp. 167–178). Cham, Switzerland: Springer. http://dx.doi.org/10.1007/978-3-319-18464-7_12

Bakshi, R., Czarnecki, D., Shaikh, Z. A., Priore, R. L., Janardhan, V., Kaliszky, Z., & Kinkel, P. R. (2000). Brain MRI lesions and atrophy are related to depression in multiple sclerosis. *NeuroReport, 11*, 1153–1158. http://dx.doi.org/10.1097/00001756-200004270-00003

Barwick, F. H., & Arnett, P. A. (2011). Relationship between global cognitive decline and depressive symptoms in multiple sclerosis. *The Clinical Neuropsychologist, 25*, 193–209. http://dx.doi.org/10.1080/13854046.2010.538435

Batista, S., Zivadinov, R., Hoogs, M., Bergsland, N., Heininen-Brown, M., Dwyer, M. G., . . . Benedict, R. H. B. (2012). Basal ganglia, thalamus and neocortical atrophy predicting slowed cognitive processing in multiple sclerosis. *Journal of Neurology, 259*, 139–146. http://dx.doi.org/10.1007/s00415-011-6147-1

Benedict, R. H. B., Hulst, H. E., Bergsland, N., Schoonheim, M. M., Dwyer, M. G., Weinstock-Guttman, B., . . . Zivadinov, R. (2013). Clinical significance of atrophy and white matter mean diffusivity within the thalamus of multiple sclerosis patients. *Multiple Sclerosis Journal, 19*, 1478–1484. http://dx.doi.org/10.1177/1352458513478675

Benedict, R. H. B., Morrow, S. A., Weinstock-Guttman, B., Cookfair, D., & Schretlen, D. J. (2010). Cognitive reserve moderates decline in information processing speed in multiple sclerosis patients. *Journal of the International Neuropsychological Society, 16*, 829–835. http://dx.doi.org/10.1017/S1355617710000688

Benedict, R. H. B., Weinstock-Guttman, B., Fishman, I., Sharma, J., Tjoa, C. W., & Bakshi, R. (2004). Prediction of neuropsychological impairment in multiple sclerosis: Comparison of conventional magnetic resonance imaging measures of atrophy and lesion burden. *Archives of Neurology, 61*, 226–230. http://dx.doi.org/10.1001/archneur.61.2.226

Bruce, J. M., Hancock, L. M., Arnett, P., & Lynch, S. (2010). Treatment adherence in multiple sclerosis: Association with emotional status, personality, and cognition. *Journal of Behavioral Medicine, 33*, 219–227. http://dx.doi.org/10.1007/s10865-010-9247-y

Byatt, N., Rothschild, A. J., Riskind, P., Ionete, C., & Hunt, A. T. (2011). Relationships between multiple sclerosis and depression. *The Journal of Neuropsychiatry and Clinical Neurosciences, 23*, 198–200. http://dx.doi.org/10.1176/jnp.23.2.jnp198

Cadden, M. H., & Arnett, P. A. (2016, February). *Cognitive reserve attenuates the effect of disability on depression in multiple sclerosis (MS)*. Paper presented at the International Neuropsychological Society, Boston, MA.

Cader, S., Cifelli, A., Abu-Omar, Y., Palace, J., & Matthews, P. M. (2006). Reduced brain functional reserve and altered functional connectivity in patients with multiple sclerosis. *Brain: A Journal of Neurology, 129*, 527–537. http://dx.doi.org/10.1093/brain/awh670

Calabrese, M., Agosta, F., Rinaldi, F., Mattisi, I., Grossi, P., Favaretto, A., . . . Filippi, M. (2009). Cortical lesions and atrophy associated with cognitive impairment in relapsing-remitting multiple sclerosis. *Archives of Neurology, 66*, 1144–1150. http://dx.doi.org/10.1001/archneurol.2009.174

Deloire, M. S. A., Salort, E., Bonnet, M., Arimone, Y., Boudineau, M., Amieva, H., . . . Brochet, B. (2005). Cognitive impairment as marker of diffuse brain abnormalities in early relapsing remitting multiple sclerosis. *Journal of Neurology, Neurosurgery and Psychiatry, 76*, 519–526. http://dx.doi.org/10.1136/jnnp.2004.045872

Dineen, R. A., Vilisaar, J., Hlinka, J., Bradshaw, C. M., Morgan, P. S., Constantinescu, C. S., & Auer, D. P. (2009). Disconnection as a mechanism for cognitive dysfunction in multiple sclerosis. *Brain: A Journal of Neurology, 132*, 239–249. http://dx.doi.org/10.1093/brain/awn275

Dobryakova, E., Rocca, M., Valsasina, P., Ghezzi, A., Colombo, B., Martinelli, V., . . . Filippi, M. (2016). Abnormalities of the executive control networking multiple sclerosis phenotypes: An fMRI effective connectivity study. *Human Brain Mapping, 37*, 2293–2304.

Egeland, J., Rund, B. R., Sundet, K., Landrø, N. I., Asbjørnsen, A., Lund, A., . . . Hugdahl, K. (2003). Attention profile in schizophrenia compared with depression: Differential effects of processing speed, selective attention and vigilance.

Acta Psychiatrica Scandinavica, 108, 276–284. http://dx.doi.org/10.1034/ j.1600-0447.2003.00146.x

Ellis, H. C., & Ashbrook, P. W. (1988). Resource allocation model of the effects of depressed mood states on memory. In K. F. J. P. Forgas (Ed.), *Affect, cognition, and social behavior* (pp. 25–43). Göttingen, Sweden: Hogrefe.

Faivre, A., Rico, A., Zaaraoui, W., Crespy, L., Reuter, F., Wybrecht, D., . . . Audoin, B. (2012). Assessing brain connectivity at rest is clinically relevant in early multiple sclerosis. *Multiple Sclerosis Journal, 18,* 1251–1258. http://dx.doi.org/ 10.1177/1352458511435930

Feinstein, A., Magalhaes, S., Richard, J. F., Audet, B., & Moore, C. (2014). The link between multiple sclerosis and depression. *Nature Reviews. Neurology, 10,* 507–517. http://dx.doi.org/10.1038/nrneurol.2014.139

Feinstein, A., O'Connor, P., Akbar, N., Moradzadeh, L., Scott, C. J., & Lobaugh, N. J. (2009). Diffusion tensor imaging abnormalities in depressed multiple sclerosis patients. *Multiple Sclerosis, 16,* 189–196. http://dx.doi.org/10.1177/ 1352458509355461

Feinstein, A., Roy, P., Lobaugh, N., Feinstein, K., O'Connor, P., & Black, S. (2004). Structural brain abnormalities in multiple sclerosis patients with major depression. *Neurology, 62,* 586–590. http://dx.doi.org/10.1212/ 01.WNL.0000110316.12086.0C

Fischer, J. S., Foley, F. W., Aikens, J. E., Ericson, G. D., Rao, S. M., & Shindell, S. (1994). What do we *really* know about cognitive dysfunction, affective disorders, and stress in multiple sclerosis? A practitioner's guide. *Journal of Neurologic Rehabilitation, 8,* 151–164. http://dx.doi.org/10.1177/136140969400800309

Genova, H. M., Cagna, C. J., Chiaravalloti, N. D., DeLuca, J., & Lengenfelder, J. (2016). Dynamic assessment of social cognition in individuals with multiple sclerosis: A pilot study. *Journal of the International Neuropsychological Society, 22,* 83–88. http://dx.doi.org/10.1017/S1355617715001137

Genova, H. M., Hillary, F. G., Wylie, G., Rypma, B., & DeLuca, J. (2009). Examination of processing speed deficits in multiple sclerosis using functional magnetic resonance imaging. *Journal of the International Neuropsychological Society, 15,* 383–393. http://dx.doi.org/10.1017/S1355617709090535

Glanz, B. I., Healy, B. C., Rintell, D. J., Jaffin, S. K., Bakshi, R., & Weiner, H. L. (2010). The association between cognitive impairment and quality of life in patients with early multiple sclerosis. *Journal of the Neurological Sciences, 290,* 75–79. http://dx.doi.org/10.1016/j.jns.2009.11.004

Goldman Consensus Group. (2005). The Goldman Consensus statement on depression in multiple sclerosis. *Multiple Sclerosis Journal, 11,* 328–337. http://dx.doi.org/ 10.1191/1352458505ms1162oa

Grech, L. B., Kiropoulos, L. A., Kirby, K. M., Butler, E., Paine, M., & Hester, R. (2015). The effect of executive function on stress, depression, anxiety, and quality of life in multiple sclerosis. *Journal of Clinical and Experimental Neuropsychology, 37,* 549–562. http://dx.doi.org/10.1080/13803395.2015.1037723

Hecke, W. V., Nagels, G., Leemans, A., Vandervliet, E., Sijbers, J., & Parizel, P. M. (2010). Correlation of cognitive dysfunction and diffusion tensor MRI measures in patients with mild and moderate multiple sclerosis. *Journal of Magnetic Resonance Imaging, 31,* 1492–1498. http://dx.doi.org/10.1002/jmri.22198

Heesen, C., Schulz, K. H., Fiehler, J., Von der Mark, U., Otte, C., Jung, R., . . . Gold, S. M. (2010). Correlates of cognitive dysfunction in multiple sclerosis. *Brain, Behavior, and Immunity, 24,* 1148–1155. http://dx.doi.org/10.1016/j.bbi.2010.05.006

Hertel, P. T. (2004). Memory for emotional and nonemotional events in depression: A question of habit? In D. R. P. Hertel (Ed.), *Memory and emotion* (pp. 186–216). New York, NY: Oxford University Press. http://dx.doi.org/10.1093/acprof:oso/9780195158564.003.0006

Hindle, J. V., Martyr, A., & Clare, L. (2014). Cognitive reserve in Parkinson's disease: A systematic review and meta-analysis. *Parkinsonism & Related Disorders, 20,* 1–7. http://dx.doi.org/10.1016/j.parkreldis.2013.08.010

Hohol, M. J., Guttmann, C. R., Orav, J., Mackin, G. A., Kikinis, R., Khoury, S. J., . . . Weiner, H. L. (1997). Serial neuropsychological assessment and magnetic resonance imaging analysis in multiple sclerosis. *Archives of Neurology, 54,* 1018–1025. http://dx.doi.org/10.1001/archneur.1997.00550200074013

Houtchens, M. K., Benedict, R. H. B., Killiany, R., Sharma, J., Jaisani, Z., Singh, B., . . . Bakshi, R. (2007). Thalamic atrophy and cognition in multiple sclerosis. *Neurology, 69,* 1213–1223. http://dx.doi.org/10.1212/01.wnl.0000276992.17011.b5

Hulst, H. E., Steenwijk, M. D., Versteeg, A., Pouwels, P. J., Vrenken, H., Uitdehaag, B. M., . . . Barkhof, F. (2013). Cognitive impairment in MS: Impact of white matter integrity, gray matter volume, and lesions. *Neurology, 80,* 1025–1032. http://dx.doi.org/10.1212/WNL.0b013e31828726cc

Jonsson, A., Andresen, J., Storr, L., Tscherning, T., Sorensen, P. S., & Ravnborg, M. (2006). Cognitive impairment in newly diagnosed multiple sclerosis patients: A 4-year follow-up study. *Journal of the Neurological Sciences, 245,* 77–85.

Kenealy, P. M., Beaumont, G. J., Lintern, T., & Murrell, R. (2000). Autobiographical memory, depression and quality of life in multiple sclerosis. *Journal of Clinical and Experimental Neuropsychology, 22,* 125–131. http://dx.doi.org/10.1076/1380-3395(200002)22:1;1-8;FT125

Kessler, R. C., Berglund, P., Demler, O., Jin, R., Koretz, D., Merikangas, K. R., . . . Wang, P. S., & the National Comorbidity Survey Replication. (2003). The epidemiology of major depressive disorder: Results from the National Comorbidity Survey Replication (NCS-R). *JAMA, 289,* 3095–3105. http://dx.doi.org/10.1001/jama.289.23.3095

Kinsinger, S. W., Lattie, E., & Mohr, D. C. (2010). Relationship between depression, fatigue, subjective cognitive impairment, and objective neuropsychological functioning in patients with multiple sclerosis. *Neuropsychology, 24,* 573–580. http://dx.doi.org/10.1037/a0019222

Kiy, G., Lehmann, P., Hahn, H. K., Eling, P., Kastrup, A., & Hildebrandt, H. (2011). Decreased hippocampal volume, indirectly measured, is associated with depressive symptoms and consolidation deficits in multiple sclerosis. *Multiple Sclerosis Journal, 17*, 1088–1097. http://dx.doi.org/10.1177/1352458511403530

Kraemer, M., Herold, M., Uekermann, J., Kis, B., Daum, I., Wiltfang, J., . . . Abdel-Hamid, M. (2013). Perception of affective prosody in patients at an early stage of relapsing–remitting multiple sclerosis. *Journal of Neuropsychology, 7*, 91–106. http://dx.doi.org/10.1111/j.1748-6653.2012.02037.x

Lazeron, R. H., Boringa, J. B., Schouten, M., Uitdehaag, B. M., Bergers, E., Lindeboom, J., . . . Polman, C. H. (2005). Brain atrophy and lesion load as explaining parameters for cognitive impairment in multiple sclerosis. *Multiple Sclerosis, 11*, 524–531. http://dx.doi.org/10.1191/1352458505ms1201oa

Louapre, C., Perlbarg, V., García-Lorenzo, D., Urbanski, M., Benali, H., Assouad, R., . . . Stankoff, B. (2014). Brain networks disconnection in early multiple sclerosis cognitive deficits: An anatomofunctional study. *Human Brain Mapping, 35*, 4706–4717. http://dx.doi.org/10.1002/hbm.22505

Mathews, A., & MacLeod, C. (2005). Cognitive vulnerability to emotional disorders. *Annual Review of Clinical Psychology, 1*, 167–195. http://dx.doi.org/10.1146/annurev.clinpsy.1.102803.143916

McDermott, L. M., & Ebmeier, K. P. (2009). A meta-analysis of depression severity and cognitive function. *Journal of Affective Disorders, 119*, 1–8. http://dx.doi.org/10.1016/j.jad.2009.04.022

Miech, R. A., & Shanahan, M. J. (2000). Socioeconomic status and depression over the life course. *Journal of Health and Social Behavior, 41*, 162–176. http://dx.doi.org/10.2307/2676303

Mike, A., Strammer, E., Aradi, M., Orsi, G., Perlaki, G., Hajnal, A., . . . Illes, Z. (2013). Disconnection mechanism and regional cortical atrophy contribute to impaired processing of facial expressions and theory of mind in multiple sclerosis: A structural MRI study. *PLoS One, 8*, e82422. http://dx.doi.org/10.1371/journal.pone.0082422

Mohr, D. C., Goodkin, D. E., Bacchetti, P., Boudewyn, A. C., Huang, L., Marrietta, P., . . . Dee, B. (2000). Psychological stress and the subsequent appearance of new brain MRI lesions in MS. *Neurology, 55*, 55–61. http://dx.doi.org/10.1212/WNL.55.1.55

Nigro, S., Passamonti, L., Riccelli, R., Toschi, N., Rocca, F., Valentino, P., . . . Quattrone, A. (2014). Structural "connectomic" alterations in the limbic system of multiple sclerosis patients with major depression. *Multiple Sclerosis Journal, 21*, 1003–1012.

Niino, M., Mifune, N., Kohriyama, T., Mori, M., Ohashi, T., Kawachi, I., . . . Kikuchi, S. (2014). Apathy/depression, but not subjective fatigue, is related with cognitive dysfunction in patients with multiple sclerosis. *BMC Neurology, 14*, 3. http://dx.doi.org/10.1186/1471-2377-14-3

Papadopoulou, A., Müller-Lenke, N., Naegelin, Y., Kalt, G., Bendfeldt, K., Kuster, P., . . . Penner, I. K. (2013). Contribution of cortical and white matter lesions to cognitive impairment in multiple sclerosis. *Multiple Sclerosis, 19*, 1290–1296. http://dx.doi.org/10.1177/1352458513475490

Patten, S. B., & Metz, L. M. (1997). Depression in multiple sclerosis. *Psychotherapy and Psychosomatics, 66*, 286–292. http://dx.doi.org/10.1159/000289150

Paty, D. W., & Ebers, G. C. (1998). *Multiple sclerosis.* Philadelphia, PA: FA Davis.

Rabinowitz, A. R., & Arnett, P. A. (2009). A longitudinal analysis of cognitive dysfunction, coping, and depression in multiple sclerosis. *Neuropsychology, 23,* 581–591. http://dx.doi.org/10.1037/a0016064

Raine, C. S., McFarland, H. F., & Hohlfeld, R. (2008). *Multiple sclerosis: A comprehensive text.* Edinburgh, Scotland: Elsevier Health Sciences.

Rao, S. M., Leo, G. J., Bernardin, L., & Unverzagt, F. (1991). Cognitive dysfunction in multiple sclerosis. I. Frequency, patterns, and prediction. *Neurology, 41,* 685–691. http://dx.doi.org/10.1212/WNL.41.5.685

Rao, S. M., Leo, G. J., Haughton, V. M., St. Aubin-Faubert, P., & Bernardin, L. (1989). Correlation of magnetic resonance imaging with neuropsychological testing in multiple sclerosis. *Neurology, 39,* 161–166. http://dx.doi.org/10.1212/WNL.39.2.161

Riccelli, R., Passamonti, L., Cerasa, A., Nigro, S., Cavalli, S. M., Chiriaco, C., . . . Quattrone, A. (2015). Individual differences in depression are associated with abnormal function of the limbic system in multiple sclerosis patients. *Multiple Sclerosis Journal, 22,* 1094–1105.

Sabatini, U., Pozzilli, C., Pantano, P., Koudriavtseva, T., Padovani, A., Millefiorini, E., . . . Lenzi, G. L. (1996). Involvement of the limbic system in multiple sclerosis patients with depressive disorders. *Biological Psychiatry, 39,* 970–975. http://dx.doi.org/10.1016/0006-3223(95)00291-X

Sadovnick, A. D., Remick, R. A., Allen, J., Swartz, E., Yee, I. M. L., Eisen, K., . . . Paty, D. W. (1996). Depression and multiple sclerosis. *Neurology, 46,* 628–632. http://dx.doi.org/10.1212/WNL.46.3.628

Scheurich, A., Fellgiebel, A., Schermuly, I., Bauer, S., Wölfges, R., & Müller, M. J. (2008). Experimental evidence for a motivational origin of cognitive impairment in major depression. *Psychological Medicine, 38,* 237–246. http://dx.doi.org/10.1017/S0033291707002206

Shen, Y., Bai, L., Gao, Y., Cui, F., Tan, Z., Tao, Y., . . . Zhou, L. (2014). Depressive symptoms in multiple sclerosis from an in vivo study with TBSS. *BioMed Research International, 2014,* 148465. http://dx.doi.org/10.1155/2014/148465

Staffen, W., Mair, A., Zauner, H., Unterrainer, J., Niederhofer, H., Kutzelnigg, A., . . . Ladurner, G. (2002). Cognitive function and fMRI in patients with multiple sclerosis: Evidence for compensatory cortical activation during an attention task. *Brain, 125,* 1275–1282. http://dx.doi.org/10.1093/brain/awf125

Stern, Y. (2002). What is cognitive reserve? Theory and research application of the reserve concept. *Journal of the International Neuropsychological Society, 8,* 448–460. http://dx.doi.org/10.1017/S1355617702813248

Strober, L. B., & Arnett, P. A. (2015). Depression in multiple sclerosis: The utility of common self-report instruments and development of a disease-specific measure. *Journal of Clinical and Experimental Neuropsychology, 37,* 722–732. http://dx.doi.org/10.1080/13803395.2015.1063591

Sumowski, J. F., Chiaravalloti, N., & DeLuca, J. (2009). Cognitive reserve protects against cognitive dysfunction in multiple sclerosis. *Journal of Clinical and Experimental Neuropsychology, 31,* 913–926. http://dx.doi.org/10.1080/13803390902740643

Sumowski, J. F., & Leavitt, V. M. (2013). Cognitive reserve in multiple sclerosis. *Multiple Sclerosis Journal, 19,* 1122–1127. http://dx.doi.org/10.1177/1352458513498834

Sundgren, M., Maurex, L., Wahlin, Å., Piehl, F., & Brismar, T. (2013). Cognitive impairment has a strong relation to nonsomatic symptoms of depression in relapsing-remitting multiple sclerosis. *Archives of Clinical Neuropsychology, 28,* 144–155. http://dx.doi.org/10.1093/arclin/acs113

Viner, R., Fiest, K. M., Bulloch, A. G. M., Williams, J. V. A., Lavorato, D. H., Berzins, S., . . . Patten, S. B. (2014). Point prevalence and correlates of depression in a national community sample with multiple sclerosis. *General Hospital Psychiatry, 36,* 352–354. http://dx.doi.org/10.1016/j.genhosppsych.2013.12.011

Zorzon, M., Zivadinov, R., Nasuelli, D., Ukmar, M., Bratina, A., Tommasi, M. A., . . . Cazzato, G. (2002). Depressive symptoms and MRI changes in multiple sclerosis. *European Journal of Neurology, 9,* 491–496. http://dx.doi.org/10.1046/j.1468-1331.2002.00442.x

5

COGNITION AND NEUROPSYCHIATRIC DISORDERS IN MULTIPLE SCLEROSIS

ANTHONY FEINSTEIN AND BENNIS PAVISIAN

The behavioral manifestations of multiple sclerosis (MS) are diverse, common, and, if left untreated, can prove profoundly disabling. Much of the attention over the years has focused on depression because it is the most frequent disorder encountered, with an incidence of 979 in 100,000 people with MS (Marrie, Fisk, et al., 2015). This chapter, however, looks elsewhere at an array of disorders that have been less extensively studied. These include anxiety in its various manifestations, bipolar affective disorder, euphoria, and pseudobulbar affect (PBA). For each of these disorders, the literature pertaining to phenomenology, prevalence, magnetic resonance imaging (MRI) brain correlates, and treatment is summarized.

http://dx.doi.org/10.1037/0000097-006
Cognition and Behavior in Multiple Sclerosis, J. DeLuca and B. M. Sandroff (Editors)
Copyright © 2018 by the American Psychological Association. All rights reserved.

ANXIETY

Anxiety is a broad descriptive term that encompasses individual symptoms and syndromal diagnoses. The study of anxiety has been relatively neglected in people with MS, as it has been in the general neuropsychiatry literature. This oversight is unfortunate because symptoms are common and add appreciably to the disability linked to MS. In a U.K. registry study of close to 8,000 people with MS, 54.1% were found to have clinically significant symptoms of anxiety (Jones et al., 2012). Those most affected were women with relapsing–remitting disease. A higher prevalence in women was also reported by Théaudin, Romero, and Feinstein (2016) in a large clinic based sample (*n* = 711) in which the overall point prevalence of anxiety deemed clinically important according to a threshold score on the Hospital Anxiety and Depression Scale (HADS) was 47.7%. Epidemiological data confirm the high comorbidity, with an incidence of 638 in 100,000 people with MS (Marrie, Fisk, et al., 2015).

Moving from symptom to syndrome, the prevalence rates of generalized anxiety disorder, panic disorder, and obsessive-compulsive disorder in people with MS were reported to be 3 times the general population estimates (Korostil & Feinstein, 2007). High rates of social anxiety disorder have also been found (Poder et al., 2008). Of note is that, should anxiety be comorbid with depression, it may increase the frequency of suicidal thinking (Quesnel & Feinstein, 2004). The clinical significance of this point is underscored by the high suicide rate in people with MS (Stenager et al., 1992; Stenager & Stenager, 1992).

When it comes to assessing anxiety in people with MS, it is important not to misconstrue symptoms of MS as those of emotional distress. Examples of symptom overlap include insomnia, difficulties with concentration, and the sensory changes that can accompany a panic attack. A useful psychometric instrument that can help tease out and quantify anxiety symptoms in people with MS is the HADS (Zigmond & Snaith, 1983), which has been validated for use in people with MS (Honarmand & Feinstein, 2009). The reasons for the high frequency of anxiety in people with MS have not been systematically addressed. Heightened expressions of anxiety have been recorded soon after the diagnosis has been given, suggesting that for some people, their distress should be seen as reactive (Janssens et al., 2003). Of note is that some (da Silva et al., 2011; Jones et al., 2012; Théaudin et al., 2016), but not all (Dahl, Stordal, Lydersen, & Midgard, 2009), studies have reported higher rates of anxiety in women with MS. All these studies, however, were descriptive and as such cannot shed light on why gender might influence the presence, and quite plausibly the expression, of anxiety. Neuroimaging is also not helpful in elucidating pathogenesis. Only one MRI study has focused on anxiety and found no correlates with any measure of regional or total lesion load or brain volume (Zorzon et al., 2001).

The anxiety treatment literature in people with MS is equally sparse. A systematic review and meta-analysis of interventions for depression and anxiety in people with MS unearthed only a single anxiety study, and this for injection phobia, where treatment proved ineffective (Fiest et al., 2016). Other studies have looked at overall psychological distress, of which anxiety was one component. In a randomized controlled trial involving people experiencing adjustment-related distress, cognitive behavior therapy (CBT) proved effective, even when administered over the telephone (Moss-Morris et al., 2013).

BIPOLAR AFFECTIVE DISORDER

The clinical features of this syndrome, previously called manic-depressive disorder, include the triad of elevated (euphoric) or irritable mood, grandiose or persecutory beliefs that can reach delusional intensity, and behavioral changes reflecting increased energy, less need for sleep, and fast or pressured speech, to mention but three features. The annual incidence per 100,000 people with MS has been estimated at 328, one third that of depression alone. Supportive epidemiological data also come from an earlier study of 702,238 residents of Monroe County, New York (Schiffer, Wineman, & Weitkamp, 1986). Working off lifetime risks for bipolar illness and MS, the authors anticipated a comorbidity rate of 5.4 but instead found double that. In all cases, the onset of MS preceded the symptoms of bipolar illness. The authors went on to conclude that their figure may have been an underestimate of the true comorbidity because cases of either disorder may not have been kept on the county's computerized record system.

In addition, indirect evidence supporting the association may be found in a study of almost 3,000 psychiatric inpatients who were screened for MS. Although only 10 patients with MS were found, they were more likely to have presented with manic or hypomanic symptoms compared with the remainder of the sample (Pine, Douglas, Charles, Davies, & Kahn, 1995). This finding is supported by data from the Swedish National Patient Register containing 16,467 people with MS and 30,761 with bipolar disorder. The risk of having MS was increased in those with a bipolar illness (hazards ratio = 1.8, $p < .0001$; Johansson et al., 2014). Finally, a systematic review of the frequency of psychiatric disorders in MS concluded that the prevalence rate for bipolar illness was 5.83%, 3 times that in the general population (Marrie, Reingold, et al., 2015).

Reasons for this elevated rate of bipolar disorder have focused on three sources: genetics, a reaction to steroids, and brain imaging. In all three categories, data are limited. Beginning with genetics, attention has centered on the determination of family histories. In the Monroe County study, five of the 10 individuals identified with bipolar disorder had a first- or second-degree relative with a significant affective illness. Although the numbers here are small, they are nevertheless suggestive of a possible genetic link. Small numbers characterized another study of 56 people with MS divided into four groups: bipolar ($n = 15$), unipolar depression ($n = 16$), no mood disorder ($n = 13$), and probably no mood disorder ($n = 12$). Two thirds of the people with MS and bipolar disorder had a relative with an affective disorder compared with only one person in the unipolar depression group and two people in the group without affective disorders, a statistically significant difference. Associations with various human leukocyte antigen subtypes were sought but not found, perhaps due to the small sample size (Schiffer et al., 1986).

The mood-altering properties of steroids and adrenocorticotropic hormones have been well described, which begs the question of to what degree has this influenced the mental state of people with MS? This was investigated retrospectively in a sample of 50 people with MS given steroids, nine of whom developed mania or hypomania during treatment. The most striking risk factors to emerge were a history of depression, either before or after the diagnosis of MS and a family history of depression, alcoholism, or both. ACTH was also considered more likely to trigger mania than prednisone.

To date there are no detailed MRI studies of people with MS and bipolar disorder. A single MRI study of psychosis in MS ($n = 10$, half of whom had a bipolar illness) revealed a more extensive hyperintense lesion area around the temporal horns compared with a matched nonpsychotic MS sample (Feinstein, Kartsounis, Miller, Youl, & Ron, 1992). However, of five manic MS subjects who underwent MRI in a later study, only one had lesions within the temporal lobes (Hutchinson, Stack, & Buckley, 1993).

In keeping with the paucity of clinical and radiological findings, there are no randomized controlled treatment studies of bipolar illness in people with MS. As such, the treating physician is forced to borrow from algorithms used in the general psychiatric population, albeit with a few caveats, given concerns of the side effects of medication in the already neurologically compromised brain. Mood-stabilizing medication is the mainstay of treatment. Lithium carbonate is reportedly effective in treating steroid-induced mania (Falk, Mahnke, & Poskanzer, 1979; Minden, Orav, & Schildkraut, 1988), but its effectiveness in MS bipolar presentations is equivocal with support for (Solomon, 1978) and against (Kwentus, Hart, Calabrese, & Hekmati, 1986). For those individuals with MS who are unable to tolerate lithium, valproic acid (Stip & Daoust, 1995) is an effective substitute. Mood-stabilizing medication alone, however, may prove insufficient in the manic individual who has become psychotic. Here the clinician will have no recourse other than to use antipsychotic medications. The second-generation medications such as olanzapine, quetiapine, and risperidone are preferable to older drugs such as chlorpromazine and haloperidol given the lower likelihood of extrapyramidal side effects. This point is particularly important when treating a person with MS who already has significant motor compromise because a combination of medication-induced sedation and further motor impairment appreciably lowers the threshold for falls.

EUPHORIA

Euphoria in people with MS may be a symptom of bipolar affective disorder, but it may also represent its own stand-alone behavioral abnormality. The early MS behavioral literature considered it one of the pathognomonic presentations of mental state change, and the 18th-century literature (for a review, see Finger, 1998) is replete with phenomenological descriptions. However, it was only in the 20th century that researchers began describing the prevalence of the disorder. Cottrell and Wilson (1926) reported that it was present in more than two thirds of their sample. They discerned four distinct variants: *euphoria sclerotica*, reflecting a persistently cheerful mood; *eutonia sclerotic*, encompassing a lack of concern over physical disability; *pes sclerotica*, indicative of an incongruous optimism for the future; and *emotional lability*. Although the validity of this classification has never been put to the test, the categories, with the exception of emotional lability, are thought to capture the essential clinical features of the syndrome. The cheerful, optimistic demeanor of the euphoric individual therefore bares a superficial resemblance to the mental state of a hypomanic patient, without displaying evidence of the physical overactivity, increased energy, and grandiose plans that characterize the latter. Euphoria is therefore best viewed as a fixed mental state, akin to a personality change and not subject to the often wild fluctuations seen in bipolar disorder. The presentation is usually readily discernible from mania or hypomania.

The studies that followed Cottrell and Wilson's (1926) landmark paper reported far more modest estimates. A comparison of people with MS and people with muscular dystrophy revealed the presence of euphoria in 26% of the former and none in the latter (Surridge, 1969). Poser (1980) reported a 24% rate, half that of Rabins et al. (1986), who applied the Cottrell and Wilson (1926) criteria to their sample. The reasons for these revised estimates were twofold. First, more careful clinical inquiry revealed that the euphoria displayed by many individuals was quite superficial and masked underlying feelings of sadness and worry. The second is that the category labeled *emotional lability* was really its own distinct behavioral syndrome, which would soon come to be called *pseudobulbar affect* or pathological laughter and crying (discussed later in the chapter). In a summary article, drawing together the extant literature, Rabins (1990) concluded that euphoria as a stand-alone behavioral change was present in a *median* of 25% of people with MS.

Subsequent studies using structured interviews and more representative samples have lowered the rates even further. There are two studies using the Neuropsychiatric Inventory (Cummings et al., 1994) that arrived at similar conclusions. In the first of these, which involved 44 people with MS and 25 healthy control subjects, euphoria was elicited in 13% of the MS group, the sixth most frequent behavioral change after (in descending order) depression (79%), agitation (40%), anxiety (37%), irritability (35%), and apathy (20%; Diaz-Olavarrieta, Cummings, Velazquez, & Garcia de la Cadena, 1999). A second study using the same methodology arrived at a prevalence of 9% (Fishman, Benedict, Bakshi, Priore, & Weinstock-Guttman, 2004). Duncan, Malcolm-Smith, Ameen, and Solms (2015) emphasized that this falloff over time in the frequency of euphoria is indicative of changing definitions rather than an actual decline in the disorder but concluded their brief review by suggesting that further work is needed to better define the true nature of the disorder.

Unlike the situation with respect to bipolar affective disorder, there is a small brain imaging literature devoted to euphoria in people with MS, and the findings fit together well. Studies have linked the behavior to greater neurological disability and more marked cognitive impairment (Fishman et al., 2004; Rabins et al., 1986; Surridge, 1969), a secondary progressive disease course (Fishman et al., 2004; Rabins et al., 1986), ventricular atrophy on computed tomography (Rabins et al., 1986), a heavy frontal lesion burden on MRI (Diaz-Olavarrieta et al., 1999; Reischies, Baum, Bräu, Hedde, & Schwindt, 1988), and more widespread lesions in general (Ron & Logsdail, 1989). In a study of 98 people with MS that included both a detailed analysis of personality constructs and brain MRI data, an association was found between euphoria on one hand and a reduction in gray matter volume and impaired cognition on the other; this relationship was mediated by personality changes that included high neuroticism and low conscientiousness (Test, 2013). Interestingly, Cottrell and Wilson (1926), in their widely cited and influential paper, concluded that euphoria was not associated with cognitive compromise, an error that has detracted from their otherwise accurate behavioral descriptions of the disorder.

There are no treatment studies of euphoria, and one may quite reasonably ask why would one want to treat individuals with advanced MS who appear untroubled by their marked disability? Here is it germane to observe that those most distressed by the situation are the family and friends who serve as caregivers and whose insight into the true nature of the disease and the impending future implications understandably give them cause for concern.

PSEUDOBULBAR AFFECT

PBA has also been called pathological laughing and crying, emotional incontinence, and excessive emotionalism. In keeping with a *Diagnostic and Statistical Manual of Mental Disorders*–style coinage, the syndrome has more recently been repackaged as Involuntary Emotional Expression Disorder and various inclusion criteria stipulated. It is now generally accepted that PBA refers to individuals who cry when not feeling sad or who laugh in the absence of mirth, or who show features of both crying and laughing in the absence of mood congruent feelings. This display of affect is considered involuntary. However, the definition of the disorder has varied historically, and as such prevalence rates have varied as well. Returning to the study by Cottrell and Wilson (1926), of the 100 patients studied, 85 were deemed to have various degrees of pathological affect. These included 71% who were smiling and laughing constantly, 19% who showed a mix of smiling and laughing, 2% whose affect switched rapidly from laughing to crying, and a further 2% who were constantly crying. The authors observed that these displays of affect were present with minimal if any provocation and persisted over time. In hindsight, it is apparent that this study had numerous methodological flaws ranging from a biased sample selection to use of a structured interview that had not been validated. The importance of the study, however, transcends the statistics that we now know to be inaccurate. Rather, it should be seen as a first, pioneering attempt that went beyond individual case reports and focused instead on describing behavioral changes in a large group of people with MS.

Fifteen years after this landmark study, a second report appeared in which 13 of 199 (6.5%) outpatients with MS, most notably those in the later stages of the disease, displayed features of uncontrollable laughter, crying, or both (Langworthy & Hesser, 1940). The phenomenon was considered part of a pseudobulbar palsy and thought to reflect a disconnection of bulbar mechanisms from higher cortical control. The authors expressed a degree of uncertainty when it came to differentiating the syndrome from euphoria and speculated that the two might be part of the same continuum. This diagnostic uncertainty would bedevil subsequent research efforts and can explain why later studies arrived at elevated prevalence rates that varied from 10% to 79% (Pratt, 1951; Sugar & Nadell, 1943; Surridge, 1969).

Poeck (1969) can be credited with bringing diagnostic rigor to the subject, irrespective of the underlying neurological disorder. He made a distinction between PBA on one hand and a number of other symptom complexes on the other that included emotional lability (episodes of crying and, less frequently, laughing that were considered excessive but nevertheless appropriate to the context in which they occurred), *Witzelsucht* (facetiousness), euphoria, and laughing or crying secondary to substance abuse, psychosis, or histrionic behavior. PBA was attributed to a release of inhibition of the motor component of facial expression. Poeck defined four components to the syndrome: a response to nonspecific stimuli, the absence of an association between affective change and the observed expression, the inability to voluntarily control facial expression, and the absence of a corresponding mood change that exceeded the period of laughing or crying.

These tight diagnostic criteria were applied by Feinstein et al. (1997) in a wide-ranging study of 152 people with MS attending a tertiary referral MS clinic. In addition, all participants were administered the Pathological Laughing and Crying Scale (PLACS; Robinson et al., 1993), which quantifies aspects of PBA including duration, relationship to external events, degree of voluntary control, inappropriateness in relation to emotions, and extent of associated distress. Of the 152 participants, 15 were found to have PBA, thereby establishing a point prevalence of 9.9%. Comparisons were then undertaken between these 15 subjects and the remainder of the sample without PBA. The PBA group had MS for 2.5 years longer than the rest of the sample and were more likely to have entered a secondary progressive stage to their illness. Type II error likely prevented these differences reaching statistical significance. Their mean Expanded Disability Status Scale score was 6.4 ($SD = 1.7$). In keeping with the tight diagnostic criteria used to define PBA, no subject in this group was considered euphoric. Moreover, scores on the Hospital Anxiety and Depression Scale did indicate the presence of clinically significant depression in those subjects who were prone to episodes of uncontrollable crying. On the other hand, the 15 subjects with PBA had a lower performance IQ (and by extension total IQ) than the remainder of the sample with further analysis of the Wechsler Adult Intelligence Scale—Revised data revealing the most marked deficits on the arithmetic, digit symbol (limited to digits backward), and picture arrangement tests.

A more detailed cognitive inquiry was completed in 11 of the 15 people with PBA, and the results were compared with 13 demographically and disease-matched people with MS who did not have PBA. The PBA group performed more poorly on the Stroop test and the Controlled Oral Word Association Test (COWAT) an index of verbal fluency, attention, and semantic memory (Feinstein, O'Connor, Gray, & Feinstein, 1999). This result was subsequently replicated in a retrospective study involving chart reviews of 153 people with MS who had been administered a detailed neuropsychological battery and a self-report measure of emotional dyscontrol, the Center for

Neurological Study—Lability Scale (CNS–LS; Hanna et al., 2016). Elevated scores on the CNS–LS, a proxy for PBA, were linked to a more impaired performance on the COWAT and greater memory deficits on the California Verbal Learning Test.

The etiology of PBA may be traced to a dysfunctional neural network connecting widely dispersed brain regions. Wilson (1924), in his classic work on the subject, highlighted two anatomical foci he considered pivotal to the pathogenesis: the bulbar nuclei in the brainstem and the motor cortex exerting a top-down, voluntary control over the bulbar nuclei. Wilson suggested that damage to the corticospinal, corticobulbar, and corticopontine tracts connecting the two regions was instrumental in generating the involuntary affect. In short, PBA was viewed as a disconnection syndrome, the bulbar nuclei becoming functionally separated from cortical control. Subsequent brain imaging work has confirmed this, while also revealing that the neural network is more diffuse than Wilson originally envisaged. For example, a detailed volumetric MRI study implicated not only the brainstem in the pathogenesis of PBA, but also bilateral inferior parietal, bilateral orbitofrontal, and medial-superior frontal regions (see Color Plate 7; Ghaffar, Chamelian, & Feinstein 2008). An elegant case report has also implicated the cerebellum, a region rich in connection to the prefrontal cortex, with PBA (Parvizi, Anderson, Martin, Damasio, & Damasio, 2001).

Before leaving the imaging findings, it is of note that the MRI data, limited as they are, add support to the phenomenological distinction between PBA and major depression. Detailed structural MRI data account for approximately 40% to 45% of the variance when it comes to explaining the development of depression (Feinstein et al., 2010). The figure rises to almost to 80% with PBA (Ghaffar et al., 2008).

PBA can be well treated. Tricyclic antidepressant medication, most notably amitriptyline in small doses (< 75 mg per day), proved effective in two thirds of subjects in a double-blind crossover trial (Schiffer, Herndon, & Rudick, 1985). Anecdotal evidence also supports the efficacy of the selective serotonin reuptake inhibitor fluoxetine (Seliger, Hornstein, Flax, Herbert, & Schroeder, 1992; Sloan, Brown, & Pentland, 1992), and a single case report demonstrated efficacy for valproic acid (Johnson & Nichols, 2015). However, the most robust evidence comes from a serendipitous discovery—namely, that a combination of dextromethorphan and quinidine can modulate involuntary laughter and crying. A randomized controlled trial of 150 people with MS and PBA randomized to dextromethorphan/quinidine ($n = 76$) and placebo ($n = 74$) revealed that the drug-treated group experienced significantly fewer episodes of laughing and crying with a concomitant improvement in quality of life (Panitch et al., 2006).

CONCLUSIONS AND FUTURE DIRECTIONS

This chapter has summarized the data relating to various neuropsychiatric syndromes associated with MS. In a disease without cure, good symptom management takes on even greater importance. First, however, the correct diagnosis must be made. Here clinicians are fortunate for they can benefit from a long history of careful inquiry that has, over the years, honed the criteria into clearly recognizable syndromes. All the disorders discussed, euphoria apart, are treatable. Which underscores yet again the need for awareness and vigilance in detecting the presence of these potentially reversible syndromes that exert such a profound effect on a person's quality of life.

REFERENCES

Cottrell, S. S., & Wilson, S. A. K. (1926). The affective symptomatology of disseminated sclerosis: A study of 100 cases. *Journal of Neurology and Psychopathology, 1*, 1–30.

Cummings, J. L., Mega, M., Gray, K., Rosenberg-Thompson, S., Carusi, D. A., & Gornbein, J. (1994). The Neuropsychiatric Inventory: Comprehensive assessment of psychopathology in dementia. *Neurology, 44*, 2308–2314. http://dx.doi.org/10.1212/WNL.44.12.2308

da Silva, A. M., Vilhena, E., Lopes, A., Santos, E., Gonçalves, M. A., Pinto, C., . . . Cavaco, S. (2011). Depression and anxiety in a Portuguese MS population: Associations with physical disability and severity of disease. *Journal of Neurological Sciences, 306*, 66–70.

Dahl, O.-P., Stordal, E., Lydersen, S., & Midgard, R. (2009). Anxiety and depression in multiple sclerosis: A comparative population-based study in Nord-Trøndelag County, Norway. *Multiple Sclerosis Journal, 15*, 1495–1501. http://dx.doi.org/10.1177/1352458509351542

Diaz-Olavarrieta, C., Cummings, J. L., Velazquez, J., & Garcia de la Cadena, C. (1999). Neuropsychiatric manifestations of multiple sclerosis. *The Journal of Neuropsychiatry and Clinical Neurosciences, 11*, 51–57.

Duncan, A., Malcolm-Smith, S., Ameen, O., & Solms, M. (2015). Changing definitions of euphoria in multiple sclerosis: A short report. *Multiple Sclerosis Journal, 21*, 776–779. http://dx.doi.org/10.1177/1352458514549400

Falk, W. E., Mahnke, M. W., & Poskanzer, D. C. (1979). Lithium prophylaxis of corticotropin-induced psychosis. *Journal of the American Medical Association, 241*, 1011–1012. http://dx.doi.org/10.1001/jama.1979.03290360027021

Feinstein, A., Feinstein, K., Gray, T., & O'Connor, P. (1997). Prevalence and neurobehavioral correlates of pathological laughing and crying in multiple sclerosis. *Archives of Neurology, 54*, 1116–1121. http://dx.doi.org/10.1001/archneur.1997.00550210050012

Feinstein, A., Kartsounis, L. D., Miller, D. H., Youl, B. D., & Ron, M. A. (1992). Clinically isolated lesions of the type seen in multiple sclerosis: A cognitive, psychiatric, and MRI follow up study. *Journal of Neurology, Neurosurgery & Psychiatry, 55*, 869–876. http://dx.doi.org/10.1136/jnnp.55.10.869

Feinstein, A., O'Connor, P., Akbar, N., Moradzadeh, L., Scott, C. J., & Lobaugh, N. J. (2010). Diffusion tensor imaging abnormalities in depressed multiple sclerosis patients. *Multiple Sclerosis, 16*, 189–196. http://dx.doi.org/10.1177/1352458509355461

Feinstein, A., O'Connor, P., Gray, T., & Feinstein, K. (1999). The effects of anxiety on psychiatric morbidity in patients with multiple sclerosis. *Multiple Sclerosis, 5*, 323–326. http://dx.doi.org/10.1191/135245899678846348

Fiest, K. M., Walker, J. R., Bernstein, C. N., Graff, L. A., Zarychanski, R., Abou-Setta, A. M., . . . CIHR Team. (2016). Systematic review and meta-analysis of interventions for depression and anxiety in persons with multiple sclerosis. *Multiple Sclerosis and Related Disorders, 5*, 12–26.

Finger, S. (1998). A happy state of mind: A history of mild elation, denial of disability, optimism, and laughing in multiple sclerosis. *Archives of Neurology, 55*, 241–250. http://dx.doi.org/10.1001/archneur.55.2.241

Fishman, I., Benedict, R. H., Bakshi, R., Priore, R., & Weinstock-Guttman, B. (2004). Construct validity and frequency of euphoria sclerotica in multiple sclerosis. *The Journal of Neuropsychiatry and Clinical Neurosciences, 16*, 350–356.

Ghaffar, O., Chamelian, L., & Feinstein, A. (2008). Neuroanatomy of pseudobulbar affect. *Journal of Neurology, 255*, 406–412.

Hanna, J., Feinstein, A., & Morrow, S. A. (2016). The association of pathological laughing and crying and cognitive impairment in multiple sclerosis. *Journal of the Neurological Sciences, 361*, 200–203.

Honarmand, K., & Feinstein, A. (2009). Validation of the Hospital Anxiety and Depression Scale for use with multiple sclerosis patients. *Multiple Sclerosis, 15*, 1518–1524. http://dx.doi.org/10.1177/1352458509347150

Hutchinson, M., Stack, J., & Buckley, P. (1993). Bipolar affective disorder prior to the onset of multiple sclerosis. *Acta Neurologica Scandinavica, 88*, 388–393. http://dx.doi.org/10.1111/j.1600-0404.1993.tb05365.x

Janssens, A. C., van Doorn, P. A., de Boer, J. B., van der Meché, F. G., Passchier, J., & Hintzen, R. Q. (2003). Impact of recently diagnosed multiple sclerosis on quality of life, anxiety, depression and distress of patients and partners. *Acta Neurologica Scandinavica, 108*, 389–395. http://dx.doi.org/10.1034/j.1600-0404.2003.00166.x

Johansson, V., Lundholm, C., Hillert, J., Masterman, T., Lichtenstein, P., Landén, M., & Hultman, C. M. (2014). Multiple sclerosis and psychiatric disorders: comorbidity and sibling risk in a nationwide Swedish cohort. *Multiple Sclerosis, 20*, 1881–1891.

Johnson, B., & Nichols, S. (2015). Crying and suicidal, but not depressed. Pseudobulbar affect in multiple sclerosis successfully treated with valproic acid: Case report and literature review. *Palliative and Supportive Care, 13,* 1797–1801. http://dx.doi.org/10.1017/S1478951514000376

Jones, K. H., Ford, D. V., Jones, P. A., John, A., Middleton, R. M., Lockhart-Jones, H., . . . Noble, J. G. (2012). A large-scale study of anxiety and depression in people with multiple sclerosis: A survey via the web portal of the UK MS Register. *PLoS ONE, 7,* e41910. http://dx.doi.org/10.1371/journal.pone.0041910

Korostil, M., & Feinstein, A. (2007). Anxiety disorders and their clinical correlates in multiple sclerosis patients. *Multiple Sclerosis, 13,* 67–72. http://dx.doi.org/10.1177/1352458506071161

Kwentus, J. A., Hart, R. P., Calabrese, V., & Hekmati, A. (1986). Mania as a symptom of multiple sclerosis. *Psychosomatics, 27,* 729–731. http://dx.doi.org/10.1016/S0033-3182(86)72623-6

Langworthy, O. R., & Hesser, F. H. (1940). Syndrome of pseudobulbar palsy: An anatomic and physiologic analysis. *Archives of Internal Medicine, 65,* 106–121. http://dx.doi.org/10.1001/archinte.1940.00190070116008

Marrie, R. A., Fisk, J. D., Tremlett, H., Wolfson, C., Warren, S., Tennakoon, A., . . . the CIHR Team in the Epidemiology and Impact of Comorbidity on Multiple Sclerosis. (2015). Differences in the burden of psychiatric comorbidity in MS vs the general population. *Neurology, 85,* 1972–1979. http://dx.doi.org/10.1212/WNL.0000000000002174

Marrie, R. A., Reingold, S., Cohen, J., Stuve, O., Trojano, M., Sorensen, P. S., . . . Reider, N. (2015). The incidence and prevalence of psychiatric disorders in multiple sclerosis: A systematic review. *Multiple Sclerosis Journal, 21,* 305–317.

Minden, S. L., Orav, J., & Schildkraut, J. J. (1988). Hypomanic reactions to ACTH and prednisone treatment for multiple sclerosis. *Neurology, 38,* 1631–1634. http://dx.doi.org/10.1212/WNL.38.10.1631

Moss-Morris, R., Dennison, L., Landau, S., Yardley, L., Silber, E., & Chalder, T. (2013). A randomized controlled trial of cognitive behavioral therapy (CBT) for adjusting to multiple sclerosis (the saMS trial): Does CBT work and for whom does it work? *Journal of Consulting and Clinical Psychology, 81,* 251–262. http://dx.doi.org/10.1037/a0029132

Panitch, H. S., Thisted, R. A., Smith, R. A., Wynn, D. R., Wymer, J. P., Achiron, A., . . . the Pseudobulbar Affect in Multiple Sclerosis Study Group. (2006). Randomized, controlled trial of dextromethorphan/quinidine for pseudobulbar affect in multiple sclerosis. *Annals of Neurology, 59,* 780–787. http://dx.doi.org/10.1002/ana.20828

Parvizi, J., Anderson, S. W., Martin, C. O., Damasio, H., & Damasio, A. R. (2001). Pathological laughter and crying: A link to the cerebellum. *Brain, 124,* 1708–1719. http://dx.doi.org/10.1093/brain/124.9.1708

Pine, D. S., Douglas, C. J., Charles, E., Davies, M., & Kahn, D. (1995). Patients with multiple sclerosis presenting to psychiatric hospitals. *Journal of Clinical Psychiatry, 56,* 297–306.

Poder, K., Ghatavi, K., Fisk, J. D., Campbell, T. L., Kisely, S., Sarty, I., . . . Bhan, V. (2008). Social anxiety in a multiple sclerosis clinic population. *Multiple Sclerosis, 15,* 393–398.

Poeck, K. (1969). Pathophysiology of emotional disorders associated with brain damage. In P. Vinken & G. Bruyn (Eds.), *Handbook of clinical neurology* (pp. 343–367). Amsterdam, The Netherlands: North Holland.

Poser, C. M. (1980). Exacerbations, activity and progression in multiple sclerosis. *Archives of Neurology, 37,* 471–474.

Pratt, R. T. C. (1951). An investigation of the psychiatric aspects of disseminated sclerosis. *Journal of Neurology, Neurosurgery, and Psychiatry, 14,* 326–335.

Quesnel, S., & Feinstein, A. (2004). Multiple sclerosis and alcohol: A study of problem drinking. *Multiple Sclerosis, 10,* 197–201.

Rabins, P. V. (1990). Euphoria in multiple sclerosis. *Neurobehavioral aspects of multiple sclerosis* (pp. 180–185). New York, NY: Oxford University Press.

Rabins, P. V., Brooks, B. R., O'Donnell, P., Pearlson, G. D., Moberg, P., Jubelt, B., . . . Folstein, M. F. (1986). Structural brain correlates of emotional disorder in multiple sclerosis. *Brain, 109,* 585–597.

Reischies, F. M., Baum, K., Bräu, H., Hedde, J. P., & Schwindt, G. (1988). Cerebral magnetic resonance imaging findings in multiple sclerosis. Relation to disturbance of affect, drive, and cognition. *Archives of Neurology, 45,* 1114–1116. http://dx.doi.org/10.1001/archneur.1988.00520340068014

Robinson, R. G., Parikh, R. M., Lipsey, J. R., Starkstein, S. E., & Price, T. R. (1993). Pathological laughing and crying following stroke: Validation of a measurement scale and a double-blind treatment study. *The American Journal of Psychiatry, 150,* 286–293. http://dx.doi.org/10.1176/ajp.150.2.286

Ron, M. A., & Logsdail, S. J. (1989). Psychiatric morbidity in multiple sclerosis: A clinical and MRI study. *Psychological Medicine, 19,* 887–895. http://dx.doi.org/10.1017/S0033291700005602

Schiffer, R. B., Herndon, R. M., & Rudick, R. A. (1985). Treatment of pathologic laughing and weeping with amitriptyline. *The New England Journal of Medicine, 312,* 1480–1482. http://dx.doi.org/10.1056/NEJM198506063122303

Schiffer, R. B., Wineman, N. M., & Weitkamp, L. R. (1986). Association between bipolar affective disorder and multiple sclerosis. *American Journal of Psychiatry, 143,* 94–95. http://dx.doi.org/10.1176/ajp.143.1.94

Seliger, G. M., Hornstein, A., Flax, J., Herbert, J., & Schroeder, K. (1992). Fluoxetine improves emotional incontinence. *Brain Injury, 6,* 267–270. http://dx.doi.org/10.3109/02699059209029668

Sloan, R. L., Brown, K. W., & Pentland, B. (1992). Fluoxetine as a treatment for emotional lability after brain injury. *Brain Injury, 6,* 315–319. http://dx.doi.org/10.3109/02699059209034945

Solomon, J. G. (1978). Multiple sclerosis masquerading as lithium toxicity. *The Journal of nervous and mental disease, 166,* 663–665.

Stenager, E. N., & Stenager, E. (1992). Suicide and patients with neurologic diseases: Methodologic problems. *Archives of Neurology, 49*, 1296–1303.

Stenager, E. N., Stenager, E., Koch-Henriksen, N., Brønnum-Hansen, H., Hyllested, K., Jensen, K., & Bille-Brahe, U. (1992). Suicide and multiple sclerosis: An epidemiological investigation. *Journal of Neurology, Neurosurgery & Psychiatry, 55*, 542–545. http://dx.doi.org/10.1136/jnnp.55.7.542

Stip, E., & Daoust, L. (1995). Valproate in the treatment of mood disorder due to multiple sclerosis. *The Canadian Journal of Psychiatry, 40*, 219–220.

Sugar, C., & Nadell, R. (1943). Mental symptoms in multiple sclerosis. *The Journal of Nervous and Mental Disease, 98*, 267–280.

Surridge, D. (1969). An investigation into some psychiatric aspects of multiple sclerosis. *The British Journal of Psychiatry, 115*, 749–764. http://dx.doi.org/10.1192/bjp.115.524.749

Test, M. (2013). Influence of personality on the relationship between gray matter volume and neuropsychiatric symptoms in multiple sclerosis. *Psychosomatic Medicine, 75*, 253–261.

Théaudin, M., Romero, K., & Feinstein, A. (2016). In multiple sclerosis anxiety, not depression, is related to gender. *Multiple Sclerosis Journal, 22*, 239–244.

Wilson, S. A. K. (1924). Some problems in neurology. *The Journal of Neurology and Psychopathology, 4*, 299–333. http://dx.doi.org/10.1136/jnnp.s1-4.16.299

Zigmond, A. A. S., & Snaith, R. P. (1983). The Hospital Anxiety and Depression Scale. *Acta Psychiatrica Scandinavica, 67*, 361–370.

Zorzon, M., de Masi, R., Nasuelli, D., Ukmar, M., Pozzi Mucelli, R., Cazzato, G., . . . Zivadinov, R. (2001). Depression and anxiety in multiple sclerosis. A clinical and MRI study in 95 subjects. *Journal of Neurology, 248*, 416–421. http://dx.doi.org/10.1007/s004150170184

6

COGNITION AND FATIGUE IN MULTIPLE SCLEROSIS

MASSIMILIANO CALABRESE AND MARCO PITTERI

Fatigue is among the most debilitating symptoms in multiple sclerosis (MS) and a main cause of reduced quality of life among MS patients, 53% to 87% of whom report significant fatigue (Strober & Arnett, 2005) that interferes with occupational status and participation in everyday activities. Fatigue is the most frequent cause of dismissal or unemployment (79.1%) compared with physical problems with legs or feet (54.9%); physical problems with arms or hands (44.8%); difficulty with memory, concentration, or thinking (34.7%); or balance or dizziness (41.5%; Simmons, Tribe, & McDonald, 2010). Given its grave impact, identification of factors associated with fatigue (e.g., disease severity, depression, and sleep disturbance) has been a main priority in research and clinical care among MS patients (e.g., Braley & Chervin, 2010; Strober & Arnett, 2005). Unfortunately, fatigue in MS remains poorly understood and often underemphasized. This is probably due to the perception of fatigue, which is a subjective phenomenon

http://dx.doi.org/10.1037/0000097-007
Cognition and Behavior in Multiple Sclerosis, J. DeLuca and B. M. Sandroff (Editors)

that has no exact definition because of the overlap between the lay notion of tiredness and its clinically relevant symptomatology.

Since the first reports of fatigue as a frequent problem in MS, its definition, accurate quantification, and etiology have been a matter of debate. Fatigue is often described as multifactorial in nature and is frequently divided into various components, such as peripheral versus central fatigue (Chaudhuri & Behan, 2000), physical versus cognitive or mental fatigue, subjective versus objective fatigue (Kluger, Krupp, & Enoka, 2013), and trait versus state fatigue (Genova et al., 2013).

In the first dichotomy, *peripheral fatigue* is related to neuromuscular disorders such as myasthenia gravis and metabolic myopathies, whereas *central fatigue* is typical of neurological disorders, such as MS. Peripheral fatigue would be related to peripheral skeletal muscle and is usually defined as a decrease in the capacity of the skeletal muscle to generate force because of action potential failure, excitation–contraction coupling failure, or impairment of cross-bridge cycling, in the presence of unchanged or increasing neural drive (Häkkinen & Komi, 1983). In contrast, *central fatigue* has been defined as a failure of physical and mental tasks that require self-motivation and internal cues in the absence of demonstrable cognitive failure or motor weakness (Chaudhuri & Behan, 2000). Central fatigue can also influence peripheral skeletal muscle as a reduction in neural drive to the muscle, resulting in a decline in force production or tension development that is independent of changes in skeletal muscle contractility (Enoka & Stuart, 1992). Therefore, to define central fatigue and distinguish it from the peripheral fatigue, it is necessary to establish the presence of both physical and mental fatigue.

The Multiple Sclerosis Council for Clinical Practice Guidelines published a consensus definition of fatigue for MS patients (1998) that defined fatigue as a "subjective lack of physical and/or mental energy that is perceived by the individual or caregiver to interfere with usual and desired activities" (p. 2). Note the emphasis on the *subjective* nature of fatigue in this definition. It should be noted that the vast literature shows that subjective and objective fatigue do not correlate (see DeLuca, 2005b). As such, reliance on only subjective fatigue may be misleading. Thus, the term *cognitive fatigue* (CF) refers to a multidimensional construct that can be defined both subjectively and objectively.

The fact that clinical and experimental studies have shown little to no relationship between self-report and actual, objective measurements of fatigue in a variety of clinical populations is a major impediment to our understanding of CF (see DeLuca, 2005a). It has been shown that CF does not always result in decreased performance over a prolonged period of time, such as during the course of a workday or during tasks that require sustained cognitive activity

(Ackerman, 2011; Ackerman & Kanfer, 2009; Hanken, Eling, & Hildebrandt, 2015; Johnson, Lange, DeLuca, Korn, & Natelson, 1997; Sandry, Genova, Dobryakova, DeLuca, & Wylie, 2014).

Moreover, subjective ratings of fatigue have shown little or no relationship to disease characteristics such as lesion load, disease duration, disease course (e.g., relapsing–remitting (RRMS) vs. progressive), or functional impairment as measured by the Expanded Disability Status Scale (EDSS; Bakshi et al., 2000; L. Krupp, 2006).

OBJECTIVE MEASURES OF CF

Although subjectively, CF can be perceived as worsening performance over time and can be objectively measured (L. B. Krupp & Elkins, 2000; Kujala, Portin, Revonsuo, & Ruutiainen, 1995; Schwid et al., 2003). For instance, the Paced Auditory Serial Addition Test (PASAT) has been used as an objective measure of CF in MS, even though its sensitivity in detecting CF varies based on scoring method (Schwid et al., 2003; Walker, Berard, Berrigan, Rees, & Freedman, 2012). As the task progresses, indeed, MS patients have significant difficulty maintaining the sustained cognitive effort required to successfully perform the task, which is inferred to reflect CF. A significant decrease in performance was noted on the second half of the task compared with the first half, indicating an inability of MS patients to maintain the required cognitive effort necessary to continuously and successfully meet the task demands over time (Morrow, Rosehart, & Johnson, 2015).

A proposed alternative way to measure fatigue was to record response time variability (RTV) during a sustained mental task. MS patients with low RTV perform repetitive cognitive tasks in a consistent manner over time (i.e., low CF); in contrast, MS patients with high RTV are unable to maintain consistent response latencies, suggesting that higher RTV is associated with CF in MS patients (Bruce, Bruce, & Arnett, 2010). High RTV is also associated with primary fatiguing disorders. Increased RTV has been documented among various fatiguing neuropsychiatric conditions, including mild cognitive impairment, traumatic brain injury, and schizophrenia (Kaiser et al., 2008; Stuss, Murphy, Binns, & Alexander, 2003). It has been hypothesized that RTV may be a cognitive marker for poor top-down attentional and executive control mechanisms (Bellgrove, Hester, & Garavan, 2004). According to this view, patients with greater RTV may have to exert more mental effort to consistently focus their attention and stay on task. This could also be true in MS patients who suffer from fatigue.

SUBJECTIVE MEASURES OF CF

Even though most assessments of CF severity have relied on self-report questionnaires, these have significant limitations (Cohen et al., 2000). First, patients are asked to rate CF without appropriately defining it. As a result, it is not clear whether patients are rating distinct symptoms. Assessments could easily be confounded by motor impairment, cognitive impairment, or depression if these measures are not adequately considered through specific assessments. Second, questionnaires are inherently subjective. Even if patients are satisfactorily rating the intended symptom, it is not clear whether they are capable of accurately rating their own fatigue any better than they could rate their own motor, cognitive, or sensory impairment. Third, the use of self-report questionnaires requires retrospective assessments of fatigue over relatively long periods. This makes self-report scales subjected to recall bias. Because of these limitations, more rigorously defined, quantifiable measures are needed for clinical evaluations and clinical trials (Schwid et al., 2003).

To summarize, correlations used to investigate the relationship between subjective and objective CF are generally not significant, suggesting that subjective and objective CF are independent. Subjective and objective CF may continuously fail to correlate because subjective sense and performance may not be the ideal measures of fatigue. Importantly, CF does not have to result in behavioral changes or performance deficits, and thus a relationship may not be supported, in large part because the intuitive assumption that CF and performance are related is inaccurate (DeLuca, 2005a).

BEHAVIORAL ISSUES

The co-occurrence of both fatigue and cognitive impairment in patients suffering from MS is not surprising given that both of these symptoms are frequent and are today recognized as hallmarks of the disease (e.g., Achiron et al., 2005; Achiron, Barak, & Rotstein, 2003; Moccia et al., 2015; Pitteri, Romualdi, Magliozzi, Monaco, & Calabrese, 2017).

A recent review (Hanken, Manousi, et al., 2015) on fatigue and cognitive performance reported that there is no evidence of a relation between fatigue and memory performance, cognitive speed/selective attention, language, or visuospatial processing, and there is only weak evidence of an association with working memory. There seems to be relatively strong evidence of an association with alertness/vigilance, however. These results suggest the existence of a relation between fatigue and alerting/vigilance only, with respect to other cognitive functions.

It is also worth citing Parmenter et al.'s (2003) study, in which it has been approached the issue of cognitive involvement on fatigue by examining MS patients' cognitive performance on two occasions: during a period of high fatigue and during a period of relatively low fatigue. No differences in performance were found in MS patients during these two conditions (Parmenter, Denney, & Lynch, 2003).

In contrast to its inconsistent relationship with cognitive variables, fatigue demonstrates a relationship with personality, depressiveness, anxiety, somatization behavior (Jiang et al., 2003), and depression (Bakshi et al., 2000), even though there are conflicting results explained by different sample size and by the use of specific/unspecific instruments for evaluation of fatigue (e.g., Pittion-Vouyovitch et al., 2006; Siegert & Abernethy, 2005).

The presence of other psychological disorders and personality traits suggest that fatigue, especially in early MS states, may also be influenced by psychological and personality-associated features that are premorbid factors not intrinsically linked with MS (Schreiber, Lang, Kiltz, & Lang, 2015; Smith, Martin-Herz, Womack, & Marsigan, 2003). Furthermore, sleep disturbance (Strober, 2015) can also contribute significantly to fatigue in MS when taking into account both biological and psychological variables (Rosenberg & Shafor, 2005; Strober & Arnett, 2005).

Taken together, these findings suggest that the relationship between cognitive measures and self-report questionnaires on fatigue may be dependent on the nature of the task as well as on the contribution of psychological (e.g., mood) and/or physiological (e.g., stress) factors that may explain some of the contrasting results reported in previous studies.

IMAGING DATA

Important results on the identification of the pathogenic mechanisms related to fatigue come from the application of functional and structural magnetic resonance imaging (MRI).

Functional MRI

In the past few years, it has been shown that increased cerebral activity, observed by functional MRI (fMRI), is associated with objective CF (DeLuca, Genova, Hillary, & Wylie, 2008; Filippi et al., 2002). For instance, DeLuca et al. (2008) noted that across performance of a sustained cognitive task, increased activation in the MS group relative to healthy control subjects was observed in the basal ganglia and the frontal and parietal areas. These findings were replicated in persons with traumatic brain injury (Kohl, Wylie, Genova, Hillary,

& DeLuca, 2009) and are consistent with the model of central CF proposed by Chaudhuri and Behan (2000). Other fMRI studies have observed a relation between cortical activation and fatigue severity (Filippi et al., 2002). Particularly, in the Filippi et al. (2002) study, fatigue scores correlated inversely with right-hand finger flexion–extension motor activation in several motor-associated regions: Greater fatigue was associated with less relative activation in these regions. Subsequent studies indicated that non–motor functions of the basal ganglia might be involved in fatigue processes, where greater activation over time in MS patients was observed over repeated sessions of a processing speed task (see DeLuca et al., 2008). One study reported that performance of a cognitively fatiguing mental task (e.g., the PASAT) altered MS patients' activation patterns on a finger–thumb opposition motor task (Tartaglia, Narayanan, & Arnold, 2008). After the mentally fatiguing task, repeating the motor task was associated with patients recruiting significantly more of bilateral cingulate gyrus and left primary sensory cortex, while activating less of the left premotor and supplementary motor area (Tartaglia et al., 2008). For the first time, a challenging mental task was shown to alter the pattern of cerebral activation on an unrelated motor task in MS patients. The authors suggested that functional reorganization of existing motor pathways allows MS patients to successfully perform tasks despite significant brain injury, but that the cost of these adaptations may be increased fatigue (Tartaglia et al., 2008).

Functional imaging studies all point to fatigue in MS patients being associated with reaching the limit of neuronal compensation. Several studies interpreted the increased cerebral activity also as "compensation" for maintaining effective cognitive functioning, which somehow allows patients to maintain adequate behavioral performance. Changes in functional activation in MS patients have often been correlated with improved cognitive performance, such as following cognitive rehabilitation; authors have thus interpreted such neuroplasticity as having a positive or "adaptive" outcome (for a review, see Tomassini et al., 2012). However, it is important to recognize that such plasticity may also be maladaptive. The term *maladaptive plasticity* may be used to refer to cerebral inefficiency in situations in which neuroplasticity is correlated with cognitive impairment or decline (Chiaravalloti et al., 2005; Hillary et al., 2003; Rocca & Filippi, 2016).

The altered cerebral activation may represent the extra "effort" (i.e., allocation of more neural resources) required to maintain the same level of performance (e.g., Christodoulou et al., 2001; DeLuca et al., 2008; Lange et al., 2005). It is possible that this extra effort may not necessarily represent "compensation" mechanisms but may actually reflect CF (Chiaravalloti et al., 2005). It is also possible that compensation itself might lead to CF. Equally, CF might require the recruitment of additional brain areas to compensate for the extra "effort" required for continued task performance. That is, compensation and fatigue are not mutually exclusive explanations for increases in brain activity in MS. Despite the large amount of data available on this topic, these interpretations are preliminary and must be viewed with caution.

Structural MRI

The Role of White Matter Damage

Several conventional and nonconventional MRI studies have tried to evaluate the relation between white matter (WM) damage and the origin of fatigue, sometimes providing conflicting results. Some authors have reported a significant, albeit modest, correlation between fatigue and T1 and T2 WM lesion load, especially in right parietal-temporal and left frontal WM (Sepulcre et al., 2009; Tedeschi et al., 2007); others have failed to find any correlation with T2 WM lesion load (Bakshi et al., 1999; van der Werf et al., 1998), gadolinium-enhancing lesions (Mainero et al., 1999), and brain atrophy (Marrie, Fisher, Miller, Lee, & Rudick, 2005). Moreover, no significant difference in the normal appearing WM (NAWM) was observed between MS patients with or without fatigue with magnetization transfer and diffusion tensor MRI (Codella et al., 2002). On the contrary, diffuse periventricular axonal injury was associated with increased fatigue in MS patients. Independent of EDSS score, T2 lesion volume, age, and disease duration, the N-acetylaspartate/creatinine ratio was significantly lower in persons with MS with high fatigue compared with those with low fatigue. This suggests that widespread axonal dysfunction could be associated with fatigue in MS (Tartaglia et al., 2004).

In line with previous findings (Bakshi et al., 1999; Codella et al., 2002; Mainero et al., 1999), Bisecco et al. (2016) found that global MRI measures (T2 lesion volume, normalized brain volume, normalized gray matter and WM volume) did not differ between fatigued and not fatigued MS patients; diffusion tensor imaging analysis revealed significantly reduced fractional anisotropy (FA) values for both patient groups compared with control subjects, but the reduced FA values occurred over the entire brain and were not limited to specific regions. No differences were observed between the two MS patient groups. The mean diffusivity values of both patient groups were significantly increased compared with control subjects, whereas there were no significant differences between them. The correlational analysis between fatigue scores and diffusion indices showed that fatigue was correlated with abnormalities (FA decrease and/or RD increase) of several tracts, in particular, with the forceps minor and the cingulum: These structures are connected to frontal areas and are involved in attention and executive functions, and they have been related to the co-occurrence of fatigue and depression (Gobbi, Rocca, Pagani, et al., 2014; Gobbi, Rocca, Riccitelli, et al., 2014) and to level of fatigue (Pardini, Bonzano, Mancardi, & Roccatagliata, 2010) in MS patients. With regard to the between-groups analysis, these results overlap with and unify previous findings (Bester et al., 2013; Pardini et al., 2010, 2015; Wilting et al., 2016) sustaining the hypothesis that fatigue severity in MS is related to the amount of microstructural damage in several WM tracts connected with frontal lobes.

Among regional approaches, the ones using diffusion tensor imaging have shown a relationship between fatigue and WM damage in specific tracts (Bester et al., 2013; Rocca et al., 2014; Wilting et al., 2016). These findings, however, also showed some discrepancies that might be explained by methodological (e.g., region of interest vs. whole-brain WM assessment) and/or clinical-demographic (e.g., MS phenotypes, coexistence of depression and sleep disorders) differences. Taken together, these observations favor a role of WM damage in developing fatigue in MS.

The Role of Prefrontal Cortex and Basal Ganglia

A significant amount of neuroimaging evidence suggests that failure of the non-motor function of the basal ganglia (Chaudhuri & Behan, 2000) might be responsible for the feeling of CF in MS subjects. fMRI studies have reported that the pattern of striatal activity in MS patients differs from that observed in healthy control subjects (DeLuca et al., 2008; Dobryakova, DeLuca, Genova, & Wylie, 2013; Genova et al., 2013). In healthy control subjects, there was a steady decrease in striatal activity across repeated blocks of a processing speed task. This decrease is consistent with the idea that healthy control subjects rely on striatal mechanisms early in task performance but rely on these mechanisms less and less as the task progresses. A different pattern was observed in the MS group. The striatal activity remained constant across the repeated blocks of the task, whereas there was a significant increase in prefrontal cortex activation. This pattern of brain activity was observed despite no differences in performance accuracy between healthy control subjects and MS patients (Dobryakova et al., 2013). These data suggest that MS patients have to recruit greater prefrontal cortex resources to maintain performance comparable to that of healthy individuals.

The role of striatum in CF has also been emphasized by several studies that demonstrated aberrant task-elicited activity related to CF, specifically affecting the thalamo–striato–cortical system (Chaudhuri & Behan, 2000; Dobryakova, Genova, DeLuca, & Wylie, 2015). Structural changes in the prefrontal cortex and basal ganglia might play a role in MS-related fatigue as well. For example, Calabrese et al. (2010) showed that the thickness of the cortical areas belonging to the striatum–thalamus–frontal cortex pathway explained up to 70% of the fatigue value changes, suggesting an association between the neurodegenerative process and the development of fatigue in RRMS patients taking place in the striatum–thalamus–frontal cortex pathway. The inclusion of posterior parietal cortex as one of the best predictors of the Modified Fatigue Impact Scale cognitive domain suggests the major role of the posterior attentional system in determining CF in RRMS (Calabrese et al., 2010).

In another study, MS patients showed altered brain responses in the thalamo–striato–cortical network during performance of a complex working memory task that challenged fatigue (Engström, Flensner, Landtblom, Ek, & Karlsson, 2013). Interestingly, brain activation in certain cortical and subcortical areas of the network (the left posterior parietal cortex and the right substantia nigra) was positively correlated to perceived fatigue ratings.

The structural and functional evidence of abnormalities in the frontal and striatal regions would be in line with the dopamine imbalance hypothesis. Striatum and prefrontal cortex, indeed, are regions heavily innervated by dopaminergic neurons, and converging evidence suggests that an imbalance in dopamine plays a key role in fatigue. Indeed, dopaminergic medication has been shown to alleviate fatigue in individuals with traumatic brain injury, with chronic fatigue syndrome, and in cancer patients, also indicating that dopamine might play an important role in fatigue perception (Dobryakova et al., 2013, 2015).

Other convergent data come from correlational studies using the PASAT. In a group of MS patients with fatigue, whole-brain analyses detected the emergence of a pattern of fronto–temporal–occipital hyperconnectivity, centered on the left superior frontal gyrus (Pravatà et al., 2016). Additional analyses of resting-state functional connectivity between the left superior frontal gyrus and two independently defined nodes of the thalamo–striato–cortical circuit revealed different fatigue-related dynamics, with the caudate showing hyperconnectivity immediately after PASAT and a delayed hypoconnectivity with the thalamus. Importantly, the severity of CF symptoms was related to both the cortico–cortical and cortico–subcortical patterns (Pravatà et al., 2016).

Moreover, in a recent fMRI study, it was suggested that impaired timing of activation of critical areas of the sensorimotor network contributed to distinguishing MS patients who report fatigue and that an abnormal recruitment of critical regions of the motor network and nonmotor connections of the basal ganglia was correlated to central fatigue in these patients (Rocca & Filippi, 2016).

Finally, increased event-related desynchronization (ERD) and reduced postmovement event-related synchronization (ERS) in the frontal regions were observed in fatigued RRMS compared with both nonfatigued RRMS and healthy control subjects (Leocani et al., 2001), and a significant direct correlation between fatigue and frontal cortex atrophy (i.e., left superior frontal gyrus and bilateral middle frontal gyri) was noticed (Sepulcre et al., 2009). A possible role of the striatum–thalamus–frontal cortex pathway in the genesis of fatigue was also suggested by the finding of a reduced metabolic activity of the putamen, the lateral and medial prefrontal cortex, the premotor cortex, and the right supplementary motor area in severely fatigued MS patients (Roelcke et al., 1997). Although no direct relation between fatigue and global atrophy has been found, several studies using voxel-based morphometry (VBM) or cortical thickness measures showed some evidence for an association of fatigue with atrophy of the frontoparietal cortex and of the basal ganglia (Calabrese et al., 2010; Pellicano et al., 2010; Sepulcre et al., 2009). Increased levels of fatigue were associated with smaller cortical volumes in the rostral and caudal middle frontal, and in parts of the pre- and postcentral regions, of the right hemisphere of MS patients (Nygaard et al., 2015). Atrophy in specific locations in MS patients experiencing fatigue appears to be related to neural regulation of the alerting/vigilance network (Hanken, Eling, & Hildebrandt, 2014).

On the basis of these data, fatigue would be neither a compensatory state nor a psychogenic trait. It would be a feeling with behavioral effects that seem related to brain atrophy or neurochemical dysfunctions: In particular, it was proposed that the failure of nonmotor function of the basal ganglia negatively affects the striatal–thalamic–frontal cortical system, resulting in fatigue (Chaudhuri & Behan, 2000).

PRINCIPAL TREATMENTS OF FATIGUE

Pharmacological Treatments

There is widespread agreement in the literature that, due to the complex, multidimensional, and highly subjective nature of MS-related fatigue, comprehensive goal-oriented management programs that incorporate multidisciplinary expertise are required, and patients need to be evaluated regularly through appropriate clinical outcome measures (Asano & Finlayson, 2014; Kos, Duportail, D'hooghe, Nagels, & Kerckhofs, 2007). Different drugs were used for treatment of fatigue in MS patients included amantadine, modafinil, and pemoline. However, results from meta-analyses and systematic reviews showed insufficient evidence to support these pharmacological agents for management of MS-related fatigue (Asano & Finlayson, 2014;

Peuckmann-Post, Elsner, Krumm, Trottenberg, & Radbruch, 2010; Taus et al., 2003).

Nutt et al. (2006) analyzed the differential profiles of antidepressants on mood, behavior, and somatic symptoms. They argued that antidepressants such as selective serotonin reuptake inhibitors (SSRIs) affect mood symptoms, whereas dopaminergic and noradrenergic drugs reduce fatigue and enhance positive affect, as we can see in reward effects and their relationship to dopamine (Dobryakova et al., 2013, 2015).

More recently, some clinical trials (Cooper, Tucker, & Papakostas, 2014; Papakostas et al., 2006) directly comparing SSRIs, bupropion, and antidepressants that enhance dopaminergic and especially noradrenergic activity showed that the general impact of both classes of antidepressants is similar for various depressive symptoms, but that bupropion reduces fatigue significantly more than the SSRIs patients with major depressive disorder.

There are also some trials with bupropion as treatment for fatigue in the context of MS (Pardini, Capello, Krueger, Mancardi, & Uccelli, 2013; Siniscalchi, Gallelli, Tolotta, Loiacono, & De Sarro, 2010) showing that lower reward responsiveness at baseline predicted higher fatigue remission rates in bupropion-treated patients compared with escitalopram-treated patients. Finally, duloxetine, an antidepressant with a strong noradrenergic profile, has also been used effectively in treating CF (Solaro et al., 2013).

Physical Activity

In the past, MS patients were advised not to participate in physical activities because it was believed to lead to worsening of symptoms or fatigue (Sutherland & Andersen, 2001). However, recent studies on exercise therapy in MS have demonstrated that it results in a substantial long-term reduction in functional limitations and enhanced quality of life and has the potential to reduce fatigue in MS patients (Andreasen, Stenager, & Dalgas, 2011; Asano & Finlayson, 2014; Latimer-Cheung et al., 2013). Some types of exercise interventions, which include endurance and resistance-training component, may have potential beneficial effects on fatigue reduction in MS patients. Although a recent meta-analysis has reported that exercise training in MS was associated with a significant reduction in fatigue with a moderate effect size (Pilutti, Greenlee, Motl, Nickrent, & Petruzzello, 2013), overall, physical activity does seem to exert consistent effects on MS-related fatigue (Motl & Sandroff, 2015), even though data for an optimal type or intensity of exercise intervention are still lacking of definitive results (Heine, van de Port, Rietberg, van Wegen, & Kwakkel, 2015).

Behavioral Interventions

There has been a growing interest in these interventions as a means of empowering patients and improving their symptoms and overall quality of life (Moss-Morris et al., 2012; van Kessel et al., 2008). A structured fatigue management program based on psychological approaches delivered by health professionals can be effective in reducing fatigue severity and increasing fatigue self-efficacy for MS patients (Asano & Finlayson, 2014). A group-based interactive program for managing MS-fatigue applying cognitive behavioral and energy effectiveness techniques to lifestyle has been useful in significantly reducing fatigue severity (P. W. Thomas et al., 2014; S. Thomas et al., 2013), even though there are results that show no efficacy in reducing the impact of fatigue compared with a placebo intervention program (Kos et al., 2007). Psychological interventions, such as mindfulness-based interventions (Simpson et al., 2014) and, particularly, cognitive behavior therapy (CBT; van Kessel et al., 2008), can be effective and clinically feasible cost-effective treatments for MS fatigue. CBT can also promote significantly greater improvements in fatigue severity and impact, and also in anxiety, depression, and quality of life (Moss-Morris et al., 2012). Education programs, energy conservation, self-management, fatigue management program, and CBT appear effective in reducing fatigue (Neill, Belan, & Ried, 2006).

Taken together, treatment evidence suggested that there is a continuing need for comprehensive, multidisciplinary, long-term management of fatigue that includes both pharmacological and nonpharmacological interventions. Nonpharmacological interventions (e.g., exercise and psychological–educational interventions) seem to have stronger and more favorable effect in reducing the impact or severity of fatigue compared with commonly prescribed drugs.

CONCLUSIONS AND FUTURE DIRECTIONS

Evaluating and treating CF remains difficult, particularly because a basic understanding of the variables that contribute to CF are not well defined. Novel insights into how and why CF manifests may ultimately lead to improved clinical treatment strategies for CF (Sandry et al., 2014).

Advancing scientific efforts to measure and validate CF requires the application of novel paradigms, specifically designed to operationalize current conceptual definitions of this hypothetical construct. Until now, a standardized measure of CF has not been developed.

The association between fatigue and cognitive reserve in MS patients should be investigated, extending previous findings that suggest fatigue does not have a direct influence on cognitive performance but is mediated by other factors (e.g., disease duration, age, educational attainment; Scarpazza et al., 2013).

Response time variability (Bruce et al., 2010) has shown a strong relationship between objective behavioral measures and self-reported CF in MS patients. These results provide insight into the underlying cognitive mechanisms associated with self-reported fatigue and open the door for the use of new methodologies in the study of CF in MS.

A useful approach may be to reconceptualize fatigue into two groups of factors (DeLuca, 2005a): (a) factors that initiate fatigue (e.g., systemic disease) and (b) factors that perpetuate or exacerbate fatigue (e.g., depression, sleep disturbance, pain, medication effects, deconditioning). These factors have been referred to as *primary fatigue* and *secondary fatigue*, respectively. Although both primary and secondary factors contribute to the feeling of fatigue, it is likely that the secondary factors are those that complicate the understanding of self-report.

Fatigue in initial stages of MS might largely be driven by factors associated with disease coping, whereas fatigue in later stages should predominantly be related with neuronal loss (atrophy) in the brain and functional consequences of brain lesions. Psychological factors (depression, anxiety, inadequate disease coping) and physical factors (disease status, disease progression) might interact in the generation of fatigue in MS (e.g., see Strober & Arnett, 2005). Thus, the dichotomy of physical and mental fatigue in MS patients and the conflicting results reported so far may be reconciled by the view of fatigue representing a complex syndrome with different mechanisms of origin.

Most studies on CF in MS have failed to show a relationship between subjective and objective measures of CF. The general notion that fatigue must result in decreased cognitive performance is not supported, although there appears to be some consistency but only in the area of alertness/vigilance.

Further, high and low levels of fatigue do not map onto changes in cognitive performance, suggesting that CF is not directly related to cognitive problems. For instance, self-reported, subjective fatigue has been shown to have no relationship with memory performance, cognitive speed/selective attention and language or visuospatial processing.

Neuroimaging evidence showed that there are different functional brain-activity patterns despite no differences in performance accuracy between healthy control subjects and MS patients, suggesting that MS patients have to recruit greater neural resources to maintain performance comparable to healthy individuals. Employment of additional resources suggests increased effort expenditure that might result in a subjective experience of CF. The increase of brain activity is correlated with the subjective sense of fatigue but is not associated with objective performance. Hence, for the first time, we have results that subjective fatigue can be related to objective measures (e.g., fMRI)—namely, brain activation—but not related to objective behavioral performance. This is the key point to keep in mind to approach future investigations of CF in MS patients.

REFERENCES

Achiron, A., Barak, Y., & Rotstein, Z. (2003). Longitudinal disability curves for predicting the course of relapsing-remitting multiple sclerosis. *Multiple Sclerosis*, *9*, 486–491. http://dx.doi.org/10.1191/1352458503ms945oa

Achiron, A., Polliack, M., Rao, S. M., Barak, Y., Lavie, M., Appelboim, N., & Harel, Y. (2005). Cognitive patterns and progression in multiple sclerosis: Construction and validation of percentile curves. *Journal of Neurology, Neurosurgery, & Psychiatry*, *76*, 744–749. http://dx.doi.org/10.1136/jnnp.2004.045518

Ackerman, P. L. (2011). 100 years without resting. In P. L. Ackerman (Ed.), *Cognitive fatigue: Multidisciplinary perspectives on current research and future applications* (pp. 11–43). Washington, DC: American Psychological Association. http://dx.doi.org/10.1037/12343-001

Ackerman, P. L., & Kanfer, R. (2009). Test length and cognitive fatigue: An empirical examination of effects on performance and test-taker reactions. *Journal of Experimental Psychology: Applied*, *15*, 163–181. http://dx.doi.org/10.1037/a0015719

Andreasen, A. K., Stenager, E., & Dalgas, U. (2011). The effect of exercise therapy on fatigue in multiple sclerosis. *Multiple Sclerosis*, *17*, 1041–1054. http://dx.doi.org/10.1177/1352458511401120

Asano, M., & Finlayson, M. L. (2014). Meta-analysis of three different types of fatigue management interventions for people with multiple sclerosis: Exercise, education, and medication. *Multiple Sclerosis International*, *2014*, 798285. http://dx.doi.org/10.1155/2014/798285

Bakshi, R., Miletich, R. S., Henschel, K., Shaikh, Z. A., Janardhan, V., Wasay, M., . . . Kinkel, P. R. (1999). Fatigue in multiple sclerosis: Cross-sectional correlation with brain MRI findings in 71 patients. *Neurology*, *53*, 1151–1153. http://dx.doi.org/10.1212/WNL.53.5.1151

Bakshi, R., Shaikh, Z. A., Miletich, R. S., Czarnecki, D., Dmochowski, J., Henschel, K., . . . Kinkel, P. R. (2000). Fatigue in multiple sclerosis and its relationship to depression and neurologic disability. *Multiple Sclerosis*, *6*, 181–185. http://dx.doi.org/10.1191/135245800701566052

Bellgrove, M. A., Hester, R., & Garavan, H. (2004). The functional neuroanatomical correlates of response variability: Evidence from a response inhibition task. *Neuropsychologia*, *42*, 1910–1916. http://dx.doi.org/10.1016/j.neuropsychologia.2004.05.007

Bester, M., Lazar, M., Petracca, M., Babb, J. S., Herbert, J., Grossman, R. I., & Inglese, M. (2013). Tract-specific white matter correlates of fatigue and cognitive impairment in benign multiple sclerosis. *Journal of the Neurological Sciences, 330,* 61–66. http://dx.doi.org/10.1016/j.jns.2013.04.005

Bisecco, A., Caiazzo, G., d'Ambrosio, A., Sacco, R., Bonavita, S., Docimo, R., . . . Gallo, A. (2016). Fatigue in multiple sclerosis: The contribution of occult white matter damage. *Multiple Sclerosis Journal, 22,* 1676–1684. http://dx.doi.org/10.1177/1352458516628331

Braley, T. J., & Chervin, R. D. (2010). Fatigue in multiple sclerosis: Mechanisms, evaluation, and treatment. *Sleep, 33,* 1061–1067. http://dx.doi.org/10.1093/sleep/33.8.1061

Bruce, J. M., Bruce, A. S., & Arnett, P. A. (2010). Response variability is associated with self-reported cognitive fatigue in multiple sclerosis. *Neuropsychology, 24,* 77–83. http://dx.doi.org/10.1037/a0015046

Calabrese, M., Rinaldi, F., Grossi, P., Mattisi, I., Bernardi, V., Favaretto, A., . . . Gallo, P. (2010). Basal ganglia and frontal/parietal cortical atrophy is associated with fatigue in relapsing–remitting multiple sclerosis. *Multiple Sclerosis, 16,* 1220–1228. http://dx.doi.org/10.1177/1352458510376405

Chaudhuri, A., & Behan, P. O. (2000). Fatigue and basal ganglia. *Journal of the Neurological Sciences, 179*(Suppl. 1–2), 34–42.

Chiaravalloti, N., Hillary, F., Ricker, J., Christodoulou, C., Kalnin, A., Liu, W.-C., . . . DeLuca, J. (2005). Cerebral activation patterns during working memory performance in multiple sclerosis using FMRI. *Journal of Clinical and Experimental Neuropsychology, 27,* 33–54. http://dx.doi.org/10.1080/138033990513609

Christodoulou, C., DeLuca, J., Ricker, J. H., Madigan, N. K., Bly, B. M., Lange, G., . . . Ni, A. C. (2001). Functional magnetic resonance imaging of working memory impairment after traumatic brain injury. *Journal of Neurology, Neurosurgery, and Psychiatry, 71,* 161–168. http://dx.doi.org/10.1136/jnnp.71.2.161

Codella, M., Rocca, M. A., Colombo, B., Rossi, P., Comi, G., & Filippi, M. (2002). A preliminary study of magnetization transfer and diffusion tensor MRI of multiple sclerosis patients with fatigue. *Journal of Neurology, 249,* 535–537. http://dx.doi.org/10.1007/s004150200060

Cohen, J. A., Fischer, J. S., Bolibrush, D. M., Jak, A. J., Kniker, J. E., Mertz, L. A., . . . Cutter, G. R. (2000). Intrarater and interrater reliability of the MS functional composite outcome measure. *Neurology, 54,* 802–806. http://dx.doi.org/10.1212/WNL.54.4.802

Cooper, J. A., Tucker, V. L., & Papakostas, G. I. (2014). Resolution of sleepiness and fatigue: A comparison of bupropion and selective serotonin reuptake inhibitors in subjects with major depressive disorder achieving remission at doses approved in the European Union. *Journal of Psychopharmacology, 28,* 118–124. http://dx.doi.org/10.1177/0269881113514878

DeLuca, J. (2005a). Fatigue, cognition, and mental effort. In J. DeLuca (Ed.), *Fatigue as a window to the brain* (pp. 37–58). Cambridge, MA: MIT Press.

DeLuca, J. (2005b). Fatigue: Its definition, its study, and its future. In J. DeLuca (Ed.), *Fatigue as a window to the brain* (pp. 319–325). Cambridge, MA: MIT Press.

DeLuca, J., Genova, H. M., Hillary, F. G., & Wylie, G. (2008). Neural correlates of cognitive fatigue in multiple sclerosis using functional MRI. *Journal of the Neurological Sciences, 270*(1-2), 28–39. http://dx.doi.org/10.1016/j.jns.2008.01.018

Dobryakova, E., DeLuca, J., Genova, H. M., & Wylie, G. R. (2013). Neural correlates of cognitive fatigue: Cortico-striatal circuitry and effort-reward imbalance. *Journal of the International Neuropsychological Society, 19*, 849–853. http://dx.doi.org/10.1017/S1355617713000684

Dobryakova, E., Genova, H. M., DeLuca, J., & Wylie, G. R. (2015). The dopamine imbalance hypothesis of fatigue in multiple sclerosis and other neurological disorders. *Frontiers in Neurology, 6*, 52. http://dx.doi.org/10.3389/fneur.2015.00052

Engström, M., Flensner, G., Landtblom, A. M., Ek, A. C., & Karlsson, T. (2013). Thalamo-striato-cortical determinants to fatigue in multiple sclerosis. *Brain and Behavior, 3*, 715–728. http://dx.doi.org/10.1002/brb3.181

Enoka, R. M., & Stuart, D. G. (1992). Neurobiology of muscle fatigue. *Journal of Applied Physiology, 72*, 1631–1648.

Filippi, M., Rocca, M. A., Colombo, B., Falini, A., Codella, M., Scotti, G., & Comi, G. (2002). Functional magnetic resonance imaging correlates of fatigue in multiple sclerosis. *NeuroImage, 15*, 559–567. http://dx.doi.org/10.1006/nimg.2001.1011

Genova, H. M., Rajagopalan, V., DeLuca, J., Das, A., Binder, A., Arjunan, A., . . . Wylie, G. (2013). Examination of cognitive fatigue in multiple sclerosis using functional magnetic resonance imaging and diffusion tensor imaging. *PLoS One, 8*, e78811. http://dx.doi.org/10.1371/journal.pone.0078811

Gobbi, C., Rocca, M. A., Pagani, E., Riccitelli, G. C., Pravatà, E., Radaelli, M., . . . Filippi, M. (2014). Forceps minor damage and co-occurrence of depression and fatigue in multiple sclerosis. *Multiple Sclerosis Journal, 20*, 1633–1640. http://dx.doi.org/10.1177/1352458514530022

Gobbi, C., Rocca, M. A., Riccitelli, G., Pagani, E., Messina, R., Preziosa, P., . . . Filippi, M. (2014). Influence of the topography of brain damage on depression and fatigue in patients with multiple sclerosis. *Multiple Sclerosis Journal, 20*, 192–201. http://dx.doi.org/10.1177/1352458513493684

Häkkinen, K., & Komi, P. V. (1983). Electromyographic and mechanical characteristics of human skeletal muscle during fatigue under voluntary and reflex conditions. *Electroencephalography and Clinical Neurophysiology, 55*, 436–444. http://dx.doi.org/10.1016/0013-4694(83)90132-3

Hanken, K., Eling, P., & Hildebrandt, H. (2014). The representation of inflammatory signals in the brain—A model for subjective fatigue in multiple sclerosis. *Frontiers in Neurology, 5*, 264. http://dx.doi.org/10.3389/fneur.2014.00264

Hanken, K., Eling, P., & Hildebrandt, H. (2015). Is there a cognitive signature for MS-related fatigue? *Multiple Sclerosis, 21*, 376–381. http://dx.doi.org/10.1177/1352458514549567

Hanken, K., Manousi, A., Klein, J., Kastrup, A., Eling, P., & Hildebrandt, H. (2015). On the relation between self-reported cognitive fatigue and the posterior hypothalamic–brainstem network. *European Journal of Neurology, 23*, 101–109.

Heine, M., van de Port, I., Rietberg, M. B., van Wegen, E. E., & Kwakkel, G. (2015). Exercise therapy for fatigue in multiple sclerosis. *Cochrane Database of Systematic Reviews, 9*, CD009956. http://dx.doi.org/10.1002/14651858.CD009956.pub2

Hillary, F. G., Chiaravalloti, N. D., Ricker, J. H., Steffener, J., Bly, B. M., Lange, G., . . . DeLuca, J. (2003). An investigation of working memory rehearsal in multiple sclerosis using fMRI. *Journal of Clinical and Experimental Neuropsychology, 25*, 965–978. http://dx.doi.org/10.1076/jcen.25.7.965.16490

Jiang, N., Sato, T., Hara, T., Takedomi, Y., Ozaki, I., & Yamada, S. (2003). Correlations between trait anxiety, personality and fatigue: Study based on the Temperament and Character Inventory. *Journal of Psychosomatic Research, 55*, 493–500. http://dx.doi.org/10.1016/S0022-3999(03)00021-7

Johnson, S. K., Lange, G., DeLuca, J., Korn, L. R., & Natelson, B. (1997). The effects of fatigue on neuropsychological performance in patients with chronic fatigue syndrome, multiple sclerosis, and depression. *Applied Neuropsychology, 4*, 145–153. http://dx.doi.org/10.1207/s15324826an0403_1

Kaiser, S., Roth, A., Rentrop, M., Friederich, H.-C., Bender, S., & Weisbrod, M. (2008). Intra-individual reaction time variability in schizophrenia, depression and borderline personality disorder. *Brain and Cognition, 66*, 73–82. http://dx.doi.org/10.1016/j.bandc.2007.05.007

Kluger, B. M., Krupp, L. B., & Enoka, R. M. (2013). Fatigue and fatigability in neurologic illnesses: Proposal for a unified taxonomy. *Neurology, 80*, 409–416. http://dx.doi.org/10.1212/WNL.0b013e31827f07be

Kohl, A. D., Wylie, G. R., Genova, H. M., Hillary, F. G., & DeLuca, J. (2009). The neural correlates of cognitive fatigue in traumatic brain injury using functional MRI. *Brain Injury, 23*, 420–432. http://dx.doi.org/10.1080/02699050902788519

Kos, D., Duportail, M., D'hooghe, M., Nagels, G., & Kerckhofs, E. (2007). Multidisciplinary fatigue management programme in multiple sclerosis: A randomized clinical trial. *Multiple Sclerosis, 13*, 996–1003. http://dx.doi.org/10.1177/1352458507078392

Krupp, L. (2006). Fatigue is intrinsic to multiple sclerosis (MS) and is the most commonly reported symptom of the disease [Editorial]. *Multiple Sclerosis, 12*, 367–368. http://dx.doi.org/10.1191/135248506ms1373ed

Krupp, L. B., & Elkins, L. E. (2000). Fatigue and declines in cognitive functioning in multiple sclerosis. *Neurology, 55*, 934–939. http://dx.doi.org/10.1212/WNL.55.7.934

Kujala, P., Portin, R., Revonsuo, A., & Ruutiainen, J. (1995). Attention related performance in two cognitively different subgroups of patients with multiple sclerosis. *Journal of Neurology, Neurosurgery, & Psychiatry, 59*, 77–82. http://dx.doi.org/10.1136/jnnp.59.1.77

Lange, G., Steffener, J., Cook, D. B., Bly, B. M., Christodoulou, C., Liu, W. C., . . . Natelson, B. H. (2005). Objective evidence of cognitive complaints in chronic fatigue syndrome: A BOLD fMRI study of verbal working memory. *NeuroImage, 26,* 513–524. http://dx.doi.org/10.1016/j.neuroimage.2005.02.011

Latimer-Cheung, A. E., Pilutti, L. A., Hicks, A. L., Martin Ginis, K. A., Fenuta, A. M., MacKibbon, K. A., & Motl, R. W. (2013). Effects of exercise training on fitness, mobility, fatigue, and health-related quality of life among adults with multiple sclerosis: A systematic review to inform guideline development. *Archives of Physical Medicine and Rehabilitation, 94,* 1800–1828.e3. http://dx.doi.org/10.1016/j.apmr.2013.04.020

Leocani, L., Colombo, B., Magnani, G., Martinelli-Boneschi, F., Cursi, M., Rossi, P., . . . Comi, G. (2001). Fatigue in multiple sclerosis is associated with abnormal cortical activation to voluntary movement—EEG evidence. *NeuroImage, 13,* 1186–1192. http://dx.doi.org/10.1006/nimg.2001.0759

Mainero, C., Faroni, J., Gasperini, C., Filippi, M., Giugni, E., Ciccarelli, O., . . . Pozzilli, C. (1999). Fatigue and magnetic resonance imaging activity in multiple sclerosis. *Journal of Neurology, 246,* 454–458. http://dx.doi.org/10.1007/s004150050382

Marrie, R. A., Fisher, E., Miller, D. M., Lee, J. C., & Rudick, R. A. (2005). Association of fatigue and brain atrophy in multiple sclerosis. *Journal of the Neurological Sciences, 228,* 161–166. http://dx.doi.org/10.1016/j.jns.2004.11.046

Moccia, M., Lanzillo, R., Palladino, R., Chang, K. C.-M., Costabile, T., Russo, C., . . . Brescia Morra, V. (2015). Cognitive impairment at diagnosis predicts 10-year multiple sclerosis progression. *Multiple Sclerosis, 22,* 659–667.

Morrow, S. A., Rosehart, H., & Johnson, A. M. (2015). Diagnosis and quantification of cognitive fatigue in multiple sclerosis. *Cognitive and Behavioral Neurology, 28,* 27–32. http://dx.doi.org/10.1097/WNN.0000000000000050

Moss-Morris, R., McCrone, P., Yardley, L., van Kessel, K., Wills, G., & Dennison, L. (2012). A pilot randomised controlled trial of an Internet-based cognitive behavioural therapy self-management programme (MS Invigor8) for multiple sclerosis fatigue. *Behaviour Research and Therapy, 50,* 415–421. http://dx.doi.org/10.1016/j.brat.2012.03.001

Motl, R. W., & Sandroff, B. M. (2015). Benefits of exercise training in multiple sclerosis. *Current Neurology and Neuroscience Reports, 15,* 62. http://dx.doi.org/10.1007/s11910-015-0585-6

Neill, J., Belan, I., & Ried, K. (2006). Effectiveness of non-pharmacological interventions for fatigue in adults with multiple sclerosis, rheumatoid arthritis, or systemic lupus erythematosus: A systematic review. *Journal of Advanced Nursing, 56,* 617–635. http://dx.doi.org/10.1111/j.1365-2648.2006.04054.x

Nutt, D. J., Baldwin, D. S., Clayton, A. H., Elgie, R., Lecrubier, Y., Montejo, A. L., . . . Tylee, A. (2006). Consensus statement and research needs: The role of dopamine and norepinephrine in depression and antidepressant treatment. *The Journal of Clinical Psychiatry, 67*(Suppl. 6), 46–49.

Nygaard, G. O., Walhovd, K. B., Sowa, P., Chepkoech, J.-L., Bjørnerud, A., Due-Tønnessen, P., . . . Harbo, H. F. (2015). Cortical thickness and surface area relate to specific symptoms in early relapsing-remitting multiple sclerosis. *Multiple Sclerosis*, *21*, 402–414. http://dx.doi.org/10.1177/1352458514543811

Papakostas, G. I., Nutt, D. J., Hallett, L. A., Tucker, V. L., Krishen, A., & Fava, M. (2006). Resolution of sleepiness and fatigue in major depressive disorder: A comparison of bupropion and the selective serotonin reuptake inhibitors. *Biological Psychiatry*, *60*, 1350–1355. http://dx.doi.org/10.1016/j.biopsych.2006.06.015

Pardini, M., Bonzano, L., Bergamino, M., Bommarito, G., Feraco, P., Murugavel, A., . . . Roccatagliata, L. (2015). Cingulum bundle alterations underlie subjective fatigue in multiple sclerosis. *Multiple Sclerosis Journal*, *21*, 442–447. http://dx.doi.org/10.1177/1352458514546791

Pardini, M., Bonzano, L., Mancardi, G. L., & Roccatagliata, L. (2010). Frontal networks play a role in fatigue perception in multiple sclerosis. *Behavioral Neuroscience*, *124*, 329–336. http://dx.doi.org/10.1037/a0019585

Pardini, M., Capello, E., Krueger, F., Mancardi, G., & Uccelli, A. (2013). Reward responsiveness and fatigue in multiple sclerosis. *Multiple Sclerosis Journal*, *19*, 233–240. http://dx.doi.org/10.1177/1352458512451509

Parmenter, B. A., Denney, D. R., & Lynch, S. G. (2003). The cognitive performance of patients with multiple sclerosis during periods of high and low fatigue. *Multiple Sclerosis*, *9*, 111–118. http://dx.doi.org/10.1191/1352458503ms859oa

Pellicano, C., Gallo, A., Li, X., Ikonomidou, V. N., Evangelou, I. E., Ohayon, J. M., . . . Bagnato, F. (2010). Relationship of cortical atrophy to fatigue in patients with multiple sclerosis. *Archives of Neurology*, *67*, 447–453. http://dx.doi.org/10.1001/archneurol.2010.48

Peuckmann-Post, V., Elsner, F., Krumm, N., Trottenberg, P., & Radbruch, L. (2010). Pharmacological treatments for fatigue associated with palliative care. *Cochrane Database of Systematic Reviews*, *11*, CD006788. http://dx.doi.org/10.1002/14651858.CD006788.pub2

Pilutti, L. A., Greenlee, T. A., Motl, R. W., Nickrent, M. S., & Petruzzello, S. J. (2013). Effects of exercise training on fatigue in multiple sclerosis: A meta-analysis. *Psychosomatic Medicine*, *75*, 575–580. http://dx.doi.org/10.1097/PSY.0b013e31829b4525

Pitteri, M., Romualdi, C., Magliozzi, R., Monaco, S., & Calabrese, M. (2017). Cognitive impairment predicts disability progression and cortical thinning in MS: An 8-year study. *Multiple Sclerosis*, *23*, 848–854. http://dx.doi.org/10.1177/1352458516665496

Pittion-Vouyovitch, S., Debouverie, M., Guillemin, F., Vandenberghe, N., Anxionnat, R., & Vespignani, H. (2006). Fatigue in multiple sclerosis is related to disability, depression and quality of life. *Journal of the Neurological Sciences*, *243*, 39–45. http://dx.doi.org/10.1016/j.jns.2005.11.025

Pravatà, E., Zecca, C., Sestieri, C., Caulo, M., Riccitelli, G. C., Rocca, M. A., . . . Gobbi, C. (2016). Hyperconnectivity of the dorsolateral prefrontal cortex following mental effort in multiple sclerosis patients with cognitive fatigue. *Multiple Sclerosis Journal, 22,* 1665–1675. http://dx.doi.org/10.1177/1352458515625806

Rocca, M. A., & Filippi, M. (2016). Functional reorganization is a maladaptive response to injury—YES. *Multiple Sclerosis, 23,* 191–193.

Rocca, M. A., Parisi, L., Pagani, E., Copetti, M., Rodegher, M., Colombo, B., . . . Filippi, M. (2014). Regional but not global brain damage contributes to fatigue in multiple sclerosis. *Radiology, 273,* 511–520. http://dx.doi.org/10.1148/radiol.14140417

Roelcke, U., Kappos, L., Lechner-Scott, J., Brunnschweiler, H., Huber, S., Ammann, W., . . . Leenders, K. L. (1997). Reduced glucose metabolism in the frontal cortex and basal ganglia of multiple sclerosis patients with fatigue: A 18F-fluorodeoxyglucose positron emission tomography study. *Neurology, 48,* 1566–1571. http://dx.doi.org/10.1212/WNL.48.6.1566

Rosenberg, J. H., & Shafor, R. (2005). Fatigue in multiple sclerosis: A rational approach to evaluation and treatment. *Current Neurology and Neuroscience Reports, 5,* 140–146. http://dx.doi.org/10.1007/s11910-005-0012-5

Sandry, J., Genova, H. M., Dobryakova, E., DeLuca, J., & Wylie, G. (2014). Subjective cognitive fatigue in multiple sclerosis depends on task length. *Frontiers in Neurology, 5,* 214.

Scarpazza, C., Braghittoni, D., Casale, B., Malagú, S., Mattioli, F., di Pellegrino, G., & Ladavas, E. (2013). Education protects against cognitive changes associated with multiple sclerosis. *Restorative Neurology and Neuroscience, 31,* 619–631.

Schreiber, H., Lang, M., Kiltz, K., & Lang, C. (2015). Is personality profile a relevant determinant of fatigue in multiple sclerosis? *Frontiers in Neurology, 6,* 2.

Schwid, S. R., Tyler, C. M., Scheid, E. A., Weinstein, A., Goodman, A. D., & McDermott, M. P. (2003). Cognitive fatigue during a test requiring sustained attention: A pilot study. *Multiple Sclerosis, 9,* 503–508. http://dx.doi.org/10.1191/1352458503ms946oa

Sepulcre, J., Masdeu, J. C., Goñi, J., Arrondo, G., Vélez de Mendizábal, N., Bejarano, B., & Villoslada, P. (2009). Fatigue in multiple sclerosis is associated with the disruption of frontal and parietal pathways. *Multiple Sclerosis, 15,* 337–344. http://dx.doi.org/10.1177/1352458508098373

Siegert, R. J., & Abernethy, D. A. (2005). Depression in multiple sclerosis: A review. *Journal of Neurology, Neurosurgery, & Psychiatry, 76,* 469–475. http://dx.doi.org/10.1136/jnnp.2004.054635

Simmons, R. D., Tribe, K. L., & McDonald, E. A. (2010). Living with multiple sclerosis: Longitudinal changes in employment and the importance of symptom management. *Journal of Neurology, 257,* 926–936. http://dx.doi.org/10.1007/s00415-009-5441-7

Simpson, R., Booth, J., Lawrence, M., Byrne, S., Mair, F., & Mercer, S. (2014). Mindfulness based interventions in multiple sclerosis—a systematic review. *BMC Neurology, 14,* 15. http://dx.doi.org/10.1186/1471-2377-14-15

Siniscalchi, A., Gallelli, L., Tolotta, G. A., Loiacono, D., & De Sarro, G. (2010). Open, uncontrolled, nonrandomized, 9-month, off-label use of bupropion to treat fatigue in a single patient with multiple sclerosis. *Clinical Therapeutics, 32,* 2030–2034. http://dx.doi.org/10.1016/j.clinthera.2010.10.012

Smith, M. S., Martin-Herz, S. P., Womack, W. M., & Marsigan, J. L. (2003). Comparative study of anxiety, depression, somatization, functional disability, and illness attribution in adolescents with chronic fatigue or migraine. *Pediatrics, 111,* e376–e381.

Solaro, C., Bergamaschi, R., Rezzani, C., Mueller, M., Trabucco, E., Bargiggia, V., . . . Cavalla, P. (2013). Duloxetine is effective in treating depression in multiple sclerosis patients: An open-label multicenter study. *Clinical Neuropharmacology, 36,* 114–116. http://dx.doi.org/10.1097/WNF.0b013e3182996400

Strober, L. B. (2015). Fatigue in multiple sclerosis: A look at the role of poor sleep. *Frontiers in Neurology, 6,* 21.

Strober, L. B., & Arnett, P. A. (2005). An examination of four models predicting fatigue in multiple sclerosis. *Archives of Clinical Neuropsychology, 20,* 631–646. http://dx.doi.org/10.1016/j.acn.2005.04.002

Stuss, D. T., Murphy, K. J., Binns, M. A., & Alexander, M. P. (2003). Staying on the job: The frontal lobes control individual performance variability. *Brain, 26,* 2363–2380. http://dx.doi.org/10.1093/brain/awg237

Sutherland, G., & Andersen, M. B. (2001). Exercise and multiple sclerosis: Physiological, psychological, and quality of life issues. *The Journal of Sports Medicine and Physical Fitness, 41,* 421–432.

Tartaglia, M. C., Narayanan, S., & Arnold, D. L. (2008). Mental fatigue alters the pattern and increases the volume of cerebral activation required for a motor task in multiple sclerosis patients with fatigue. *European Journal of Neurology, 15,* 413–419. http://dx.doi.org/10.1111/j.1468-1331.2008.02090.x

Tartaglia, M. C., Narayanan, S., Francis, S. J., Santos, A. C., De Stefano, N., Lapierre, Y., & Arnold, D. L. (2004). The relationship between diffuse axonal damage and fatigue in multiple sclerosis. *Archives of Neurology, 61,* 201–207. http://dx.doi.org/10.1001/archneur.61.2.201

Taus, C., Solari, A., D'Amico, R., Branãs, P., Hyde, C., Giuliani, G., & Pucci, E. (2003). Amantadine for fatigue in multiple sclerosis. *The Cochrane Database of Systematic Reviews, 2,* CD002818. http://dx.doi.org/10.1002/14651858.CD002818

Tedeschi, G., Dinacci, D., Lavorgna, L., Prinster, A., Savettieri, G., Quattrone, A., . . . Alfano, B. (2007). Correlation between fatigue and brain atrophy and lesion load in multiple sclerosis patients independent of disability. *Journal of the Neurological Sciences, 263,* 15–19. http://dx.doi.org/10.1016/j.jns.2007.07.004

Thomas, P. W., Thomas, S., Kersten, P., Jones, R., Slingsby, V., Nock, A., . . . Hillier, C. (2014). One year follow-up of a pragmatic multi-centre randomised controlled trial of a group-based fatigue management programme (FACETS) for people with multiple sclerosis. *BMC Neurology, 14,* 109. http://dx.doi.org/10.1186/1471-2377-14-109

Thomas, S., Thomas, P. W., Kersten, P., Jones, R., Green, C., Nock, A., . . . Hillier, C. (2013). A pragmatic parallel arm multi-centre randomised controlled trial to assess the effectiveness and cost-effectiveness of a group-based fatigue management programme (FACETS) for people with multiple sclerosis. *Journal of Neurology, Neurosurgery, & Psychiatry, 84*, 1092–1099. http://dx.doi.org/10.1136/jnnp-2012-303816

Tomassini, V., Matthews, P. M., Thompson, A. J., Fuglø, D., Geurts, J. J., Johansen-Berg, H., . . . Palace, J. (2012). Neuroplasticity and functional recovery in multiple sclerosis. *Nature Reviews. Neurology, 8*, 635–646. http://dx.doi.org/10.1038/nrneurol.2012.179

van der Werf, S. P., Jongen, P. J. H., Lycklama à Nijeholt, G. J., Barkhof, F., Hommes, O. R., & Bleijenberg, G. (1998). Fatigue in multiple sclerosis: Inter-relations between fatigue complaints, cerebral MRI abnormalities and neurological disability. *Journal of the Neurological Sciences, 160*, 164–170. http://dx.doi.org/10.1016/S0022-510X(98)00251-2

van Kessel, K., Moss-Morris, R., Willoughby, E., Chalder, T., Johnson, M. H., & Robinson, E. (2008). A randomized controlled trial of cognitive behavior therapy for multiple sclerosis fatigue. *Psychosomatic Medicine, 70*, 205–213. http://dx.doi.org/10.1097/PSY.0b013e3181643065

Walker, L. A. S., Berard, J. A., Berrigan, L. I., Rees, L. M., & Freedman, M. S. (2012). Detecting cognitive fatigue in multiple sclerosis: Method matters. *Journal of the Neurological Sciences, 316*, 86–92. http://dx.doi.org/10.1016/j.jns.2012.01.021

Wilting, J., Rolfsnes, H. O., Zimmermann, H., Behrens, M., Fleischer, V., Zipp, F., & Gröger, A. (2016). Structural correlates for fatigue in early relapsing remitting multiple sclerosis. *European Radiology, 26*, 515–523. http://dx.doi.org/10.1007/s00330-015-3857-2

7

PERSONALITY AND BEHAVIORAL PROBLEMS IN MULTIPLE SCLEROSIS

CHIARA CONCETTA INCERTI, ORNELLA ARGENTO,
AND UGO NOCENTINI

This chapter is divided into two sections: The first explores personality disorders in patients with multiple sclerosis (MS), starting with definitions of personality, character, and temperament, followed by data on the occurrence of those disorders and on the relationships identified with various aspects and consequences of the illness (anatomical and functional damage, mood disorders, cognitive disorders, fatigue, stress, quality of life, etc.).

The second section describes several behavioral alterations and primarily reports data on what can be considered the consequences of dysfunctional behavior. The topics explored in the two subchapters may seem somewhat separate. In reality, personality, character, and temperament manifest in our actions and interactions and significantly influence our decisions, attitudes, ability to respond to the difficulties of life, and management of relations with others. Only recently has research been published on topics such as the influence of personality on behavior in patients with MS. These two sections of

http://dx.doi.org/10.1037/0000097-008
Cognition and Behavior in Multiple Sclerosis, J. DeLuca and B. M. Sandroff (Editors)

this chapter can provide important information on how to help these patients in their difficult life course.

PERSONALITY IN MS

Personality can be described in various ways. A rather complete definition describes it as "that pattern of characteristic thoughts, feelings and behaviors that distinguishes one person from another and that persists over time and in situations" (Phares & Chaplin, 1997, p. 9). According to various theories, personality consists of traits or personal characteristics that are rather stable over time, understood as tendencies to process information, express emotions and affection, and act and react in a relatively constant way regardless of variations in the context. Different from personality, character is associated with evaluative and moral aspects, whereas temperament represents individual emotional predisposition. This distinction is less sharp in Cloninger's theory (Cloninger, Przybeck, Dragan, & Wetzel, 1994) in which the personality would be the result of interaction between temperament and character.

When personality traits are structured in an excessively rigid and maladaptive way, causing clinically significant discomfort and involving the major life areas of the individual, we are speaking of personality disorders. These include paranoid, schizoid, schizotypal, antisocial, borderline, histrionic, narcissistic, avoidant, dependent, and obsessive-compulsive disorders.

There have been increasing reports in the literature of comorbidity among neuropsychiatric symptoms and MS; some symptoms precede illness onset, and others are reactive or associated with specific moments of the illness (Stathopoulou, Christopoulos, Soubasi, & Gourzis, 2010). Personality changes are included among these disorders. Recently, clinicians and researchers have shown increasing interest in the psychological aspects of MS. Indeed, they are considered to be an important element in the symptom picture of MS, both independently and due to their potential impact on many aspects of the everyday life of patients with MS.

The personality changes in MS patients could have different origins: anatomical and functional damage caused by the illness to various structures of the central nervous system (e.g., demyelination, atrophy), deficits provoked by the illness (e.g., cognitive deterioration), stress connected with the illness and its consequences, or collateral effects of pharmacological therapy, psychosocial factors (e.g., stigmatization, poor self-esteem). All of these factors can result in loss of emotional control that may manifest as euphoria, apathy, irritability, agitation, or disinhibition.

In patients with MS, personality and personality alterations have been evaluated with various instruments originating from different theories, including the Neuroticism Extraversion Openness—Personality Inventory (NEO–PI; McCrae & Costa, 1985), the Millon Clinical Multiaxial Inventory (MCMI–III; Millon, 1997), the Temperament and Character Inventory (TCI; Cloninger et al., 1994), and the Minnesota Multiphasic Personality Inventory (MMPI and MMPI–II; Hathaway & McKinley, 1989).

The NEO–PI and its various revisions, including the shortened NEO–FFI version and the NEO–PI–R (Costa & McCrae, 1992), are the instruments most used in research on MS (Benedict et al., 2008, 2013; Incerti, Magistrale, et al., 2015) because they allow identification of a patient's major personality traits. The NEO–PI is a self-report questionnaire based on the five-factor personality model, according to which five traits or five basic dimensions that are stable over time are the basis of personality. These include neuroticism, extraversion, openness, agreeableness, and conscientiousness. *Neuroticism* is the degree of emotional reactivity and propensity toward negative moods, such as pessimism, irritability, instability, and anxiety. *Extraversion* is the degree of dependence on external stimuli. *Openness* refers to personal disposition to look for new cultural stimuli and to thoughts external to one's own context of reference; it is at the base of creativity and the production of new ideas. *Agreeableness* refers to one's predisposition to establish positive social relations through empathy, interest, and care for others. Finally, conscientiousness is characterized by attributes such as precision, reliability, accuracy, and the ability to direct one's energy to achieve success. Research carried out with the NEO–PI in patients with MS has shown a greater presence of low levels of conscientiousness and high levels of neuroticism with respect to healthy control subjects (Benedict et al., 2013; Incerti, Magistrale, et al., 2015).

An instrument widely used in clinical practice for the psychodiagnostic evaluation of personality disorders is the MCMI–III (Millon, 1997). This questionnaire provides a description of personality traits as well as an estimate of the severity of disturbances. In particular, the MCMI–III scales produce a rather complete image of the patient's psychic world; indeed, they simultaneously provide information on both personality characteristics and main clinical syndromes such as anxiety, somatoform, dysthymia, and major depression.

Only Incerti, Argento, et al. (2015) have used this instrument in a personality study in MS. This study reported scores over the cutoff (>85) on the MCMI–III Histrionic and Narcissistic scale. However, the elevation of these scales is not indicative of a histrionic or narcissistic personality disorder because diagnoses would require the application of more diagnostic instruments, such as clinical interview and other self-reported questionnaires.

Furthermore, the study included only MS patients because MCMI–III is not applicable to healthy subjects.

Cloninger et al.'s (1994) TCI is a questionnaire based on a dimensional psychobiological model. According to this model, personality functioning depends on the interaction among four important neurotransmitters and their relative receptors, which can determine an individual's main behaviors and responses to the environment. In particular, the TCI investigates seven main personality traits that refer to temperament and character. As stated earlier, in the Cloninger's view, temperament and character interact to form personality. The temperament dimensions are Novelty Seeking, Harm Avoidance, Reward Dependence, and Persistence; the character dimensions are Self-Directedness, Cooperativeness, and Self-Transcendence. The questionnaire also provides subscales for each of these primary dimensions. Studies using the TCI in MS patients found greater sensitivity to negative stimuli (Harm Avoidance), less reactivity to positive events (Reward Dependence), lower levels of self-directionality, and high levels of neuroticism compared with healthy control subjects (Christodoulou et al., 1999; Gazioglu et al., 2014).

The MMPI is a well-known instrument widely applied in clinical practice because it examines a wide spectrum of potential psychological problems. In addition to the validity and clinical scales (i.e., the main scales of the test), the questionnaire also provides supplementary and content scales that provide additional psychological detail. Many studies have examined the suitability of the MMPI (both the original and MMPI–2) in neurological populations, proposing interesting solutions (such as statistical correction) to problems regarding its use in such populations (e.g., Gervais, Ben-Porath, Wygant, & Green, 2007; Incerti et al., 2017; Larrabee, 2003; Meyerink, Reitan, & Selz, 1988). In fact, some MMPI items refer to symptoms (such as generalized weakness, paresis, numbness, and concentration difficulties) that are compatible with neurological problems but may also reflect a neurotic state in nonneurological population. Other authors used the MMPI to assess defense mechanisms in MS patients (Hyphantis et al., 2008; Stathopoulou et al., 2010) or to examine a symptom picture and personality description of these patients (Reznikova, Terent'eva, & Kataeva, 2007; Stathopoulou et al., 2010) and obtained results consistent with those found when other instruments were used.

The studies carried out with the above-mentioned instruments highlighted that in patients with MS, the presence of high level of neuroticism and low levels of extraversion, agreeableness, and conscientiousness were linked to specific locations of cerebral damage (Benedict et al., 2008) or to problems connected with MS (e.g., fatigue, depression, work stress, cognitive impairment, quality of life). Other studies confirmed the presence of high neuroticism and low conscientiousness in patients with MS (Benedict et al., 2013).

Prevalence of Personality Disorders in Patients With MS

There are no conclusive data regarding the incidence and prevalence of personality disorders in patients with MS. Considering the available data, some studies that have looked at more general aspects of personality have found an increase in irritability and apathy in 20% to 40% of MS patients (Kaplan, Sadock, & Grebb, 1994; Mitsonis, Potagas, Zervas, & Sfagos, 2009).

Other studies applied instruments more specifically suited for the detection of personality disorders: one study (using the revised Personality Disorder Questionnaire) in 20 MS patients, 24 depressed subjects, 35 subjects with chronic fatigue syndrome, and 35 control subjects showed different percentages of personality disorders among the groups. In MS, 25% demonstrated paranoia and a further 25% demonstrated borderline personality disorder (Johnson, DeLuca, & Natelson, 1996). In a different sample of 77 MS patients, Incerti, Argento, et al. (2015; using the MCMI–III) found 20.8% of subjects with elevation in the narcissistic scale and 15.6% with elevation in the histrionic scale. Another study involving 55 patients with MS and 56 healthy control subjects (using the Structured Clinical Interview for the *Diagnostic and Statistical Manual of Mental Disorders* Axis II disorders) found a significant difference between patients and healthy controls in the frequency of personality disorders (46% in MS patients and 14% in control group), with a predominance of obsessive-compulsive and avoidant personality disorders in MS patients (Uca et al., 2016).

The foregoing data provide a rather partial account regarding the real frequency of personality disorders in MS patients. Furthermore, it is possible that cultural differences may result in a bias in the prevalence of some personality characteristics (e.g., emotion expression) over others (Kaplan et al., 1994; Mitsonis et al., 2009), depending on the geographic location of a given study. Of note, international data on cultural differences in personality characteristics in MS are scarce, although future study is warranted to capture a more complete scope of the prevalence and pattern of personality disorders in this population.

Anatomical, Functional, and Cognitive Correlates of Personality Profiles in MS

Increasing interest in the personality profiles found in patients with MS led several researchers to undertake in-depth studies of the anatomical correlates of these profiles. In particular, they investigated correlations with metabolic activity and structural cerebral aspects and reported some interesting results (Benedict et al., 2008, 2013; Reznikova et al., 2007).

Reznikova et al. (2007) analyzed cerebral metabolic activity in patients with MS with different personality profiles and found significant correlations between reduced metabolism of several cerebral areas and variants of maladjusted personality (neurotic, psychotic, and mixed). The cerebral structures most involved in pathological personality profiles were the frontal, parietal, and temporal lobes and the structures belonging to the limbic and reticular system. Thus, these cerebral structures (i.e., both cortical and subcortical) may have a role in determining personality styles. Other studies confirm the role of the frontal lobe in personality variations (Benedict, Carone, & Bakshi, 2004) and also show links among cognitive deterioration, personality changes, and cerebral atrophy in MS patients.

The personality–brain connection was explored in a review by Benedict, Carone, and Bakshi (2004). On the basis of cognitive and emotional impairment (which manifests with unmotivated euphoria and disinhibition), they identified the presence of cerebral atrophy, particularly of subcortical areas, which was confirmed by concomitant ventricular expansion. The same review showed that the presence of several personality traits (i.e., high levels of neuroticism and low levels of empathy, agreeableness, and conscientiousness) is characteristic of subjects with cognitive impairment.

Finally, subsequent studies showed a correlation between gray matter volume and low levels of conscientiousness and high levels of neuroticism, which is typically associated with euphoric-type behavioral alterations (Benedict et al., 2013).

The literature cited thus far shows a tight link between particular personality traits and cognitive impairment. The strong association among executive function (shown by the Wisconsin Card Sorting Test—Perseverative Responses and Booklet Category Test—Errors) and visual learning (Brief Visuospatial Memory Test—Recall) deficits and several personality traits can be considered a clue that frontal and temporal lobe dysfunction is at the base of the particular personality profiles seen in MS patients (Benedict, Priore, Miller, Munschauer, & Jacobs, 2001).

Taken together, the available data regarding personality profiles/disturbances and brain structure damage/dysfunction in MS patients are insufficient, and this area requires further research. Some cerebral areas, particularly the frontal regions, could play a crucial role in determining the predominance of some personality traits in MS patients. Because frontal damage also plays an important role in cognitive deficits in MS patients, the reciprocal influence of personality and cognition should be clarified in the framework of the attempt of connecting structural damage, functional impairment, and personality profiles.

Personality and Fatigue

Fatigue is among the most frequent symptoms in patients with MS, resulting in significant disability (DeLuca, 2007; Schreiber, Lang, Kiltz, &

Lang, 2015). Fatigue can be defined as "a subjective lack of physical and/or mental health that is perceived by the individual or caregiver to interfere with usual and desired activities" (Multiple Sclerosis Council for Clinical Practice Guidelines, 1998, p. 1), and occurs at all phases of the illness. Although a great deal of research has focused on fatigue in MS, there is no consensus on its definition, characteristics, or causes, making it difficult to identify and treat the problem.

Personality characteristics have been examined in research on possible causes of fatigue in MS. Studies have reported that the personality characteristics most connected with elevated fatigue are neuroticism and low levels of extraversion (Kiltz et al., 2009; Merkelbach, König, & Sittinger, 2003; Penner et al., 2007); these are often associated with irritability, inhibition, anger, depression, and pathological coping strategies, further complicating the issue (Kiltz et al., 2009). This connection has been further supported by longitudinal research (Lang et al., 2011).

The absence of premorbid history limits the validity of subjective questionnaires. The difficulty in separating some personality traits from the depressive component further confounds the correlations between personality traits and fatigue. Finally, the information captured by subjective questionnaires could be biased by the patient's unconscious perception of a certain symptom. Another limitation is the lack of instruments able to provide an objective detection of fatigue, probably because of the difficulty in its definition. This aspect was confirmed by a study in recently diagnosed MS patients that identified psychological components (i.e., specific personality characteristics such as defensive style and the strength of the self) as possible indicators of exhaustion of resources to cope with physical and psychological stress related to the illness (Hyphantis et al., 2008). Another recent study examining the link between personality and fatigue and the role of motivation showed that reward for completing a task reduced several effects of fatigue (Pardini, Cappello, Krueger, Mancardi, & Uccelli, 2013).

In conclusion, although some studies in patients with MS have found that various aspects of personality (as well as psychoemotional factors such as anxiety, depression, anger, and stress) are correlated with fatigue, there is still no unitary view able to explain the role of personality characteristics with respect to the origin of fatigue in patients with MS.

Personality, Depression, and Anxiety

Depression and anxiety are among the psychoemotional disorders found most often in MS patients (Feinstein, 2004; Feinstein, O'Connor, Gray, & Feinstein, 1999; Nocentini, Caltagirone, & Tedeschi, 2012). Studies of personality in MS patients confirmed the strong relationship with depression; in fact, the latter is related both to reported high levels of neuroticism (Gazioglu et al., 2014; Reznikova et al., 2007; Schreiber et al., 2015) and specific patterns of neurotic personality (Christodoulou et al., 1999; Larrabee, 2003). According to recent studies, depression could be one of the key elements in determining personality changes in patients with MS. In particular, Gazioglu et al. (2014) showed the influence of depression in elevating scores of several TCI scales; by contrast, Uca et al. (2016) reported that the personality disorders in MS patients might be at the base of other psychological disorders, such as anxiety and depression.

Unlike depression, where studies have attempted to examine its influence on personality, anxiety has been investigated as a generic element without using detailed and specific instruments. This complicates our understanding of the relationship between anxiety and personality. Clarifying the relationship among depression, anxiety, and personality and how much one influences the other will likely be a major goal of future research in the area of personality research in patients with MS. At the moment, this aspect is difficult to understand and varies depending on one's point of view. In fact, from a psychological perspective, if we consider that personality tends to remain constant over time, depression could be an expression of dysfunctional personality; however, if personality changes are considered to be a consequence of cerebral damage, depression could also become part of the same interpretation, creating confusion about the link between personality and depression.

Other Possible Relations Between Personality and Aspects of MS: Stress and Quality of Life

In addition to the issues described previously, changes in personality can also have an impact on other important factors, such as stress and quality of life. Recently, stress has been identified as one factor that may negatively affect the clinical disease course in patients with MS, increasing the possibility of relapses (Karagkouni, Alevizos, & Theoharides, 2013). Other than a secondary component of a broader topic, only one study investigated stress and personality together in MS patients. Incerti, Magistrale, et al. (2015) explored one aspect of stress—stress associated with work—and found a positive correlation between work stress and several specific personality traits, such as high levels of neuroticism and low levels of extraversion and conscientiousness.

Similar to stress, there is a paucity of research on quality of life and personality change in MS patients, often examined as a subcomponent in larger studies. These studies tend to show a relationship between personality changes and quality of life, health, and general well-being. For instance, a recent study recognized the role of several aspects of personality, such as introversion and neurosis, in determining perception of a rather low quality of life (Zarbo et al., 2016).

Recently, Strober (2017) reported an association between a specific type of personality, Type D (distressed personality, characterized by a greater tendency to experience negative emotions and sometimes by difficulty sharing and expressing these types of emotions, which predisposes these subjects to various forms of somatization), that is often encountered in patients with MS, which was associated with lowered overall quality of life (Strober, 2017).

Despite the relative paucity of studies, taken together the results show a consistent connection between some personality characteristics and stress and quality of life, likely having everyday life consequences such as personal relationships, employment status, and social roles.

Treatments

Currently, there is no specific therapy for treating personality disorders in patients with MS. Identifying the possible causes of personality changes could help address elective therapies. Indeed, this is particularly important: Besides the possibility of helping patients reduce psychological disorders connected with the crystallization of particular personality traits, an effective treatment of these disorders could positively influence many other aspects of the illness.

At the moment, the nonpharmacological approaches available are psychotherapy, family therapy, and social support. An integrated application of these approaches would likely lead to more lasting results (Stathopoulou et al., 2010).

Regarding psychotherapy, different approaches (e.g., psychodynamic, behavioral, cognitive, psychoanalytic) have shown some promise in helping patients identify solutions for their own psychological distress, for example, on emotions, maladjusted behaviors, negative cognitive evaluation, or unconscious psychic aspects (Hart, Vella, & Mohr, 2008).

There is currently no specific pharmacological treatment for personality disorders. Such approaches have been used exclusively to treat various psychiatric disorders that may be present in patients with MS, perhaps related to an underlying personality disorder.

Thus, whatever the origin of personality disorders in MS patients, profound psychological changes can reduce individual psychological resources and alter family and social relationships, affecting every aspect of their lives. Future research is needed to identify suitable treatments for personality disorders and their consequences in persons with MS.

BEHAVIORAL SYMPTOMS IN MS

Behavioral symptoms (BS) can be referred to as a self-regulation disorder in how people control their thoughts, feelings, and behaviors (Feinstein, 2007). BS, such as apathy and anger, are well recognized in patients with MS; however, the most frequently studied are cognitive or psychiatric symptoms because they have a more direct influence on patients' lives. A wide range of behavioral disorders that can also have a significant impact on patients' quality of life, psychosocial functioning, employment, and therapeutic adherence have yet to be amply studied. One reason for this paucity may be that many BS do not appear to be directly linked to the pathological process of MS or may be viewed as less relevant than other disturbances. What follows is a brief presentation of the more prominently reported BS in patients with MS and some of their consequences. In this section, we do not consider mood disorders, such as anxiety and depression, fatigue, pseudobulbar affect, euphoria, and inappropriateness, because they are treated elsewhere in this and others chapters of this volume.

Apathy

Apathy is a neurobehavioral symptom characterized by a lack of motivation independent from emotional distress, intellectual impairment, or diminished levels of consciousness (Marin, 1991). It has been considered a behavioral disorder consisting of deficits in goal-directed actions, decrement in goal-directed thought content, and emotional indifference associated with flat affect (Marin, 1991). Many studies have reported the presence of apathy in MS patients, as a characterizing symptom, within multisymptom assessment methods. There is a growing interest in apathy in MS as a symptom itself, independent from its comorbidity with other psychiatric symptoms, such as depression and anxiety. In fact, recent systematic reviews on BS in MS have shown that a substantial percentage of MS patients experience apathy during the course of their pathology. In an early investigation, the incidence of apathy reported was roughly 10% (Surridge, 1969), whereas more recent studies have evidenced an incidence ranging from 20% to 35% (Figved et al., 2005; Paparrigopoulos, Ferentinos, Kouzoupis, Koutsis, & Papadimitriou, 2010).

Uncertainties concerning the prevalence of apathy in MS may be a result of using nonspecific assessment tools, such as the Neuropsychiatric Inventory or the Frontal Systems Behavior Scale (Chiaravalloti & DeLuca, 2003; Figved et al., 2005). An effort to address this issue has been suggested by Raimo et al. (2014), who proposed validating the Apathy Evaluation Scale (AES) in patients with MS. Their validation study resulted in three apathy-related factors: the cognitive apathy factor, the general apathy factor, and the behavioral–emotional factor. These three factors were consistent with the previous literature showing a significant association between apathy and cognitive dysfunctions in particular executive dysfunction in MS patients (Figved et al., 2008; Niino et al., 2014). Regarding the pathological process underlying apathy, demyelinating lesions affecting frontal-subcortical circuits and limbic structures, in particular, the medial frontal-anterior cingulate circuit, have been proposed to underlie this disturbance (Cummings et al., 1994).

Anger

Anger is universally considered one of the fundamental emotions (Ekman, 1992). Its impact on interpersonal relationships and its connection with violence and aggression is well documented and may result in a range of problematic behaviors. The presence of anger in MS patients has been widely highlighted by clinicians in both qualitative and quantitative studies (Edwards, Barlow, & Turner, 2008; Kalb, 2007; Langdon & Thompson; 1999; Mohr & Cox, 2001; Nocentini et al., 2009). Facing MS can generate a complex field of feelings; among these, anger is also one of the most difficult to deal with and likely the most lasting and frequent.

Within this framework, clinicians and health professionals serve an important role in paying special attention to how anger is assessed in MS patients and how it is reported by patients. Recently, several studies have outlined the importance of the period surrounding MS diagnosis and the relevance of appropriate communication between MS patients and health professionals (Thorne, Harris, Mahoney, Con, & McGuinness, 2004; White, White, & Russell, 2007).

Another source of anger for MS patients is the unpredictability of the course of the disease and its symptoms. This seems particularly evident in both MS patients and their relatives in reaction to relapses (Kalb, 2005; LaRocca, 2005).

Only two studies have used specific instruments to investigate anger characteristics in MS. Langdon and Thompson (1999) found higher levels of anger in MS patients compared with the general population. Nocentini et al. (2009) reported higher levels of withheld anger and lower levels of anger control, suggesting that features of anger in MS patients differ from the healthy population. This study also showed that anger was independent from age, education, disease duration, disease course, disability, and fatigue but linked to mood and anxiety measures (Nocentini et al., 2009). These authors also suggested that anger in MS was not a reaction to physical disability but likely a consequence of the demyelinating disease process.

More recently, two neuroimaging studies confirmed the presence of functional differences between MS patients and healthy control subjects in processing anger (Jehna et al., 2011; Passamonti et al., 2009). Passamonti et al. (2009) reported that during an emotional facial recognition task, MS subjects showed elevated activity compared with the healthy control group in the ventrolateral prefrontal cortex and a lack of functional connectivity between two prefrontal areas (ventrolateral and medial prefrontal cortex), two posterior regions (cuneus/precuneus and superior parietal cortex) and the amygdala, a subcortical brain structure involved in fight-or-flight responses (LeDoux, 2003). Further, Jehna et al. (2011) found that MS patients had increased activation in the posterior cingulate cortex and precuneus during the recognition of facial expressions of anger and disgust compared with controls at equivalent performance (Jehna et al., 2011).

Anger in MS patients represents a recurring issue that has to be considered both in clinical settings and with regard to its impact on the family environment. Numerous variables need to be taken into account in future studies of anger in MS, including personality, coping styles, and fatigue.

Consequences of BS in MS: Falls, Domestic, and Driving Accidents

Research over the past 20 years has shown that MS patients experience a greater number of falls and physical injuries compared with matched healthy subjects. Fall-related injuries in particular have received the greatest attention because they are frequently reported by patients. According to incidence studies, at least 50% of MS patients experience single or multiple falls over a 2- to 6-month period (Cattaneo et al., 2002; Peterson, Cho, von Koch, & Finlayson, 2008). This may be underestimated because Matsuda et al. (2011) found that only 51% of MS patients who experience falls refer these injuries to health care staff. Falls negatively affect quality of life not only for MS patients (restricting daily activities and independence) but also for caregivers and represent a significant economic burden for national health care systems (Finlayson, Peterson, & Cho, 2006). Thus, the prediction and the prevention of fall risks are critical for adequate patient care.

Several factors have been proposed to be associated with fall risk in MS. These include sensory integration impairments during standing balance (Kasser, Jacobs, Foley, Cardinal, & Maddalozzo, 2011; Prosperini, Fortuna, Giannì, Leonardi, & Pozzilli, 2013), altered stability limits during leaning (Karst, Venema, Roehrs, & Tyler, 2005), muscle weakness in the lower extremities that are associated with changes in gait speed and standing sway (Chung, Remelius, Van Emmerik, & Kent-Braun, 2008) as well as forgetfulness, fatigue (Prosperini et al., 2013), urinary incontinence (Sosnoff et al., 2011), and inefficient use of assistive devices (Cattaneo et al., 2002; Coote, Hogan, & Franklin, 2013). Recently, there has been increasing interest on the role of cognitive dysfunction as a risk factor linked to the higher incidence of falls in MS. In particular, worse information processing speed and verbal memory performance have been found to be associated with higher frequencies of falls (D'Orio et al., 2012; Sosnoff et al., 2013). It has been suggested that cognitive rehabilitation may have a positive influence on falls frequency in patients with MS (Kalron, 2014).

One study showed that patients with MS experience significantly more domestic accidents, such as bumps and near falls, than healthy control subjects and that these accidents appear to be related to bowel/bladder dysfunction, fatigue, and reduced reasoning ability (Argento et al., 2014).

There are now several studies documenting increased frequency of driving difficulties in persons with MS. In particular, patients with MS are involved in significantly more accidents and commit significantly more traffic offenses than control subjects (Knecht, 1977) and are more frequently referred to health care systems because they seem to be more vulnerable to driving-related injuries (Ryan et al., 2009). Disease duration and levels of disability were seemingly unrelated to driving-related skills (Shawaryn, Schultheis, Garay, & DeLuca, 2002). Conversely, cognitive deficits have been found to negatively affect driving-related skills in MS patients. Schultheis, Garay, and DeLuca (2001) showed that MS patients with cognitive impairment and minimal physical disability perform significantly worse on tasks assessing driving-related skills and have significantly more car crashes than cognitively preserved patients, even when driving less frequently (Schultheis, Garay, Millis, & DeLuca, 2002). Deficits in information processing speed, memory, and executive functioning have been identified as the most relevant cognitive impairments in predicting the driving safety in MS patients (Lincoln & Radford, 2008). Furthermore, a recent study showed that the number of car violations in MS patients was predicted by the thalamic brain atrophy (Dehning, Kim, Nguyen, Shivapour, & Denburg, 2014).

It is interesting to note that in all studies of falls, domestic accidents, and driving studies, an important role has been attributed to cognitive efficiency. This is in line with recent research on cognitive-motor interference (CMI) in patients with MS. CMI can be defined as the changes in behavior when cognitive and a motor tasks are simultaneously performed (Wajda & Sosnoff, 2015). The mutual influence of a cognitive and a motor task is generally assessed with dual-task methodology and has been found to decrease the performance in one or both the tasks (Plummer & Eskes, 2015). Because MS patients may have both cognitive and motor impairments, the impact of CMI on their everyday activities has been shown to be greater than in healthy subjects (Hamilton et al., 2009), as reported in some studies. These results may explain the increased amount found in falls and domestic and driving accidents. Unfortunately, the real impact of the CMI in MS patients is still in its infancy (Leone, Patti, & Feys, 2015), but future studies may clarify discrepancies and guide the development of rehabilitation and prevention programs to avoid injuries in this population. Self-awareness of motor and cognitive deficits should also be a goal of future research because it may play an important role in reducing the risk of physical injuries (Ryan et al., 2009).

In summary, the occurrence of physical injuries in MS patients appears to be the consequence of a complex interaction of various factors, significantly affecting quality of life in MS patients.

CONCLUSIONS AND FUTURE DIRECTIONS

This chapter summarized the primary data on personality disorders and the consequences of behavioral alterations in MS patients. Despite the importance of these topics for MS patients and their families, it is only recently that they have received greater attention both clinically and in research. Like other consequences of MS, personality factors and behavioral disorders are the result of a variety of complex factors. This is particular true for personality disorders, which present an intriguing challenge for researchers and clinicians alike. As discussed in this chapter, some theories of personality suggest that once psychoemotional development has matured, personality is considered stable. However, even if the basic aspects of personality are difficult to modify once established, it may also be true that life events, such as a disabling disease, can heighten aspects of personality more than others. In the case of central nervous system pathologies, it is reasonable to ask the following: What happens if alterations occur in the cerebral structures that underlie personality? It is unclear when the pathological process that characterizes MS begins, but it is certainly before diagnosis. If pathological processes modify cerebral structures during personality development, one could reasonably expect that personality can be altered by the disease itself. Unfortunately, there is little to no research on how brain damage may alter personality development in MS. Personality development is a complex interaction between genetically predetermined traits and the individual's life experiences. MS may play an as-yet-undefined role in personality development and is an important topic for future research.

The consequences of behavioral alterations in MS patients is also the result of a complex interaction of various factors that must be taken into account when considering the disabling impact of MS (Ryan et al., 2009). Increasing the patient awareness of factors that may lead to behavioral alterations may result in the reduction of some risk factors (e.g., walking while performing other tasks, driving) or in specific environments (e.g., home) that may be dangerous or make patients more vulnerable to injuries (Argento et al., 2014; Ryan et al., 2009). On the other hand, physical disability and cognitive impairment alone are not the only variables responsible for physical injuries in MS patients. The proper identification of all these aspects, together with the specific ways that they influence patients' behaviors, should be an important goal for future clinical and research studies and for the development of adequate rehabilitation and preventing programs.

REFERENCES

Argento, O., Incerti, C. C., Pisani, V., Magistrale, G., Di Battista, G., Romano, S., . . . Nocentini, U. (2014). Domestic accidents and multiple sclerosis: An exploratory study of occurrence and possible causes. *Disability and Rehabilitation, 36,* 2205–2209. http://dx.doi.org/10.3109/09638288.2014.895429

Benedict, R. H. B., Carone, D. A., & Bakshi, R. (2004). Correlating brain atrophy with cognitive dysfunction, mood disturbances, and personality disorder in multiple sclerosis. *Journal of Neuroimaging, 14*(Suppl.), 36S–45S. http://dx.doi.org/10.1111/j.1552-6569.2004.tb00277.x

Benedict, R. H. B., Hussein, S., Englert, J., Dwyer, M. G., Abdelrahman, N., Cox, J. L., . . . Zivadinov, R. (2008). Cortical atrophy and personality in multiple sclerosis. *Neuropsychology, 22,* 432–441. http://dx.doi.org/10.1037/0894-4105.22.4.432

Benedict, R. H. B., Priore, R. L., Miller, C., Munschauer, F., & Jacobs, L. (2001). Personality disorder in multiple sclerosis correlates with cognitive impairment. *The Journal of Neuropsychiatry and Clinical Neurosciences, 13,* 70–76. http://dx.doi.org/10.1176/jnp.13.1.70

Benedict, R. H. B., Schwartz, C. E., Duberstein, P., Healy, B., Hoogs, M., Bergsland, N., . . . Zivadinov, R. (2013). Influence of personality on the relationship between gray matter volume and neuropsychiatric symptoms in multiple sclerosis. *Psychosomatic Medicine, 75,* 253–261. http://dx.doi.org/10.1097/PSY.0b013e31828837cc

Cattaneo, D., De Nuzzo, C., Fascia, T., Macalli, M., Pisoni, I., & Cardini, R. (2002). Risks of falls in subjects with multiple sclerosis. *Archives of Physical Medicine and Rehabilitation, 83,* 864–867. http://dx.doi.org/10.1053/apmr.2002.32825

Chiaravalloti, N. D., & DeLuca, J. (2003). Assessing the behavioral consequences of multiple sclerosis: An application of the Frontal Systems Behavior Scale (FrSBe). *Cognitive and Behavioral Neurology, 16,* 54–67. http://dx.doi.org/10.1097/00146965-200303000-00007

Christodoulou, C., Deluca, J., Johnson, S. K., Lange, G., Gaudino, E. A., & Natelson, B. H. (1999). Examination of Cloninger's basic dimensions of personality in fatiguing illness: Chronic fatigue syndrome and multiple sclerosis. *Journal of Psychosomatic Research, 47,* 597–607. http://dx.doi.org/10.1016/S0022-3999(99)00063-X

Chung, L. H., Remelius, J. G., Van Emmerik, R. E., & Kent-Braun, J. A. (2008). Leg power asymmetry and postural control in women with multiple sclerosis. *Medicine and Science in Sports and Exercise, 40,* 1717–1724. http://dx.doi.org/10.1249/MSS.0b013e31817e32a3

Cloninger, C. R., Przybeck, T. R., Dragan, M. S., & Wetzel, R. D. (1994). *The Temperament and Character Inventory (TCI): A guide to its development and use* (pp. 19–28). St. Louis, MO: Center for Psychobiology of Personality, Washington University.

Coote, S., Hogan, N., & Franklin, S. (2013). Falls in people with multiple sclerosis who use a walking aid: Prevalence, factors, and effect of strength and balance interventions. *Archives of Physical Medicine and Rehabilitation, 94,* 616–621. http://dx.doi.org/10.1016/j.apmr.2012.10.020

Costa, P. T., & McCrae, R. R. (1992). *Professional manual: Revised NEO Personality Inventory (NEO–PI–R) and NEO Five-Factor Inventory (NEO–FFI).* Odessa, FL: Psychological Assessment Resources.

Cummings, J. L., Mega, M., Gray, K., Rosenberg-Thompson, S., Carusi, D. A., & Gornbein, J. (1994). The Neuropsychiatric Inventory: Comprehensive assessment of psychopathology in dementia. *Neurology, 44,* 2308–2314. http://dx.doi.org/10.1212/WNL.44.12.2308

Dehning, M., Kim, J., Nguyen, C. M., Shivapour, E., & Denburg, N. L. (2014). Neuropsychological performance, brain imaging, and driving violations in multiple sclerosis. *Archives of Physical Medicine and Rehabilitation, 95,* 1818–1823. http://dx.doi.org/10.1016/j.apmr.2014.05.022

DeLuca, J. (2007). Fatigue, cognition and mental effort. In J. DeLuca (Ed.), *Fatigue as a window to the brain* (pp. 37–57). Cambridge, MA: The MIT Press.

D'Orio, V. L., Foley, F. W., Armentano, F., Picone, M. A., Kim, S., & Holtzer, R. (2012). Cognitive and motor functioning in patients with multiple sclerosis: Neuropsychological predictors of walking speed and falls. *Journal of the Neurological Sciences, 316,* 42–46. http://dx.doi.org/10.1016/j.jns.2012.02.003

Edwards, R. G., Barlow, J. H., & Turner, A. P. (2008). Experiences of diagnosis and treatment among people with multiple sclerosis. *Journal of Evaluation in Clinical Practice, 14,* 460–464. http://dx.doi.org/10.1111/j.1365-2753.2007.00902.x

Ekman, P. (1992). Are there basic emotions? *Psychological Review, 99,* 550–553. http://dx.doi.org/10.1037/0033-295X.99.3.550

Feinstein, A. (2004). The neuropsychiatry of multiple sclerosis. *Canadian Journal of Psychiatry, 49,* 157–163. http://dx.doi.org/10.1177/070674370404900302

Feinstein, A. (2007). *The clinical neuropsychiatry of multiple sclerosis.* Cambridge, England: Cambridge University Press. http://dx.doi.org/10.1017/CBO9780511543760

Feinstein, A., O'Connor, P., Gray, T., & Feinstein, K. (1999). The effects of anxiety on psychiatric morbidity in patients with multiple sclerosis. *Multiple Sclerosis Journal, 5,* 323–326. http://dx.doi.org/10.1191/135245899678846348

Figved, N., Benedict, R., Klevan, G., Myhr, K. M., Nyland, H. I., Landrø, N. I., . . . Aarsland, D. (2008). Relationship of cognitive impairment to psychiatric symptoms in multiple sclerosis. *Multiple Sclerosis Journal, 14*, 1084–1090. http://dx.doi.org/10.1177/1352458508092262

Figved, N., Klevan, G., Myhr, K. M., Glad, S., Nyland, H., Larsen, J. P., . . . Aarsland, D. (2005). Neuropsychiatric symptoms in patients with multiple sclerosis. *Acta Psychiatrica Scandinavica, 112*, 463–468. http://dx.doi.org/10.1111/j.1600-0447.2005.00624.x

Finlayson, M. L., Peterson, E. W., & Cho, C. C. (2006). Risk factors for falling among people aged 45 to 90 years with multiple sclerosis. *Archives of Physical Medicine and Rehabilitation, 87*, 1274–1279. http://dx.doi.org/10.1016/j.apmr.2006.06.002

Gazioglu, S., Cakmak, V. A., Ozkorumak, E., Usta, N. C., Ates, C., & Boz, C. (2014). Personality traits of patients with multiple sclerosis and their relationship with clinical characteristics. *Journal of Nervous and Mental Disease, 202*, 408–411. http://dx.doi.org/10.1097/NMD.0000000000000114

Gervais, R. O., Ben-Porath, Y. S., Wygant, D. B., & Green, P. (2007). Development and validation of a Response Bias Scale (RBS) for the MMPI–2. *Assessment, 14*, 196–208. http://dx.doi.org/10.1177/1073191106295861

Hamilton, F., Rochester, L., Paul, L., Rafferty, D., O'Leary, C. P., & Evans, J. J. (2009). Walking and talking: An investigation of cognitive-motor dual tasking in multiple sclerosis. *Multiple Sclerosis Journal, 15*, 1215–1227. http://dx.doi.org/10.1177/1352458509106712

Hart, S. L., Vella, L., & Mohr, D. C. (2008). Relationships among depressive symptoms, benefit-finding, optimism, and positive affect in multiple sclerosis patients after psychotherapy for depression. *Health Psychology, 27*, 230–238. http://dx.doi.org/10.1037/0278-6133.27.2.230

Hathaway, S. R., & McKinley, J. C. (1989). *MMPI–2. Manual for Administration and Scoring*. Minneapolis: University of Minnesota Press.

Hyphantis, T. N., Christou, K., Kontoudaki, S., Mantas, C., Papamichael, G., Goulia, P., . . . Mavreas, V. (2008). Disability status, disease parameters, defense styles, and ego strength associated with psychiatric complications of multiple sclerosis. *International Journal of Psychiatry in Medicine, 38*, 307–327. http://dx.doi.org/10.2190/PM.38.3.g

Incerti, C. C., Argento, O., Pisani, V., Magistrale, G., Sabatello, U., Caltagirone, C., & Nocentini, U. (2017). A more in-depth interpretation of MMPI–2 in MS patients by using Harris and Lingoes subscales. *Applied Neuropsychology. Adult, 24*, 439–445.

Incerti, C. C., Argento, O., Pisani, V., Mannu, R., Magistrale, G., Battista, G. D., . . . Nocentini, U. (2015). A preliminary investigation of abnormal personality traits in MS using the MCMI–III. *Applied Neuropsychology: Adult, 22*, 452–458. http://dx.doi.org/10.1080/23279095.2014.979489

Incerti, C. C., Magistrale, G., Argento, O., Pisani, V., Di Battista, G., Ferraro, E., . . . Nocentini, U. (2015). Occupational stress and personality traits in multiple sclerosis: A preliminary study. *Multiple Sclerosis and Related Disorders, 4*, 315–319. http://dx.doi.org/10.1016/j.msard.2015.06.001

Jehna, M., Langkammer, C., Wallner-Blazek, M., Neuper, C., Loitfelder, M., Ropele, S., . . . Enzinger, C. (2011). Cognitively preserved MS patients demonstrate functional differences in processing neutral and emotional faces. *Brain Imaging and Behavior, 5*, 241–251. http://dx.doi.org/10.1007/s11682-011-9128-1

Johnson, S. K., DeLuca, J., & Natelson, B. H. (1996). Personality dimensions in the chronic fatigue syndrome: A comparison with multiple sclerosis and depression. *Journal of Psychiatric Research, 30*, 9–20. http://dx.doi.org/10.1016/0022-3956(95)00040-2

Kalb, R. (2005). When MS joins the family. *Multiple sclerosis: A guide for families* (3rd ed.). New York, NY: Demos Medical.

Kalb, R. (2007). The emotional and psychological impact of multiple sclerosis relapses. *Journal of the Neurological Sciences, 256*(Suppl. 1), S29–S33. http://dx.doi.org/10.1016/j.jns.2007.01.061

Kalron, A. (2014). The relationship between specific cognitive domains, fear of falling, and falls in people with multiple sclerosis. *BioMed Research International, 2014*, 281760. http://dx.doi.org/10.1155/2014/281760

Kaplan, H. I., Sadock, B. J., & Grebb, J. A. (1994). Mental disorders due to a general medical condition. In H. I. Kaplan & B. J. Sadock (Eds.), *Synopsis of psychiatry: Behavioral sciences clinical psychiatry.* Philadelphia, PA: Lippincott Williams & Wilkins.

Karagkouni, A., Alevizos, M., & Theoharides, T. C. (2013). Effect of stress on brain inflammation and multiple sclerosis. *Autoimmunity Reviews, 12*, 947–953. http://dx.doi.org/10.1016/j.autrev.2013.02.006

Karst, G. M., Venema, D. M., Roehrs, T. G., & Tyler, A. E. (2005). Center of pressure measures during standing tasks in minimally impaired persons with multiple sclerosis. *Journal of Neurologic Physical Therapy, 29*, 170–180. http://dx.doi.org/10.1097/01.NPT.0000282314.40230.40

Kasser, S. L., Jacobs, J. V., Foley, J. T., Cardinal, B. J., & Maddalozzo, G. F. (2011). A prospective evaluation of balance, gait, and strength to predict falling in women with multiple sclerosis. *Archives of Physical Medicine and Rehabilitation, 92*, 1840–1846. http://dx.doi.org/10.1016/j.apmr.2011.06.004

Kiltz, K., Lang, M., Flachenecker, P., Meissner, H., Koehler, A., Freidel, M., . . . Schreiber, H., for the NTD Study Group on Multiple Sclerosis. (2009). Physical, cognitive and psychological dimensions of fatigue in patients with relapsing-remitting multiple sclerosis a multicentre study. *Multiple Sclerosis Journal, 15*, S116–S117.

Knecht, J. (1977). The multiple sclerosis patient as a driver [in German]. *Schweizerische Medizinische Wochenschrift, 107*, 373–378.

Lang, C., Lang, M., Flachenecker, P., Meissner, H., Freidel, M., Herbst, H., . . . Schreiber, H. (2011). Fatigue, cognition and personality in patients with relapsing-remitting multiple sclerosis (RRMS)—A longitudinal study. *Multiple Sclerosis Journal, 17*, S179.

Langdon, D. W., & Thompson, A. J. (1999). Multiple sclerosis: A preliminary study of selected variables affecting rehabilitation outcome. *Multiple Sclerosis Journal, 5*, 94–100. http://dx.doi.org/10.1191/135245899678847220

LaRocca, N. (2005). Emotional and cognitive issues. In R. Kalb (Ed.), *Multiple sclerosis: A guide for families* (3rd ed.). New York, NY: Demos Medical.

Larrabee, G. J. (2003). Exaggerated MMPI–2 symptom report in personal injury litigants with malingered neurocognitive deficit. *Archives of Clinical Neuropsychology, 18*, 673–686. http://dx.doi.org/10.1093/arclin/18.6.673

LeDoux, J. (2003). The emotional brain, fear, and the amygdala. *Cellular and Molecular Neurobiology, 23*, 727–738. http://dx.doi.org/10.1023/A:1025048802629

Leone, C., Patti, F., & Feys, P. (2015). Measuring the cost of cognitive-motor dual tasking during walking in multiple sclerosis. *Multiple Sclerosis Journal, 21*, 123–131. http://dx.doi.org/10.1177/1352458514547408

Lincoln, N. B., & Radford, K. A. (2008). Cognitive abilities as predictors of safety to drive in people with multiple sclerosis. *Multiple Sclerosis Journal, 14*, 123–128. http://dx.doi.org/10.1177/1352458507080467

Marin, R. S. (1991). Apathy: A neuropsychiatric syndrome. *The Journal of Neuropsychiatry and Clinical Neurosciences, 3*, 243–254. http://dx.doi.org/10.1176/jnp.3.3.243

Matsuda, P. N., Shumway-Cook, A., Bamer, A. M., Johnson, S. L., Amtmann, D., & Kraft, G. H. (2011). Falls in multiple sclerosis. *PM & R, 3*, 624–632. http://dx.doi.org/10.1016/j.pmrj.2011.04.015

McCrae, R. R., & Costa, P. T. (1985). *The NEO personality inventory manual.* Odessa, FL: Psychological Assessment Resources.

Merkelbach, S., König, J., & Sittinger, H. (2003). Personality traits in multiple sclerosis (MS) patients with and without fatigue experience. *Acta Neurologica Scandinavica, 107*, 195–201. http://dx.doi.org/10.1034/j.1600-0404.2003.02037.x

Meyerink, L. H., Reitan, R. M., & Selz, M. (1988). The validity of the MMPI with multiple sclerosis patients. *Journal of Clinical Psychology, 44*, 764–769. http://dx.doi.org/10.1002/1097-4679(198809)44:5<764::AID-JCLP2270440517>3.0.CO;2-Y

Millon, T. (1997). *Millon Clinical Multiaxial Inventory—III.* Bloomington, MN: Pearson Assessments.

Mitsonis, C. I., Potagas, C., Zervas, I., & Sfagos, K. (2009). The effects of stressful life events on the course of multiple sclerosis: A review. *International Journal of Neuroscience, 119*, 315–335. http://dx.doi.org/10.1080/00207450802480192

Mohr, D. C., & Cox, D. (2001). Multiple sclerosis: Empirical literature for the clinical health psychologist. *Journal of Clinical Psychology, 57*, 479–499. http://dx.doi.org/10.1002/jclp.1042

Multiple Sclerosis Council for Clinical Practice Guidelines. (1998). *Fatigue and multiple sclerosis: Evidence based management strategies for fatigue in multiple sclerosis.* Washington, DC: Paralyzed Veterans of America.

Niino, M., Mifune, N., Kohriyama, T., Mori, M., Ohashi, T., Kawachi, I., . . . Kikuchi, S. (2014). Apathy/depression, but not subjective fatigue, is related with cognitive dysfunction in patients with multiple sclerosis. *BMC Neurology, 14,* 3. http://dx.doi.org/10.1186/1471-2377-14-3

Nocentini, U., Caltagirone, C., & Tedeschi, G. (Eds.). (2012). *Neuropsychiatric dysfunction in multiple sclerosis.* Milan, Italy: Springer Science & Business Media. http://dx.doi.org/10.1007/978-88-470-2676-6

Nocentini, U., Tedeschi, G., Migliaccio, R., Dinacci, D., Lavorgna, L., Bonavita, S., . . . Caltagirone, C. (2009). An exploration of anger phenomenology in multiple sclerosis. *European Journal of Neurology, 16,* 1312–1317. http://dx.doi.org/10.1111/j.1468-1331.2009.02727.x

Paparrigopoulos, T., Ferentinos, P., Kouzoupis, A., Koutsis, G., & Papadimitriou, G. N. (2010). The neuropsychiatry of multiple sclerosis: Focus on disorders of mood, affect and behaviour. *International Review of Psychiatry, 22,* 14–21. http://dx.doi.org/10.3109/09540261003589323

Pardini, M., Capello, E., Krueger, F., Mancardi, G., & Uccelli, A. (2013). Reward responsiveness and fatigue in multiple sclerosis. *Multiple Sclerosis Journal, 19,* 233–240. http://dx.doi.org/10.1177/1352458512451509

Passamonti, L., Cerasa, A., Liguori, M., Gioia, M. C., Valentino, P., Nisticò, R., . . . Fera, F. (2009). Neurobiological mechanisms underlying emotional processing in relapsing-remitting multiple sclerosis. *Brain: A Journal of Neurology, 132,* 3380–3391. http://dx.doi.org/10.1093/brain/awp095

Penner, I. K., Bechtel, N., Raselli, C., Stöcklin, M., Opwis, K., Kappos, L., & Calabrese, P. (2007). Fatigue in multiple sclerosis: Relation to depression, physical impairment, personality and action control. *Multiple Sclerosis Journal, 13,* 1161–1167. http://dx.doi.org/10.1177/1352458507079267

Peterson, E. W., Cho, C. C., von Koch, L., & Finlayson, M. L. (2008). Injurious falls among middle aged and older adults with multiple sclerosis. *Archives of Physical Medicine and Rehabilitation, 89,* 1031–1037. http://dx.doi.org/10.1016/j.apmr.2007.10.043

Phares, E. J., & Chaplin, W. F. (1997). *Introduction to personality* (4th ed.). New York, NY: Longman.

Plummer, P., & Eskes, G. (2015). Measuring treatment effects on dual-task performance: A framework for research and clinical practice. *Frontiers in Human Neuroscience, 9,* 225. http://dx.doi.org/10.3389/fnhum.2015.00225

Prosperini, L., Fortuna, D., Giannì, C., Leonardi, L., & Pozzilli, C. (2013). The diagnostic accuracy of static posturography in predicting accidental falls in people with multiple sclerosis. *Neurorehabilitation and Neural Repair, 27,* 45–52. http://dx.doi.org/10.1177/1545968312445638

Raimo, S., Trojano, L., Spitaleri, D., Petretta, V., Grossi, D., & Santangelo, G. (2014). Apathy in multiple sclerosis: A validation study of the apathy evaluation scale. *Journal of the Neurological Sciences, 347*, 295–300. http://dx.doi.org/10.1016/j.jns.2014.10.027

Reznikova, T. N., Terent'eva, I. Y., & Kataeva, G. V. (2007). Variants of personality maladaptation in patients with multiple sclerosis. *Neuroscience and Behavioral Physiology, 37*, 747–754. http://dx.doi.org/10.1007/s11055-007-0077-5

Ryan, K. A., Rapport, L. J., Telmet Harper, K., Fuerst, D., Bieliauskas, L., Khan, O., & Lisak, R. (2009). Fitness to drive in multiple sclerosis: Awareness of deficit moderates risk. *Journal of Clinical and Experimental Neuropsychology, 31*, 126–139. http://dx.doi.org/10.1080/13803390802119922

Schreiber, H., Lang, M., Kiltz, K., & Lang, C. (2015). Is personality profile a relevant determinant of fatigue in multiple sclerosis? *Frontiers in Neurology, 6*, 2. http://dx.doi.org/10.3389/fneur.2015.00002

Schultheis, M. T., Garay, E., & DeLuca, J. (2001). The influence of cognitive impairment on driving performance in multiple sclerosis. *Neurology, 56*, 1089–1094. http://dx.doi.org/10.1212/WNL.56.8.1089

Schultheis, M. T., Garay, E., Millis, S. R., & DeLuca, J. (2002). Motor vehicle crashes and violations among drivers with multiple sclerosis. *Archives of Physical Medicine and Rehabilitation, 83*, 1175–1178. http://dx.doi.org/10.1053/apmr.2002.34279

Shawaryn, M. A., Schultheis, M. T., Garay, E., & DeLuca, J. (2002). Assessing functional status: Exploring the relationship between the multiple sclerosis functional composite and driving. *Archives of Physical Medicine and Rehabilitation, 83*, 1123–1129. http://dx.doi.org/10.1053/apmr.2002.33730

Sosnoff, J. J., Balantrapu, S., Pilutti, L. A., Sandroff, B. M., Morrison, S., & Motl, R. W. (2013). Cognitive processing speed is related to fall frequency in older adults with multiple sclerosis. *Archives of Physical Medicine and Rehabilitation, 94*, 1567–1572. http://dx.doi.org/10.1016/j.apmr.2013.02.009

Sosnoff, J. J., Boes, M. K., Sandroff, B. M., Socie, M. J., Pula, J. H., & Motl, R. W. (2011). Walking and thinking in persons with multiple sclerosis who vary in disability. *Archives of Physical Medicine and Rehabilitation, 92*, 2028–2033. http://dx.doi.org/10.1016/j.apmr.2011.07.004

Stathopoulou, A., Christopoulos, P., Soubasi, E., & Gourzis, P. (2010). Personality characteristics and disorders in multiple sclerosis patients: Assessment and treatment. *International Review of Psychiatry, 22*, 43–54. http://dx.doi.org/10.3109/09540261003589349

Strober, L. B. (2017). Personality in multiple sclerosis (MS): Impact on health, psychological well-being, coping, and overall quality of life. *Psychology Health & Medicine, 22*, 152–161.

Surridge, D. (1969). An investigation into some psychiatric aspects of multiple sclerosis. *The British Journal of Psychiatry, 115*, 749–764. http://dx.doi.org/10.1192/bjp.115.524.749

Thorne, S. E., Harris, S. R., Mahoney, K., Con, A., & McGuinness, L. (2004). The context of health care communication in chronic illness. *Patient Education and Counseling, 54,* 299–306. http://dx.doi.org/10.1016/j.pec.2003.11.009

Uca, A. U., Uguz, F., Kozak, H. H., Turgut, K., Tekin, G., Altas, M., & Akpinar, Z. (2016). Personality disorders in patients with multiple sclerosis: Prevalence and association with depressive and anxiety disorders and clinical features. *Neurology Asia, 21,* 55–61

Wajda, D. A., & Sosnoff, J. J. (2015). Cognitive-motor interference in multiple sclerosis: A systematic review of evidence, correlates, and consequences. *BioMed Research International, 2015,* 720856. http://dx.doi.org/10.1155/2015/720856

White, C. P., White, M., & Russell, C. S. (2007). Multiple sclerosis patients talking with healthcare providers about emotions. *The Journal of Neuroscience Nursing, 39,* 89–101. http://dx.doi.org/10.1097/01376517-200704000-00005

Zarbo, I. R., Minacapelli, E., Falautano, M., Demontis, S., Carpentras, G., & Pugliatti, M. (2016). Personality traits predict perceived health-related quality of life in persons with multiple sclerosis. *Multiple Sclerosis Journal, 22,* 551–558. http://dx.doi.org/10.1177/1352458515594045

8

COGNITION AND ACTIVITIES OF DAILY LIVING IN MULTIPLE SCLEROSIS

YAEL GOVEROVER

Most patients with multiple sclerosis (MS) suffer from some form of physical disability (e.g., lower or upper extremity weakness, change in muscle tone). However, 43% to 70% of patients with MS also experience cognitive impairment (Chiaravalloti & DeLuca, 2008), which, in turn, may negatively affect personal, occupational, and social functioning (Arnett & Strober, 2011; Goverover, Chiaravalloti, & DeLuca, 2016; Goverover, Strober, Chiaravalloti, & DeLuca, 2015). The link between cognitive skills and performance of everyday life activities has been clearly established (e.g., Goverover, Genova, Hillary, & DeLuca, 2007; Kalmar, Gaudino, Moore, Halper, & DeLuca, 2008). For example, persons with MS who have impaired processing speed are more likely to be unemployed and have problems performing daily activities such as cooking (Goverover, Strober, Chiaravalloti, & DeLuca, 2015), and money management (Goverover, Haas, & DeLuca, 2016).

http://dx.doi.org/10.1037/0000097-009
Cognition and Behavior in Multiple Sclerosis, J. DeLuca and B. M. Sandroff (Editors)

The human functioning taxonomy provided by the *International Classification of Functioning, Disability, and Health* (ICF; World Health Organization, 2001) provides an organization of the flow of the link between cognition and performance of activities of daily living (ADLs; see Figure 8.1). The *ICF* identifies three main domains of function: (a) the functions and structures of the body, (b) performance of activities, and (c) participation, referring to involvement in a life situation. Disability can be described as impairments, limitations, and restrictions in any of these three domains, and diverse research has been focusing on the relationship between these three domains (e.g., Goverover et al., 2015). The link between the three domains is not linear but dynamic, with environmental and personal factors serving as moderators of these relationships. However, much controversy surrounds how function is being assessed in research and in practice. In this chapter, the link between body functions, specific to cognition in MS, and performance of activities is discussed, with an emphasis on measurement issues. Participation is not discussed in this specific chapter but in other chapters that focus on involvement in employment, community integration, and quality of life.

Health care professionals often measure a person's functional status by their ability or inability to perform daily self-care activities or ADLs. The concept of ADLs was originally proposed in the 1950s by Katz (Katz, Down,

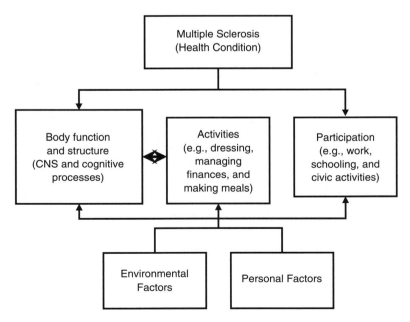

Figure 8.1. The International Classification of Functioning, Disability, and Health model.

Cash, & Grotz, 1970). ADLs are generally grouped into three main types: basic ADLs (BADLs), instrumental ADLs (IADLs), and advanced ADLs (AADLs; American Occupational Therapy Association, 2013).

BADLs (also referred to as personal ADLs) are tasks that are considered fundamental to self-care, including bathing, dressing, feeding, toileting, transferring, and continence. IADLs are those activities that may affect individuals' ability to live independently but are not necessary for personal daily functioning. IADLs usually require both motor and cognitive skills for successful completion and include more complex everyday tasks, such as using the phone, shopping, driving, and managing finances. AADLs represent the highest level of functional tasks and include working, traveling, and attending community services such as church, for example. Completion of these activities requires the successful integration of multiple lesser tasks. Thus, activities at this level may be the first to be affected by changes in health conditions.

Because ADLs tend to follow a hierarchical pattern, clinicians can efficiently assess functional status by inquiring about the most complex levels first. For example, in BADLs, eating is considered to be the easiest and bathing the most difficult (Gerrard, 2013). Thus, a person with MS who experiences problems in the most basic ADLs will most likely have difficulty with the most complex tasks.

Cognition is central to successful engagement in the activities that give life meaning (American Occupational Therapy Association, 2013). Many adults with MS experience cognitive impairments that limit their ability to perform the activities and roles that ensure the safety, independence, and life satisfaction to which most people aspire. Despite the extensive research on the prevalence and impact of cognitive impairments in MS, understanding exactly how these deficits continue to affect everyday performance remains elusive. This chapter focuses on the latest research findings of related to cognitive dysfunction and its impact on daily life in adults with MS. First, the effect of MS on performance of ADLs is presented, including the applications of traditional neuropsychological tests. Second, studies that examine the relationship between cognitive performance and performance of ADLs are discussed, including innovative performance-based test instruments that emphasize ecological validity. The chapter concludes with future directions in this area of practice and research.

ADLs AND MS

Impairments in BADLs, IADLs, and AADLs have been noted in individuals with MS. For example, in a cohort of 166 individuals with MS, only 52% were independent in personal ADLs, with even fewer being independent in IADLs (30%; Einarsson, Gottberg, Fredrikson, von Koch, & Holmqvist, 2006). Additionally, only 35% reported having a normal frequency of social and lifestyle activity participation (which could be considered AADLs), which means that 65% reported having problems in AADLs. Thus, the three types of ADLs were found to be greatly affected in upward of two thirds of people with MS.

In a 10-year follow-up of a population-based study in Stockholm, Chruzander et al. (2013) found that the proportion of the study sample with cognitive impairments, affective symptomatology, and impaired social/lifestyle activities remained stable over the years, whereas the proportion suffering from disability in walking, manual dexterity, and BADLs increased (based on the Barthel Index and the Katz Extended ADL Index; Katz et al., 1970; Mahoney & Barthel, 1965). The proportion of persons with MS who were dependent in BADLs and IADLs increased from 44% to 73% and from 66% to 73%, respectively, over the 10 years. Importantly, MS-related impairments in such ADLs, which are vital life activities, are associated with decreased quality of life and well-being in other research studies (Goverover et al., 2005; Goverover, O'Brien, Moore, & DeLuca, 2010).

Basak, Unver, and Demirkaya (2015) examined the relationship between ADLs and self-care in MS patients who had the disease for the 10 years. The majority of participants were found to be mildly dependent in performing their ADLs, with self-care levels identified as "medium" for 79.1% of the sample, which means that they needed slight help to complete their BADLs. Additionally, longer disease duration was associated with higher dependency levels. Thus, persons with MS may gradually need more help related to ADLs as the disease progresses.

Ytterberg, Johansson, Andersson, Widén Holmqvist, and von Koch (2008) examined variations in functioning and disability, with regard to cognition, manual dexterity, walking, energy, mood, ADLs, and social/lifestyle activities, every 6 months during a 2-year period in 200 persons with MS. Results indicating significant variations in ADLs and social/lifestyle activities were consistent with the 10-year study (i.e., Basak et al., 2015) on ADL trajectory in MS in which nearly all the functions that were studied worsened significantly over the 2-year period, but there was no general deterioration in the sample.

In sum, longitudinal studies using more specific instruments to assess impairments, activity limitations, and participation restrictions in MS are scarce (e.g., Huijbregts, Kalkers, de Sonneville, de Groot, & Polman, 2006). These studies found that individuals with MS have limitations performing both BADLs and IADLs. They may be independent in BADLs but limited in IADLs because their performance requires both motor and cognitive skills (Månsson & Lexell, 2004). Therefore, it is crucial to assess ADLs (i.e.,

BADLs, IADLs, and AADLs) in persons with MS. The studies that were published illustrate the importance of systematic and regular multidimensional assessment of functioning and disability in MS.

ASSESSMENT OF ADLs

Historically, neuropsychological tests were largely used to establish impairment levels related to cognition, but in recent years, interest has grown regarding how neuropsychological test performance relates to everyday functioning (Ruff, 2003). How these tests are interpreted and related to everyday functional activity is an important question. For example, rehabilitation professionals are frequently asked to make inferences about their patients' ability to complete such IADLs as driving, shopping, and preparing meals based on performance scores of neuropsychological tests. This predictive use of neuropsychological testing is based on the link between cognition and functional activities and the need for an efficient way to estimate whether problems can be anticipated in everyday ADLs (Yantz, Johnson-Greene, Higginson, & Emmerson, 2010). One could ask, what would be the best way to measure ADLs and to what assessment of ADLs should we link neuropsychological assessment? However, the development of an in vivo assessment of ADLs remains one of the biggest challenges.

During the 1990s, neuropsychologists developed several tests in an attempt to reflect on everyday situations, such as the Test of Everyday Attention (Robertson, Ward, Ridgeway, & Nimmo-Smith, 1996) and the Behavioral Assessment of the Dysexecutive Syndrome (Wilson, Alderman, Burgess, Emslie, & Evans, 1996). For example, the Test of Everyday Attention was designed to assess attention using stimuli related to everyday life activities, such as searching symbols on a map or counting how many floors an elevator went down or up; the test has good face validity, but it evaluates attention in the same way as the traditional tests did. The only change was the stimuli: Instead of searching and finding numbers on a large piece of paper filled with various shapes and numbers, participants were asked to find a symbol on a map. These newer tests were not reflective and valid measures of everyday life activities, and momentum toward adopting either of these measures has been limited (Yantz et al., 2010).

Another way to assess ADLs is through self- or proxy report or actual performance of the specific activity. Activities are typically scored by the level of assistance the person requires to complete the activity (Goverover et al., 2010). The Functional Independence Measure (FIM; Keith, Granger, Hamilton, & Sherwin, 1987) is one example of a common functional measure of BADLs. With the FIM, the level of patients' disability indicates the burden of caring for them, and items are observed and scored by a health professional on the basis of how much assistance is required for the individual to carry out ADLs. However, the FIM detects mainly activity limitations and amount of assistance required performing BADLs related to the motor impairments (e.g., upper body dressing, toilet transfer) and fewer limitations stemming from cognitive impairments (e.g., social interaction, memory, and problem-solving).

Another common assessment tool used to rank independence in BADLs is the Barthel Index (Mahoney & Barthel, 1965). It is composed of 10 items related to grooming, toilet use, walking, and other items related to performance of BADLs. It is important to note that although the FIM and the Barthel Index are the best researched measures of BADLs, they may not be sensitive to the subtle but important changes in function of persons with MS. Both use a standardized assessment format that does not take into consideration people's individual factors or contextual differences. Additionally, the questions are very general and may not be sufficiently sensitive for detecting small functional changes.

As previously mentioned, IADLs require both motor and cognitive skills for successful completion, and thus are more complicated to assess. A number of IADL assessment tools exist, with the Lawton IADL scale (Lawton & Brody, 1969) being the most widely used. This self-report scale includes eight questions related to IADL performance levels; however, because participants can provide quite general responses, this tool does not always provide an accurate assessment of functional status. For example, for the item "manages financial matters independently," responses can range from *independent*, to *needs help*, to 3 = *incapable of handling money*. Some people do not need or want to handle financial matters, and thus any of these three responses may not necessarily reflect their actual performance. In response to the item about managing laundry, participants can answer *does personal laundry completely*; *launders small items, rinses stockings*; or *all laundry must be done by others*. However, if the participant chose the third option because the laundry is always done by someone else, such as a housekeeper, spouse, or child, their answer still does not reflect why the person does not do his or her laundry. Still, as mentioned earlier, the Lawton and Brody IADL scale is among the most common used assessments to assess IADLs, probably due to its ease of administration and simplification of the IADL construct.

Regarding self-report, interviews and questionnaires are prone to bias for several reasons. Self-report is often inaccurate, especially when a person has little if any experience with a specific task (e.g., the financial example given earlier), impaired self-awareness, or false perception of one's skill level. The accuracy of informant reporting can also vary depending on how close the informant is to the patient, the informant's stress and depressive levels, and the presence of any cognitive impairment. For example, if a significant other needs to rate an item such as, "My family member performs activities that are appropriate to the time of day (sleeps at night, alert during the day)" but does not want to accept the illness, she might convince herself that if the significant other sleeps too much during the day, it is normal behavior. This caregiver may report no problems despite this being incorrect. On the other hand, if a significant other is depressed and anxious, he may report less appropriate behavior or activity then what the patient actually presents. Furthermore, if no caregiver is present, the patient is often excluded from studies focusing on everyday functioning, resulting in biased sampling due to the exclusion of people who are single and oversampling of married patients (Sadek, Stricker, Adair, & Haaland, 2011).

Performance-based assessment of everyday functioning is studied far less frequently than questionnaire-based methods, and only a few investigations have focused on assessing the IADLs in people with MS using this type of assessment (e.g., Doble, Fisk, Fisher, Ritvo, & Murray, 1994; Goverover et al., 2005, 2010; Kalmar et al., 2008), and existing performance-based assessments are, in turn, also limited. For example, Doble et al. (1994) examined the relationship between Assessment of Motor and Process Skills scores (AMPS; Fisher, 1993; an objective, performance-based assessment tool designed to measure personal ADLs and IADLs) and standard clinical ratings on the Expanded Disability Status Scale (EDSS; Kurtzke, 1983), as well as the relationship between AMPS scores and the subjective ratings of general health status on the Sickness Impact Profile (SIP; Pollard, Bobbitt, Bergner, Martin, & Gilson, 1976). Results indicated that MS participants who would not have been expected to have IADL difficulties based on the ratings of neurological impairments (i.e., the EDSS or the SIP) actually were impaired on the AMPS. Correlations were significant between the subjective ratings from the SIP and the motor—but not the process skills—components of the AMPS. It should be noted, however, that only those occupational therapists who have completed a specific training program can administer the AMPS; thus, its use in practice and research is limited.

One of the first studies focusing on IADLs in MS patients (Goverover et al., 2005) examined the relationship between performance of IADLs measured by the Executive Function Performance Test (EFPT; Baum et al., 2008), which is composed of five subtests: preparing a simple and a complex meal, managing finance, using the telephone, and washing hands, with self-report of functional status. Results indicated that self-reports of everyday functional activities did not correlate with actual everyday life performance in persons with MS but did correlate with emotional distresses. Perhaps more important, the EFPT performance was significantly worse for the MS group compared with a healthy control group, especially in the subtests of managing finance and using the telephone. In a second study (Kalmar et al., 2008), neuropsychological scores were significantly associated with the EFPT performance. Thus, the EFPT is a sensitive tool to discriminate between healthy control subjects and persons with MS; however, it is geared toward assessing executive function skills rather than performance of various kinds of ADLs that require more than just executive functions (e.g., memory, attention). Additionally, the EFPT is based on a sample of behaviors representing ADLs.

In another study, the same authors (Goverover et al., 2007) used the Timed Instrumental Activities of Daily Living (TIADL; Owsley, McGwin, Sloane, Stalvey, & Wells, 2001) and found that MS participants required significantly more time to complete this test compared with healthy participants. However, it should be emphasized that the scoring of the TIADL is based on how much time it takes to complete a simple IADL task, such as locating food items on a small shelf, read ingredients on a can of food, or counting change. Thus, similar to the EFPT that focuses on executive functions while performing IADLs, the TIADL assesses one aspect of cognitive functioning: processing speed in performance of IADLs.

Thus, although those studies provide useful information about the functional performance of persons with MS, these performance-based assessment tools (examples of some of these are provided is Table 8.1) have limitations, including safety concerns (e.g., when to ask a person to operate a stove or to walk when stability is an issue), time or space restrictions (e.g., many tests require a kitchen), or patients' physical or medical conditions (e.g., if a person is bound to bed, she may not be able to cook but may be able to order food using a computer). Additionally, administration of some tools (e.g., AMPS) requires special training for both administration and scoring. Most existing instruments use primarily kitchen-based activities, which may be biased by gender or experience. For example, if a person always cooks, he will not show any impairment because his skill level may be procedural. Lastly, many of the performance-based assessments are not detailed or sensitive enough to capture the complexity of daily functioning in persons diagnosed with MS. One such example would be the TIADL, which assesses IADL performance but takes into account only the time it took a person to complete the task and errors that were made, not why the errors were made.

Virtual reality (VR), a more contemporary method to assess ADLs, uses innovative assessment and rehabilitation tools. It presents significant advantages when applied to rehabilitation of patients with MS. These advantages include patient motivation, adaptability, and variability based on patient baseline, transparent data storage, online remote data access, economy of scale, and potentially reduced medical costs. It creates an easy-to-use environment in terms of scoring, recording performance, and giving feedback to participants. VR also has the capacity to create environments that may

TABLE 8.1

Sample of Performance-Based Instruments of IADL

Assessment	Description	Designed for
Assessment of Motor and Process Skills (Fisher, 1993)	Test a person in a relevant and familiar environment as they perform two of their own choice ADL tasks chosen from more than 120 internationally standardized tasks. It is an assessment of observation of the quality of a person's ADL performance. The quality of the person's ADL performance is assessed by observing the degree to which a person's ADL performances are free of increased clumsiness or physical effort, decreased efficiency, safety risk, and/or need for assistance.	Children and adults with developmental, neurological, and/or musculo-skeletal disorders
Executive Function Performance Test (Baum et al., 2008; Goverover et al., 2005)	This performance-based standardized assessment of cognitive function uses four to six IADLs of simple cooking (oatmeal preparation); telephone use; medication management; and bill payment.	Designed for patients with stroke; has been used with MS, adolescents, adults, and older adults
Timed Instrumental Activities of Daily Living test (Owsley et al., 2001)	Measures the time required and accuracy to complete five ADLs. These five tasks include counting out correct change with coins, locating a telephone number in a telephone book, locating ingredients on cans of food (three times), locating two food items on a grocery shelf, and locating and reading the directions on medicine bottles (2 times). If participants completed the tasks correctly, then time needed to complete the task was used. If errors were committed, the error adds a time penalty.	Community-dwelling older healthy control subjects; recently used in MS
Kitchen Task Assessment (Baum & Edwards, 1993)	This test rates the level of cognitive support required for a person to complete the task of making cooked pudding from a commercial package (i.e., independence, verbal cues, physical assistance, or totally incapable). It can be used to record changes in performance over time.	Older clients with senile dementia of the Alzheimer's type across all stages of the disease
Revised Observed Tasks of Daily Living (Diehl et al., 2005)	This performance-based test of everyday problem-solving includes nine tasks, representing medication use, telephone use, and financial management.	Community-dwelling older healthy control subjects; has recently been used with brain injury and schizophrenia
Everyday Problems Test (Willis & Marsiske, 1993)	This test assesses cognitive IADLs with 32 sets of common comprehension and reasoning questions, such as reading medication labels, recipes, and telephone bills	Community-dwelling older healthy control subjects; recently has been used with MS

Note. There are many more measurement tools designed to assess IADL; this table provides a sample of available instruments. ADLs = activities of daily living; HC = healthy control participants; IADLs = instrumental activities of daily living; MS = multiple sclerosis.

be impossible to create in real-life situations, such as driving on a highway (Burdea, 2003) for practice and research. Yet VR is not without its risks or other limitations. For example, it is a representation rather than an actual performance of a task. Whenever possible, assessing performance in the real environment (such as an office) is more realistic than a simulated environment. Also, to use the VR environment, a researcher or clinician must have access to special equipment and help to install it, making it an expensive assessment. What would be ideal is the ability to assess actual everyday life performance. For example, Actual Reality (discussed later in the chapter).

ASSOCIATION BETWEEN COGNITION AND ADLs

In general, neuropsychological performance only explains a moderate portion of variance on performance on real-world tasks of function in persons with MS (i.e., global composite measures of functional outcome; Higginson, Arnett, & Voss, 2000). For example, one study (Higginson et al., 2000) examined the relative efficacy of tests specifically designed with ecological validity in mind versus standard clinical tests assessing memory and attention to predict functional disability in MS patients. Results indicated that tests of memory (Rivermead Behavioural Memory Test; Wilson, Cockburn, & Baddeley, 1985) and attention (Test of Everyday Attention; Robertson, Ward, Ridgeway, & Nimmo-Smith, 1996) that were developed with ecological validity in mind were better predictors of functional disability than memory questionnaires (e.g., Memory Rating Scale; Rao, Hammeke, McQuillen, Khatri, & Lloyd, 1984) and neuropsychological tests of memory and attention (e.g., the California Verbal Learning Test; Delis, Kramer, Kaplan, & Ober, 1987) commonly used in assessing MS patients.

Kalmar et al. (2008) examined the role of cognitive dysfunction assessed by traditional neuropsychological measures, on performance of IADLs by individuals with MS. In that study, 74 adults with MS and 35 healthy control subjects underwent neuropsychological testing and the EFPT. In individuals with MS, cognitive performance based on neuropsychological testing was related to performance on the EFPT. A linear regression model indicated that executive control, in particular, significantly predicted IADL performance, explaining approximately 35% of the variance in everyday life activities. Thus, an assessment tool was needed that would capture a wide range of cognitive skills, such as those presented in MS.

The Internet and other automated tasks are becoming a vital part of everyday life, offering an opportunity for inclusiveness. Internet technologies have the potential to give persons with disabilities the means to live more equitably within the global community in a manner previously not possible by making the world more accessible (Internet Society, 2012). Additionally, more and more people with disabilities are using the Internet to help them function independently in their daily lives—for example, by using social networks, shopping online, or finding needed information. Kraft et al. (2009) administered a survey to 2,352 people with MS living in the United States. Their goal was to better understand attitudes toward and awareness and usage of technology among MS participants. Their results showed that participants with MS were highly technology-reliant, with technology playing a central role in their lives, providing them connections to the resources they need and the people who matter to them, giving them access to information and tools related to treatment, and helping them stay employed and engaged. People with MS who presented more severe symptoms agreed that technology plays a vital role in helping them live with MS. However, awareness of computer-related accessible technology was fairly low, and usage rates were even lower. Respondents reported lack of information as the primary barrier to linking those with MS to the accessible technologies that could greatly improve their quality of life. Thus, the use of computers and technology can improve patient quality of life; therefore, we thought to create an IADL assessment that will rely primarily on Internet and computer use. This approach for assessment is called Actual Reality (AR).

One way to assess actual everyday life functional activity is through Internet use. The AR assessment was designed specifically to use the Internet to assess actual everyday-life IADL performance of persons with disabilities, including MS (Goverover et al., 2010). The AR assessment covers a wide range of cognitive processes required to perform everyday life tasks, such as using actual websites to purchase airline tickets, pizza, and cookies. For example, in the AR task of purchasing cookies using the Internet, participants are asked to use an actual website to purchase cookies as a child's birthday present; for the pizza task, participants are asked to order pizza for a party that night from the website of a popular vendor's website. After a tutorial on basic computer use, participants are instructed to use any of the materials provided (e.g., pen, paper, calendar) and to complete the task as independently as possible. Scoring of the AR is based on rater observation that is focused on errors while performing the AR task, cues given or not given to remedy the errors, and actions the persons make to complete the task (e.g., choose the correct pizza, do not exceed a certain price). One of the biggest advantages of the AR is that anyone can perform an AR assessment as currently conceptualized, with little to no potential physical risk.

In the first study to examine the use of the AR, Goverover et al. (2010) asked both MS and healthy control participants to access the Internet to purchase airline tickets for a round-trip flight to Orlando, Florida. They were also administered the Minimal Assessment of Cognitive Functioning in Multiple

Sclerosis (Benedict et al., 2006) and completed questionnaires to assess quality of life (Functional Assessment of Multiple Sclerosis; Cella et al., 1996), functional status (Functional Behavior Profile; Baum & Edwards, 2000), and prior Internet experience. The MS group displayed significantly more difficulty than the healthy control group in accurately and independently completing the AR task (number of cues needed to complete the task), primarily due to cognitive impairment. Self-report of quality of life and everyday functional abilities did not correlate with AR performance in the MS group, but the self-report measures were significantly associated with affective symptomatology. Measures of processing speed and verbal and visual memory were significantly associated with most AR variables. The primary importance of this study is that performance of AR was found to be associated with cognition, and cognitive performance explained between 40% to 50% of the variance in AR performance (Figure 8.2).

In a follow-up study (Goverover, Chiaravalloti, & DeLuca, 2016), 41 individuals with MS and 32 healthy control participants were presented with the AR tasks of accessing the Internet to purchase an airline ticket or cookies. All participants underwent the Brief International Cognitive Assessment for Multiple Sclerosis (BICAMS; Langdon et al., 2012) and completed questionnaires to assess quality of life, affect symptomatology, and prior

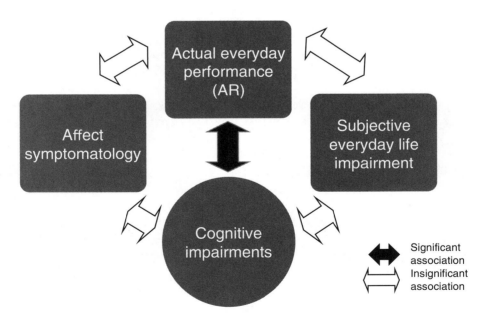

Figure 8.2. Relationship among Actual Reality, cognitive impairments, and self-report of functional performance.

Internet experience. Participants with MS performed significantly worse on the BICAMS and the AR assessment than the healthy control participants. Better BICAMS performance was associated with more independent AR performance and predicted 17% to 24% of variance in AR performance. Self-reports of quality of life did not correlate with AR or BICAMS performance.

In a recent study (Goverover & DeLuca, in press), a third AR task, purchasing pizza online, was added to the airline ticket and cookies tasks. This study established the basic psychometrics for the AR tests: interrater and test–retest reliability and discriminant and concurrent validity of the three AR tasks. Additionally, it showed that processing speed (measured by the Symbol Digit Modalities Test; Smith, 1982) score was the most consistent cognitive variable associated across the three AR tasks.

Cooking activity is also common in the world of IADL assessment. It is one of the IADLs that is important for individuals' sense of life satisfaction (Johnston, Goverover, & Dijkers, 2005). However, few studies have systematically assessed the impact of cognitive impairment on functional cooking skills in individuals with MS. Goverover et al. (2015) examined the variables associated with cooking and employment in 72 people with MS. Participants underwent a comprehensive neuropsychological test battery assessing memory, executive function, visual perception, and processing speed; they also completed questionnaires assessing activity, participation, fatigue, and affective symptoms. Results indicated that processing speed was the only variable that was consistently significantly related to both cooking and employment, affirming that it is a primary cognitive factor in MS and its influence on everyday life activity.

Managing one's own finances is an IADL that is crucial to functioning independently in today's society (Hoskin, Jackson, & Crowe, 2005a, 2005b). Money management is a complex, cognitively demanding task that involves planning (to save, spend, invest, etc.), carrying out these plans, prioritizing, avoiding impulses that contradict these plans, and being able to adjust plans in response to changing circumstances (Hoskin et al., 2005a). Therefore, we recently examined whether MS patients have more problems managing finances than healthy control subjects and, if so, which cognitive skills might contribute to that (Goverover, Haas, & DeLuca, 2016). Money management was assessed by self-report (money management questionnaire) and by AR. Results indicated that individuals with MS did, indeed, report and demonstrate more problems managing money than healthy control subjects. Impaired cognitive functioning significantly correlated with these difficulties. Specifically, processing speed was the only significant predictor, and it explained a significant amount of the variance (18%) in managing finance. Of note, visual memory, working memory, verbal memory, and executive functions were also significantly associated with managing finances in MS.

Importantly, cognitive impairment in MS also has significant consequences for employment (e.g., Strober, Chiaravalloti, Moore, & DeLuca, 2014), which in turn would also affect managing finances and financial status. These data are presented in other chapters of this volume.

In sum, several studies have now looked at a variety of tasks that have explored the relationship between neuropsychological measures and performance on a functional tasks in people with MS and whether people with MS would exhibit more problems performing IADLs than their healthy control counterparts. These studies show that neuropsychological test performance is linked significantly to performance of various tasks of everyday life. These include areas such as paying attention, remembering what we see or hear, expressing ourselves and understanding what other people say, being oriented to our surroundings so that we can travel from place to place, juggling multiple tasks, and reasoning through problems. Furthermore, people with MS seem to present more problems completing IADLs than healthy control subjects. Importantly, patient self-report of cognitive impairment typically does not correlate well with objective neuropsychological tests or with actual everyday life functional activity (e.g., AR). It is also important to remember that neuropsychological test performance only predicted part of the variance associated with everyday functional performance. Thus, more variables need to be taken into account when studying ADLs, such as personality, environmental context, life situation, psychological resources, family, among others. Moreover, independence in ADLs and successful performance of cognitive tests can be masked by mood-related issues, such as depression or anxiety. Therefore, it is important to evaluate day-to-day functioning; if an activity limitation is noticed, a full evaluation should be conducted.

CONCLUSIONS AND FUTURE DIRECTIONS

Recently, attention to the assessment and treatment of functional disability has increased. It is widely understood that impairments in ADLs, including independent living skills, social function, vocational functioning, and self-care, are present in people with MS. It is also clear that assessment of these skills can pose substantial challenges, such as avoiding bias and reduced validity in the data. Self-report and informant reports of ADLs each have certain advantages but appear to be inferior to direct assessment of skills with performance-based measures. However, studies using performance-based measures to assess ADLs have various limitations, as mentioned earlier. Even though the field of functional cognition or assessment of IADLs has some performance-based alternatives to assess ADLs, most studies to date have used self-report measures or nothing at all. For example, a recent systematic review (Goverover, Chiaravalloti, O'Brien, & DeLuca, 2017) regarding the efficacy of cognitive rehabilitation in MS found few studies, if any, that examine the efficacy of assessments of an intervention on ADLs. To date, the field of practice and research related to MS has some assessments to offer (e.g., AR, EFPT) that might be used with persons with MS.

Research suggests that persons with MS exhibit more problems performing IADLs compared with healthy control subjects due to challenges related to their cognitive abilities, vision, speech, and dexterity, and a low percentage of the MS patients have found ways to adapt to these challenges. However, in MS, the use of performance-based objective measures to assess ADLs is scarce. Looking at Figure 8.1 and at the study by Kraft et al. (2009) exemplifies the connections among impairments, activity limitation, and participation restriction. Kraft et al. noted that the noninstitutionalized MS population is highly technology-reliant and that technology seems to play a central role in their lives by providing them connections to the resources they need and the people who matter to them, giving them access to information and tools related to treatment, and helping them stay employed and engaged. Additionally, patients with more severe symptoms are even more likely to benefit from such technology. However, those with more severe symptoms may need more adaptations (environmental and contextual support); unfortunately, awareness of computer-related accessible technologies was fairly low in these participants, and usage rates were even lower. Thus, more attention is needed to observe task performance and perform an analysis to determine the underlying skills necessary for successful performance of a desired task.

Another direction that professionals in the field need to consider is the changes currently occurring in the field of clinical rehabilitation, which places greater emphasis on changing and predicting functional limitations. Thus, the development and adoption of measures that take into consideration real-world behaviors should be strongly considered, at least for patients who are generally high functioning and have only mild to moderate cognitive dysfunction. Better prediction of limitations in MS patients' everyday functioning and efficacy of treatment should help improve treatment planning and patient management and, as such, may lead to better care for individuals suffering from the potentially devastating effects of MS.

REFERENCES

American Occupational Therapy Association. (2013). *About occupational therapy.* Retrieved from http://aota.org/Consumers.aspx

Arnett, P. A., & Strober, L. B. (2011). Cognitive and neurobehavioral features in multiple sclerosis. *Expert Review of Neurotherapeutics, 11,* 411–424. http://dx.doi.org/10.1586/ern.11.12

Basak, T., Unver, V., & Demirkaya, S. (2015). Activities of daily living and self-care agency in patients with multiple sclerosis for the first 10 years. *Rehabilitation Nursing, 40,* 60–65. http://dx.doi.org/10.1002/rnj.153

Baum, M. C., Connor, L. T., Morrison, T., Hahn, M., Dromerick, A. W., & Edwards, D. F. (2008). Reliability, validity, and clinical utility of the Executive Function Performance Test: A measure of executive function in a sample of people with stroke. *American Journal of Occupational Therapy, 62,* 446–455. http://dx.doi.org/10.5014/ajot.62.4.446

Baum, M. C., & Edwards, D. F. (1993). Cognitive performance in senile dementia of the Alzheimer's type: The Kitchen Task Assessment. *American Journal of Occupational Therapy, 47,* 431–436.

Baum, M. C., & Edwards, D. F. (2000). Documenting productive behaviors. Using the functional behavior profile to plan discharge following stroke. *Journal of Gerontological Nursing, 26,* 34–43. http://dx.doi.org/10.3928/0098-9134-20000401-07

Benedict, R. H. B., Cookfair, D., Gavett, R., Gunther, M., Munschauer, F., Garg, N., & Weinstock-Guttman, B. (2006). Validity of the minimal assessment of cognitive function in multiple sclerosis (MACFIMS). *Journal of the International Neuropsychological Society, 12,* 549–558. http://dx.doi.org/10.1017/S1355617706060723

Burdea, G. C. (2003). Virtual rehabilitation—benefits and challenges. *Methods of Information in Medicine, 42,* 519–523.

Cella, D. F., Dineen, K., Arnason, B., Reder, A., Webster, K. A., Karabatsos, G., . . . Stefoski, D. (1996). Validation of the functional assessment of multiple sclerosis quality of life instrument. *Neurology, 47,* 129–139. http://dx.doi.org/10.1212/WNL.47.1.129

Chiaravalloti, N. D., & DeLuca, J. (2008). Cognitive impairment in multiple sclerosis. *The Lancet Neurology, 7,* 1139–1151. http://dx.doi.org/10.1016/S1474-4422(08)70259-X

Chruzander, C., Johansson, S., Gottberg, K., Einarsson, U., Fredrikson, S., Holmqvist, L. W., & Ytterberg, C. (2013). A 10-year follow-up of a population-based study of people with multiple sclerosis in Stockholm, Sweden: Changes in disability and the value of different factors in predicting disability and mortality. *Journal of the Neurological Sciences, 332,* 121–127. http://dx.doi.org/10.1016/j.jns.2013.07.003

Delis, D. C., Kramer, J. H., Kaplan, E., & Ober, B. A. (1987). *CVLT adult version: California Verbal Learning Test Manual, version 1.* San Antonio, TX: Psychological Corporation.

Diehl, M., Marsiske, M., Horgas, A. L., Rosenberg, A., Saczynski, J. S., & Willis, S. L. (2005). The revised observed tasks of daily living: A performance-based assessment of everyday problem solving in older adults. *Journal of Applied Gerontology, 24,* 211–230. http://dx.doi.org/10.1177/0733464804273772

Doble, S. E., Fisk, J. D., Fisher, A. G., Ritvo, P. G., & Murray, T. J. (1994). Functional competence of community-dwelling persons with multiple sclerosis using the assessment of motor and process skills. *Archives of Physical Medicine and Rehabilitation, 75*, 843–851. http://dx.doi.org/10.1016/0003-9993(94)90107-4

Einarsson, U., Gottberg, K., Fredrikson, S., von Koch, L., & Holmqvist, L. W. (2006). Activities of daily living and social activities in people with multiple sclerosis in Stockholm County. *Clinical Rehabilitation, 20*, 543–551. http://dx.doi.org/10.1191/0269215506cr953oa

Fisher, A. G. (1993). The assessment of IADL motor skills: An application of many-faceted Rasch analysis. *American Journal of Occupational Therapy, 47*, 319–329. http://dx.doi.org/10.5014/ajot.47.4.319

Gerrard, P. (2013). The hierarchy of the activities of daily living in the Katz Index in residents of skilled nursing facilities. *Journal of Geriatric Physical Therapy, 36*, 87–91. http://dx.doi.org/10.1519/JPT.0b013e318268da23

Goverover, Y., Chiaravalloti, N., & DeLuca, J. (2016). Brief International Cognitive Assessment for Multiple Sclerosis (BICAMS) and performance of everyday life tasks: Actual reality. *Multiple Sclerosis Journal, 22*, 544–550. http://dx.doi.org/10.1177/1352458515593637

Goverover, Y., Chiaravalloti, N., O'Brien, A., & DeLuca, J. (2017, September 25). Evidence-based cognitive rehabilitation for persons with multiple sclerosis: An updated review of the literature from 2007 to 2016. *Archives of Physical Medicine & Rehabilitation.* Advance online publication. http://dx.doi.org/10.1016/j.apmr.2017.07.021

Goverover, Y., & DeLuca, J. (in press). Assessing everyday life functional activity using Actual Reality™ in persons with MS. *Rehabilitation Psychology.*

Goverover, Y., Genova, H. M., Hillary, F. G., & DeLuca, J. (2007). The relationship between neuropsychological measures and the Timed Instrumental Activities of Daily Living task in multiple sclerosis. *Multiple Sclerosis, 13*, 636–644. http://dx.doi.org/10.1177/1352458506072984

Goverover, Y., Haas, S., & DeLuca, J. (2016). Money management activities in persons with multiple sclerosis. *Archives of Physical Medicine and Rehabilitation, 97*, 1901–1907. http://dx.doi.org/10.1016/j.apmr.2016.05.003

Goverover, Y., Kalmar, J., Gaudino-Goering, E., Shawaryn, M., Moore, N. B., Halper, J., & DeLuca, J. (2005). The relation between subjective and objective measures of everyday life activities in persons with multiple sclerosis. *Archives of Physical Medicine and Rehabilitation, 86*, 2303–2308. http://dx.doi.org/10.1016/j.apmr.2005.05.016

Goverover, Y., O'Brien, A. R., Moore, N. B., & DeLuca, J. (2010). Actual reality: A new approach to functional assessment in persons with multiple sclerosis. *Archives of Physical Medicine and Rehabilitation, 91*, 252–260. http://dx.doi.org/10.1016/j.apmr.2009.09.022

Goverover, Y., Strober, L., Chiaravalloti, N., & DeLuca, J. (2015). Factors that moderate activity limitation and participation restriction in people with multiple sclerosis. *American Journal of Occupational Therapy, 69*, 6902260020p1–9. http://dx.doi.org/10.5014/ajot.2015.014332

Higginson, C. I., Arnett, P. A., & Voss, W. D. (2000). The ecological validity of clinical tests of memory and attention in multiple sclerosis. *Archives of Clinical Neuropsychology, 15,* 185–204. http://dx.doi.org/10.1093/arclin/15.3.185

Hoskin, K. M., Jackson, M., & Crowe, S. F. (2005a). Can neuropsychological assessment predict capacity to manage personal finances? A comparison between brain impaired individuals with and without administrators. *Psychiatry, Psychology and Law, 12,* 56–67. http://dx.doi.org/10.1375/pplt.2005.12.1.56

Hoskin, K. M., Jackson, M., & Crowe, S. F. (2005b). Money management after acquired brain dysfunction: The validity of neuropsychological assessment. *Rehabilitation Psychology, 50,* 355–365. http://dx.doi.org/10.1037/0090-5550.50.4.355

Huijbregts, S. C., Kalkers, N. F., de Sonneville, L. M., de Groot, V., & Polman, C. H. (2006). Cognitive impairment and decline in different MS subtypes. *Journal of the Neurological Sciences, 245,* 187–194. http://dx.doi.org/10.1016/j.jns.2005.07.018

Internet Society. (2012). *Internet accessibility: Internet use by persons with disabilities: Moving forward.* Retrieved from http://www.internetsociety.org/doc/internet-accessibility-internet-use-persons-disabilities-moving-forward

Johnston, M. V., Goverover, Y., & Dijkers, M. (2005). Community activities and individuals' satisfaction with them: Quality of life in the first year after traumatic brain injury. *Archives of Physical Medicine and Rehabilitation, 86,* 735–745. http://dx.doi.org/10.1016/j.apmr.2004.10.031

Kalmar, J. H., Gaudino, E. A., Moore, N. B., Halper, J., & DeLuca, J. (2008). The relationship between cognitive deficits and everyday functional activities in multiple sclerosis. *Neuropsychology, 22,* 442–449. http://dx.doi.org/10.1037/0894-4105.22.4.442

Katz, S., Down, T. D., Cash, H. R., & Grotz, R. C. (1970). Progress in the development of the index of ADL. *The Gerontologist, 10,* 20–30.

Keith, R. A., Granger, C. V., Hamilton, B. B., & Sherwin, F. S. (1987). The functional independence measure: A new tool for rehabilitation. *Advances in Clinical Rehabilitation, 1,* 6–18.

Kraft, G. H., Kennedy, P., Lowenstein, N., Rumrill, P. D., Stewart, T., & Young, M. (2009). Staying connected. *International Journal of MS Care, 11,* 1–16. http://dx.doi.org/10.7224/1537-2073-11.S1.1

Kurtzke, J. F. (1983). Rating neurologic impairment in multiple sclerosis: An expanded disability status scale (EDSS). *Neurology, 33,* 1444–1452. http://dx.doi.org/10.1212/WNL.33.11.1444

Langdon, D. W., Amato, M. P., Boringa, J., Brochet, B., Foley, F., Fredrikson, S., . . . Benedict, R. H. B. (2012). Recommendations for a brief international cognitive assessment for multiple sclerosis (BICAMS). *Multiple Sclerosis Journal, 18,* 891–898. http://dx.doi.org/10.1177/1352458511431076

Lawton, M. P., & Brody, E. M. (1969). Assessment of older people: Self-maintaining and instrumental activities of daily living. *The Gerontologist, 9,* 179–186. http://dx.doi.org/10.1093/geront/9.3_Part_1.179

Mahoney, F. I., & Barthel, D. W. (1965). Functional evaluation: The Barthel Index. *Maryland State Medical Journal, 14,* 61–65.

Månsson, E., & Lexell, J. (2004). Performance of activities of daily living in multiple sclerosis. *Disability and Rehabilitation, 26,* 576–585. http://dx.doi.org/10.1080/09638280410001684587

Owsley, C., McGwin, G., Jr., Sloane, M. E., Stalvey, B. T., & Wells, J. (2001). Timed instrumental activities of daily living tasks: Relationship to visual function in older adults. *Optometry and Vision Science, 78,* 350–359. http://dx.doi.org/10.1097/00006324-200105000-00019

Pollard, W. E., Bobbitt, R. A., Bergner, M., Martin, D. P., & Gilson, B. S. (1976). The Sickness Impact Profile: Reliability of a health status measure. *Medical Care, 14,* 146–155. http://dx.doi.org/10.1097/00005650-197602000-00004

Rao, S. M., Hammeke, T. A., McQuillen, M. P., Khatri, B. O., & Lloyd, D. (1984). Memory disturbance in chronic progressive multiple sclerosis. *Archives of Neurology, 41,* 625–631. http://dx.doi.org/10.1001/archneur.1984.04210080033010

Robertson, I. H., Ward, T., Ridgeway, V., & Nimmo-Smith, I. (1996). The structure of normal human attention: The test of everyday attention. *Journal of the International Neuropsychological Society, 2,* 525–534. http://dx.doi.org/10.1017/S1355617700001697

Ruff, R. M. (2003). A friendly critique of neuropsychology: Facing the challenges of our future. *Archives of Clinical Neuropsychology, 18,* 847–864. http://dx.doi.org/10.1016/j.acn.2003.07.002

Sadek, J. R., Stricker, N., Adair, J. C., & Haaland, K. Y. (2011). Performance-based everyday functioning after stroke: Relationship with IADL questionnaire and neurocognitive performance. *Journal of the International Neuropsychological Society, 17,* 832–840. http://dx.doi.org/10.1017/S1355617711000841

Smith, A. (1982). *Symbol Digit Modalities Test: Manual.* Los Angeles, CA: Western Psychological Services.

Strober, L., Chiaravalloti, N., Moore, N., & DeLuca, J. (2014). Unemployment in multiple sclerosis (MS): Utility of the MS Functional Composite and cognitive testing. *Multiple Sclerosis, 20,* 112–115. http://dx.doi.org/10.1177/1352458513488235

Willis, S. L., & Marsiske, M. (1993). *Manual for the Everyday Problems Test.* University Park: The Pennsylvania State University.

Wilson, B. A., Alderman, N., Burgess, P. W., Emslie, H., & Evans, J. (1996). *Behavioural assessment of the dysexecutive syndrome.* Fareham, England: Thames Valley Test Company.

Wilson, B. A., Cockburn, J., & Baddeley, A. (1985). *The Rivermead Behavioural Memory Test* (pp. 34–36). Fareham, England: Thames Valley Test Company.

World Health Organization. (2001). *International classification of functioning, disability and health (ICF).* Geneva, Switzerland: Author.

Yantz, C. L., Johnson-Greene, D., Higginson, C., & Emmerson, L. (2010). Functional cooking skills and neuropsychological functioning in patients with stroke: An ecological validity study. *Neuropsychological Rehabilitation, 20,* 725–738. http://dx.doi.org/10.1080/09602011003765690

Ytterberg, C., Johansson, S., Andersson, M., Widén Holmqvist, L., & von Koch, L. (2008). Variations in functioning and disability in multiple sclerosis. A two-year prospective study. *Journal of Neurology, 255,* 967–973. http://dx.doi.org/10.1007/s00415-008-0767-0

9

COGNITION AND EMPLOYMENT IN MULTIPLE SCLEROSIS

LAUREN B. STROBER

It is well appreciated that multiple sclerosis (MS) has a grave impact on individuals' social, familial, and occupational roles. With regard to the latter, rates of unemployment in MS range from 24% to 80% (Julian, Vella, Vollmer, Hadjimichael, & Mohr, 2008; LaRocca, Kalb, Kendall, & Scheinberg, 1982) with approximately only 40% of individuals with MS employed (Kobelt, Berg, Lindgren, Fredrikson, & Jönsson, 2006). These rates are in stark contrast to reports that approximately 90% to 96% of individuals with MS are gainfully employed prior to their diagnosis (LaRocca et al., 1982; Pompeii, Moon, & McCrory, 2005). Given the age of disease onset, individuals with MS are typically in the prime of their careers and making important decisions regarding future employment and family life. Given the known physical and mental health benefits of employment and its overarching role on well-being and quality of life, it is imperative that individuals with MS do their best to maintain their employment, and that practitioners and allied services help

Portions of this work were funded by the National Institutes of Health NCMRR K23 HD069494.

http://dx.doi.org/10.1037/0000097-010
Cognition and Behavior in Multiple Sclerosis, J. DeLuca and B. M. Sandroff (Editors)

their patients accomplish this goal. This chapter is a review of what is known about the benefits of employment, in general, as well as among individuals with MS. The factors, including cognition, that have been shown to account for the high rates of unemployment in MS are explored, and the chapter concludes with a discussion of future directions and the need for study with regard to employment issues in MS.

COSTS AND BENEFITS ASSOCIATED WITH EMPLOYMENT STATUS

It is well known that unemployment in the general population is associated with a host of negative outcomes. Unemployment has been linked to poorer overall physical health, increased mental health problems, engagement in negative health-related behaviors, increased mortality, and even a greater suicide rate (Harris, Harris, & Shortus, 2010; Janlert, 1997; Lin, Shah, & Svoboda, 1995; Linn, Sandifer, & Stein, 1985; Lundin, Lundberg, Hallsten, Ottosson, & Hemmingsson, 2010). These decreases in health correspond with increased utilization of general and mental health care (Jin, Shah, & Svoboda, 1995; Linn et al., 1985). Such findings suggest that individuals simply become "sick" following loss of employment. When there is a pre-existing health condition, such as MS, it is possible that these outcomes may be more detrimental as patients may simply become "sicker." Reports among individuals with MS suggest that this may be the case, wherein unemployed individuals with MS report significantly lower scores on physical and mental health outcomes than employed persons with the disease (Solari & Radice, 2001). Moreover, as stated above, unemployed individuals have also been shown to engage in increasing negative health-related behaviors such as smoking and alcohol use; this has been shown in MS as well (Strober & Arnett, 2016). Some of these consequences of unemployment are seen in only a short time period (e.g., 6 months) (Linn et al., 1985) and suggest that among individuals with a disability, even short-term unemployment can have significant mental and physical health implications and may also produce a barrier for reemployment.

In contrast, investigations consistently report improvements in mental and physical health following reemployment. In particular, a 1-year longitudinal investigation of individuals who left work for a medical illness found that those that returned to work demonstrated greater improvements in physical and mental health than those that did not return (Pattani, Constantinovici, & Williams, 2004). Similarly, reemployment within 6 months is associated with increases in physical and mental health, with effect sizes ranging from .11 to .66; the largest effects being for mental health, social functioning, and role limitations due to emotional or physical problems (Schuring, Mackenbach, Voorham, & Burdorf, 2011).

While the evidence is clear that employment is associated with physical and mental health, being gainfully employed is also an integral part of one's identity, self-esteem, and value system. Women actively engaged in the workforce are more confident (Clausen & Gilens, 1990) and more emotionally stable (Roberts & Chapman, 2000). It has also been shown that those invested in a career have higher self-esteem (Baruch & Barnett, 1986), and that those whose work is more complex are likely to be more intellectually flexible, take more personal responsibility, have greater self-esteem, are more likely to engage in intellectually demanding leisure activities, and are more receptive to innovation and change (Miller, Schooler, Kohn, & Miller, 1979). Such attributes can be particularly important for women who are managing an unpredictable, chronic illness such as MS.

These benefits of employment are certainly seen in the descriptions provided by individuals with MS and are likely to be beneficial to their overall well-being, health, and quality of life (QOL). When specifically asked, approximately 40% of unemployed individuals with MS report wanting to return to work (Johnson & Fraser, 2005; Pompeii et al., 2005) and consider work as having much more benefit than mere financial gain, stating that it is a way of being part of society. Johnson et al. (2004) also found that individuals with MS view work as important to their identity, self-esteem, and social contact, with many describing it as "therapeutic" (Johnson et al., 2004). Finally, many have demonstrated a significant association between employment in MS and health-related as well as overall QOL (Krokavcova et al., 2010; Miller & Dishon, 2006; Pack, Szirony, Kushner, & Bellaw, 2014; Patti et al., 2007; Solari & Radice, 2001). Similarly, Pack and colleagues (2014) reported that employed individuals rate their overall QOL one third of a standard deviation higher than those unemployed. Thus, maintenance of employment in MS is likely to have a substantial impact on ones' QOL, health status, social support, and illness management and is a likely contributor to overall well-being in the long term. However, to achieve this, one must consider the hurdles that individuals with MS report with regard to employment.

UNEMPLOYMENT IN MS

Reports as early as the 1960s suggested a high (nearly 70%) unemployment rate among individuals with MS (Bauer, Firnhaber, & Winkler, 1965). Subsequent reports in the late 1970s and early 1980s indicated that unemployment was a "significant but potentially treatable problem in MS" (Scheinberg et al., 1981, p. 61), with reports of unemployment ranging from

45% to 80% (LaRocca, Kalb, Scheinberg, & Kendall, 1985; Rozin, Schiff, Kahana, & Soffer, 1975; Scheinberg et al., 1981). Over the past 50 years, these rates have remained fairly stable, ranging from 40% to 80% (see Table 9.1).

Such high rates of unemployment are striking given again that many individuals with MS are in the prime of their careers. Moreover, while MS is often progressive and presumably prevents individuals from maintaining employment later in the disease process, reports of unemployment have been shown to be as high as 70% to 80% within only the first 5 years of diagnosis, a time at which disability may be rather minimal for many (Kornblith, LaRocca, & Baum, 1986). Given this fact, efforts to identify the factors associated with such early departure from the workforce have been a top priority

TABLE 9.1
Rates of Unemployment Reported
Over the Past Five Decades (1965–2015)

Author, year	Sample size (N)	Rate of unemployment (%)
Bauer et al., 1965	258	69
Rozin et al., 1975	172	45
Scheinberg et al., 1981	257	80
LaRocca et al., 1982	312	77
Kornblith et al., 1986	949	80
Jackson et al., 1991	210	76
Edgley et al., 1991	602	67
Beatty et al., 1995	102	63
Solari & Radice, 2001	251	41
Busche et al., 2003	96	48
Smith & Arnett, 2005	50	42
O'Connor et al., 2005	100	64
Phillips & Stuifberg, 2006	176	45
Julian et al., 2008	8,867	56
Uccelli et al., 2009	1,141	39
Simmons et al., 2010	667	64
Honarmand et al., 2011	106	61
Morrow et al., 2010	97	45
Krokavcova et al., 2010	184	56
Strober et al., 2012	111	42
Krause et al., 2013	87	45
Moore et al., 2013	169	43
Strober et al., 2014	77	48
van Der Hiele et al., 2014	44	43
Pack et al., 2014	1,171	55
Cadden & Arnett, 2015	53	38
Honan et al., 2015	111	44
van der Hiele et al., 2015	55	64
Strober & Arnett, 2015	68	40

and area of investigation over the past approximately 30 years. Reports as far back as the early 1980s suggested that physical disability was not enough to account for the high rate of unemployment in an otherwise highly functioning population (Scheinberg et al., 1981). In one of the seminal studies of employment in MS around that time, LaRocca and colleagues (1985) confirmed that disability level, age, gender, and education only account for 14% of the variance in predicting employment status among their sample in which 77% were unemployed (see Figure 9.1). Such findings suggest that 86% of the variance is unexplained.

It was proposed then that premorbid personality, coping style, characteristics of the workplace, and social support systems were likely to contribute to the probability of an individual with MS staying employed. Nearly 2 decades later, Rätsep, Kallasmaa, Pulver, and Gross-Paju (2000) asserted that psychosocial disability remains unexplained solely by disease severity or sociodemographic variables, and recommended that more attention be given to the role that personality and coping has on the adjustment to MS, including employment status (Rätsep et al., 2000). While more recent work has investigated these latter factors, there is abundant literature examining the demographic and disease-related factors associated with unemployment in MS, which we review first.

Disease and Demographic Factors Associated With Unemployment in MS

Men with MS are more likely to be unemployed than women—the rate of unemployment among men is approximately 4.8 times higher than for women with MS (Raggi et al., 2016; Simmons, Tribe, & McDonald, 2010). Older age (Busche, Fisk, Murray, & Metz, 2003; Krokavcova et al., 2010; O'Connor, Cano, Ramió i Torrentà, Thompson, & Playford, 2005) and less education have also been shown to be predictive of job loss (Flensner, Landtblom, Söderhamn, & Ek, 2013; Lunde et al., 2014; Smith & Arnett,

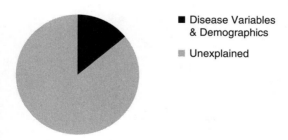

■ Disease Variables & Demographics

▨ Unexplained

Figure 9.1. Variance accounted for in predicting employment status in 1985.

2005). When examining certain disease characteristics, individuals with MS with greater disability level (Busche et al., 2003; Honarmand, Akbar, Kou, & Feinstein, 2011; Julian et al., 2008; Smith & Arnett, 2005) and/or a progressive course are more likely to be unemployed than those with a relapsing-remitting course (Julian et al., 2008; Morales-Gonzáles et al., 2004; Pompeii et al., 2005); a longer disease duration also has been shown to play a role (Busche et al., 2003; Julian et al., 2008; Putzki et al., 2009). Other disease factors shown to influence rates of unemployment in MS include poor balance and difficulty walking (O'Connor et al., 2005), bladder/bowel incontinence, heat sensitivity (Simmons et al., 2010), and fatigue—with fatigue being the greatest culprit (Dyck & Jongbloed, 2000; Edgley, Sullivan, & Dehoux, 1991; Simmons et al., 2010; see Table 9.2).

TABLE 9.2
Primary Reasons (%) Cited by Individuals With MS
for Work Difficulties of Leaving the Workforce

Symptom(s)	1980[a]	1985[b]	1991[c]	2003[d]	2005[e]	2007[d]
Fatigue	9.3	13.9	50.3	79.1	28	69.5
Lower extremity physical problems				54.9		43.8
Upper extremity physical problems				44.8		39.4
General physical difficulties/ limitations	52.7	27.5				
Muscle weakness			42.9		15	
Cognitive difficulties			8.3	34.7	12	36.7
Balance or dizziness				41.5	40	31.2
Mobility/walking difficulties			52.4		45	
Heat sensitivity				34.1		30.0
Bowel/bladder problems			40.7	28.3	14	23.1
Pain				20.8	9	23.3
Visual problems	15.9	7.4	22.6	23.5	12	17.1
Tremor				15.7		14.9
Non-pain sensations symptoms				16.1		13.1
Speaking difficulties				9.7	1	9.7
Handwriting					26	
Coordination difficulties					11	
Emotional difficulties	1.6	2.8	13		1	
Transportation difficulties	12.1	7.9			48	
Other (mostly marriage and/or pregnancy)	37.4	15.6				

Note. Data from the following studies: [a]Scheinberg et al., 1981; [b]LaRocca et al., 1985; [c]Jackson, Quaal, & Reeves, 1991; [d]Simmons, Tribe, & McDonald, 2010; [e]O'Connor et al., 2005.

Cognitive Factors Associated With Unemployment in MS

As can be seen in Table 9.2, cognitive impairment is a primary reason for work difficulties. More specifically, deficits in information processing speed and memory have been shown to greatly contribute to individuals leaving the workforce or sustaining changes in work status (Honan, Brown, & Batchelor, 2015; Strober, Chiaravalloti, Moore, & DeLuca, 2014). Among the handful of studies that have included a comprehensive assessment of factors contributing to lack of employment status, cognitive functioning, impairments in processing speed, and memory have consistently reigned as the most significant culprits (accounting for an additional 5% to 20% of the variance in predicting employment status), above and beyond disease and demographic factors (Honan et al., 2015; Morrow et al., 2010; L. Strober et al., 2012, 2014). Specifically, one measure of information processing speed, the Symbol Digit Modalities Test (SDMT), has been shown to account for the greatest amount of variance in employment status—ranging from 5% to 20% of the variance. Effect sizes for differences in SDMT scores between employed and unemployed persons with MS were also found to be significantly large—ranging from $d = 0.80$ to 0.88 across these four recent studies. More striking is that this effect size is consistent with a 9- to 10-point difference on the SDMT across the four study populations. More recently, Campbell, Rashid, Cercignani, and Langdon (2017) found an even greater effect size of 1.39, which was associated with a difference of 13 or more points on the SDMT. Moreover, when examining cognitive performance on a recommended neuropsychological test battery, the SDMT reigned as the most salient predictor of employment status. With regard to learning and memory, performance on simple word list learning tasks, such as the California Verbal Learning Test (CVLT), have been shown to differentiate those who are working and those that are no longer employed. In fact, Morrow and colleagues (2010) sought to determine if "clinically meaningful decline" in cognition would predict changes in employment status among individuals with MS. To accomplish this, they followed 97 employed individuals over a year's time and compared neuropsychological testing at baseline and follow-up between individuals who reported no change in their employment status and those who reported a deterioration. Individuals who reported a deterioration in work status demonstrated a significant decline on measures of learning, memory, and processing speed. In contrast, those who reported no change in their work status demonstrated an improvement on those measures. The authors further contend that a decline of 4 points on the SDMT and 2 points on total learning on the CVLT-Second Edition (CVLT-II) distinguished those who remained employed and those who progressed to work disability. Thus, although fairly large differences on cognitive testing (e.g., 9–13 points on the SDMT) may distinguish those who are working from those who are not working, small changes on an individual basis may be clinically meaningful when it comes to changes in employment status in MS.

Others have examined the role of executive functioning on work difficulties or unemployment in MS. More specifically, it has been hypothesized that executive functions, such as multitasking, organization, planning, or working memory, would play a large role in the ability to maintain employment. It was shown in a fairly small sample ($N = 30$) that individuals who cut back on their working hours performed worse on a multitasking test than those who were able to maintain their working hours (Morse, Schultheis, McKeever, & Leist, 2013). In another study, van der Hiele and colleagues (2015) found that unemployed persons with MS reported greater difficulties in organization, planning, and sustained attention and were more easily distracted than their employed counterparts. However, on objective testing of executive functions, the only difference between employed and unemployed individuals was the number of correct sorts of the Wisconsin Card Sorting Test.

In sum, changes or difficulties in processing speed and/or learning and memory and, to a lesser extent, executive function, are most likely accountable for individuals having difficulty at work and/or leaving the workforce. Efforts to ameliorate and/or treat these cognitive impairments are likely to assist individuals with MS in maintaining their employment. Moreover, given what we know of cognitive reserve in MS (Sumowski, Chiaravalloti, & DeLuca, 2009), and the role of occupational attainment, early intervention(s) aimed at assuring that individuals with MS achieve their occupational goals may mitigate further cognitive decline. Related to this, consideration should be given to the association of cognitive functioning and employment status when examining cognitive outcomes, such as cognitive reserve. Study samples that are biased toward either employed or unemployed participants may not be most representative of the MS population as a whole and may over- or underestimate cognitive functioning in MS. Finally, the majority of investigations examining employment issues in MS have been retrospective. Future prospective, longitudinal studies that examine cognitive functioning over time, and how this relates to employment difficulties and/or departure from the workforce (and subsequent follow-up), are warranted in hopes of having a better understanding as to how cognitive functioning contributes to employment status in MS over the course of the illness. Nonetheless, what can be gleaned from the present literature is that cognitive difficulties can contribute an additional 20% of explained variance above disease and demographic variables, when attempting to understand the factors associated with unemployment in MS. More specifically, upon closer look of the investigations conducted so far, it is estimated that upward of 43% of the variance in employment status can now be accounted for by demographics, disease variables, and cognition (see Figure 9.2).

This is an overall decrease in unexplained variance from the reported figure of 86% in 1985, but still leaves approximately 57% of the variance unexplained. We turn now to a brief discussion of other factors worthy of consideration when examining employment issues in MS. These factors have received less attention but are otherwise worthy of investigation.

Person-Specific Factors as Contributors to Unemployment in MS

As stated earlier, one of the first seminal studies examining the predictors of unemployment in MS suggested that further consideration be given to the role of factors such as personality, coping, and features of the workplace. More recently, research has identified that personality, namely persistence or conscientiousness, was a significant predictor of employment status, above and beyond disease severity and cognitive impairment (Strober et al., 2012). In fact, personality independently accounted for 4% of the variance in employment status, compared with 15% for disease severity and 5% for SDMT performance (see Figure 9.3).

The finding that persistence, a facet of conscientiousness, was predictive of employment status is not surprising as persistence is viewed as the degree to which individuals are industrious, hardworking, persistent, and stable, despite frustration and fatigue (Benjamin et al., 2000). Highly persistent individuals are considered ambitious and perfectionistic and demonstrate a determination and tenacity to achieve a goal (Judge, Higgins, Thoresen, & Barrick, 1999). Moreover, earlier work suggests that conscientiousness, as rated by an informant, was predictive of work status in MS (Benedict et al., 2005). More recently, another investigation demonstrated that other facets

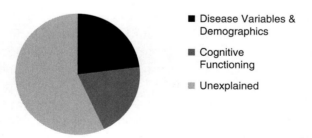

■ Disease Variables & Demographics

■ Cognitive Functioning

▨ Unexplained

Figure 9.2. Variance accounted for in predicting employment status in present day across several studies.

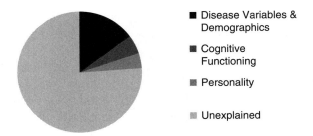

Figure 9.3. Variance accounted for in predicting employment status by demographics, disease variables, cognitive functioning, and personality. Data from Strober et al., 2012.

of personality may play a role in employment status. Specifically, individuals with MS who endorsed having a "Type D or distressing" personality, as evident by high neuroticism and social discomfort, were more likely to report feeling as if they needed to leave the workforce. In fact, compared to individuals who were remaining employed, individuals considering leaving the workforce were nearly twice as likely to have these personality traits as those who intended to continue working (Strober, 2017).

With regard to coping, it has also been reported that coping styles may differentiate those who are employed from those who are not. Unemployed women with MS are seemingly more likely to engage in maladaptive coping, such as behavioral disengagement and substance use (Strober & Arnett, 2016). Most recently, it has also been shown that avoidant coping, such as denial, is a predictor of shorter time to disability among individuals with MS who were, on average, fairly early on in the disease process (Grytten et al., 2017). Finally, when examining the role of workplace factors, employed women described their work as being a positive event in their lives. Indeed, job security and fellow coworkers were considered to be an uplift (Strober & Arnett, 2016). This latter finding supports the contention that individuals with MS perceive their work colleagues and the support they may receive from them as a benefit; this is consistent with earlier work in which individuals with MS report that working provides great social support (Johnson et al., 2004). Findings suggest that, although certain demographics, disease factors, and cognitive impairment(s) are significant contributors to changes in employment status in MS, there are other more mutable psychological factors that may also play a role in determining who with MS stays in the workforce and who is more likely to leave. Consideration of these factors seems imperative when assisting individuals with MS in making informed decisions regarding employment. Moreover, interventions aimed at addressing these factors (e.g., coping) are likely to have a substantial impact not only on employment, but overall functioning and adjustment to MS. Further investigations examining the contribution of these factors and the outcomes of intervention aimed at ameliorating them are also warranted and are likely the next step in understanding the multitude of factors associated with employment in MS.

CONCLUSIONS AND FUTURE DIRECTIONS

In conclusion, employment serves as a great proxy for overall QOL and plays a significant role on physical health, mental well-being, self-esteem, and purpose in life. Rates of unemployment in MS are high and can be attributed to a host of factors, many of which warrant intervention. Specifically, interventions aimed at ameliorating fatigue and cognitive impairment may hold the most merit followed by vocational rehabilitation/workplace accommodations addressing issues such as mobility issues, heat sensitivity, bowel/bladder issues, and balance concerns. Consideration of other psychological factors, such as personality, coping, and self-efficacy, will also likely yield a greater understanding of the multitude of person-specific factors influencing employment in MS. It is hoped that the present chapter alerts practitioners, researchers, and patients to the importance of such, implores researchers to consider these factors when investigating employment issues in MS, and enlightens clinicians when making informed decisions with their patients. Finally, efforts should be made to implement greater vocational rehabilitation services for individuals with MS, potentially early on in the disease process and as routine care, in hopes that we can assure that individuals can meet their career goals and remain in the workforce for as long as possible.

REFERENCES

Baruch, G. K., & Barnett, R. C. (1986). Role quality, multiple role involvement, and psychological well-being in midlife women. *Journal of Personality and Social Psychology, 51,* 578–585. http://dx.doi.org/10.1037/0022-3514.51.3.578

Bauer, H. J., Firnhaber, W., & Winkler, W. (1965). Prognostic criteria in multiple sclerosis. *Annals of the New York Academy of Sciences, 122,* 542–551. http://dx.doi.org/10.1111/j.1749-6632.1965.tb20234.x

Beatty, W. W., Blanco, C. R., Wilbanks, S. L., Paul, R. H., & Hames, K. A. (1995). Demographic, clinical, and cognitive characteristics of multiple sclerosis patients who continue to work. *Neurorehabilitation and Neural Repair, 9*, 167–173. http://dx.doi.org/10.1177/154596839500900306

Benedict, R. H. B., Wahlig, E., Bakshi, R., Fishman, I., Munschauer, F., Zivadinov, R., & Weinstock-Guttman, B. (2005). Predicting quality of life in multiple sclerosis: Accounting for physical disability, fatigue, cognition, mood disorder, personality, and behavior change. *Journal of the Neurological Sciences, 231*, 29–34. http://dx.doi.org/10.1016/j.jns.2004.12.009

Benjamin, J., Osher, Y., Lichtenberg, P., Bachner-Melman, R., Gritsenko, I., Kotler, M., . . . Ebstein, R. P. (2000). An interaction between the catechol O-methyltransferase and serotonin transporter promoter region polymorphisms contributes to tridimensional personality questionnaire persistence scores in normal subjects. *Neuropsychobiology, 41*, 48–53. http://dx.doi.org/10.1159/000026632

Busche, K. D., Fisk, J. D., Murray, T. J., & Metz, L. M. (2003). Short term predictors of unemployment in multiple sclerosis patients. *The Canadian Journal of Neurological Sciences/Le Journal Canadien des Sciences Neurologiques, 30*, 137–142.

Cadden, M., & Arnett, P. (2015). Factors associated with employment status in individuals with multiple sclerosis. *International Journal of MS Care, 17*, 284–291. http://dx.doi.org/10.7224/1537-2073.2014-057

Campbell, J., Rashid, W., Cercignani, M., & Langdon, D. (2017). Cognitive impairment among patients with multiple sclerosis: Associations with employment and quality of life. *Postgraduate Medical Journal, 93*, 143–147. http://dx.doi.org/10.1136/postgradmedj-2016-134071

Clausen, J. A., & Gilens, M. (1990). Personality and labor force participation across the life course: A longitudinal study of women's careers. *Sociological Forum, 5*, 595–618.

Dyck, I., & Jongbloed, L. (2000). Women with multiple sclerosis and employment issues: A focus on social and institutional environments. *Canadian Journal of Occupational Therapy, 67*, 337–346. http://dx.doi.org/10.1177/000841740006700506

Edgley, K., Sullivan, M. J., & Dehoux, E. (1991). A survey of multiple sclerosis: II. Determinants of employment status. *Canadian Journal of Rehabilitation.*

Flensner, G., Landtblom, A.-M., Söderhamn, O., & Ek, A.-C. (2013). Work capacity and health-related quality of life among individuals with multiple sclerosis reduced by fatigue: A cross-sectional study. *BMC Public Health, 13*, 224. http://dx.doi.org/10.1186/1471-2458-13-224

Grytten, N., Skår, A. B., Aarseth, J. H., Assmus, J., Farbu, E., Lode, K., . . . Myhr, K. M. (2017). The influence of coping styles on long-term employment in multiple sclerosis: A prospective study. *Multiple Sclerosis Journal, 23*, 1008–1017. http://dx.doi.org/10.1177/1352458516667240

Harris, M. F., Harris, E., & Shortus, T. D. (2010). How do we manage patients who become unemployed? *The Medical Journal of Australia, 192*, 98–101.

Honan, C. A., Brown, R. F., & Batchelor, J. (2015). Perceived cognitive difficulties and cognitive test performance as predictors of employment outcomes in people with multiple sclerosis. *Journal of the International Neuropsychological Society, 21,* 156–168. http://dx.doi.org/10.1017/S1355617715000053

Honarmand, K., Akbar, N., Kou, N., & Feinstein, A. (2011). Predicting employment status in multiple sclerosis patients: The utility of the MS functional composite. *Journal of Neurology, 258,* 244–249. http://dx.doi.org/10.1007/s00415-010-5736-8

Jackson, M. F., Quaal, C., & Reeves, M. A. (1991). Effects of multiple sclerosis on occupational and career patterns. *Axone, 13,* 16–17, 20–22.

Janlert, U. (1997). Unemployment as a disease and diseases of the unemployed. *Scandinavian Journal of Work, Environment & Health, 23*(Suppl. 3), 79–83.

Jin, R. L., Shah, C. P., & Svoboda, T. J. (1995). The impact of unemployment on health: A review of the evidence. *CMAJ: Canadian Medical Association Journal, 153,* 529–540.

Johnson, K. L., & Fraser, R. T. (2005). Mitigating the impact of multiple sclerosis on employment. *Physical Medicine and Rehabilitation Clinics of North America, 16,* 571–582. http://dx.doi.org/10.1016/j.pmr.2005.01.004

Johnson, K. L., Yorkston, K. M., Klasner, E. R., Kuehn, C. M., Johnson, E., & Amtmann, D. (2004). The cost and benefits of employment: A qualitative study of experiences of persons with multiple sclerosis. *Archives of Physical Medicine and Rehabilitation, 85,* 201–209. http://dx.doi.org/10.1016/S0003-9993(03)00614-2

Judge, T. A., Higgins, C. A., Thoresen, C. J., & Barrick, M. R. (1999). The big five personality traits, general mental ability, and career success across the life span. *Personnel Psychology, 52,* 621–652. http://dx.doi.org/10.1111/j.1744-6570.1999.tb00174.x

Julian, L. J., Vella, L., Vollmer, T., Hadjimichael, O., & Mohr, D. C. (2008). Employment in multiple sclerosis: Exiting and re-entering the work force. *Journal of Neurology, 255,* 1354–1360. http://dx.doi.org/10.1007/s00415-008-0910-y

Kobelt, G., Berg, J., Lindgren, P., Fredrikson, S., & Jönsson, B. (2006). Costs and quality of life of patients with multiple sclerosis in Europe. *Journal of Neurology, Neurosurgery & Psychiatry, 77,* 918–926. http://dx.doi.org/10.1136/jnnp.2006.090365

Kornblith, A. B., La Rocca, N. G., & Baum, H. M. (1986). Employment in individuals with multiple sclerosis. *International Journal of Rehabilitation Research, 9,* 155–165. http://dx.doi.org/10.1097/00004356-198606000-00006

Krause, I., Kern, S., Horntrich, A., & Ziemssen, T. (2013). Employment status in multiple sclerosis: Impact of disease-specific and non-disease-specific factors. *Multiple Sclerosis Journal, 19,* 1792–1799. http://dx.doi.org/10.1177/1352458513485655

Krokavcova, M., Nagyova, I., Van Dijk, J. P., Rosenberger, J., Gavelova, M., Middel, B., . . . Groothoff, J. W. (2010). Self-rated health and employment status in patients with multiple sclerosis. *Disability and Rehabilitation, 32,* 1742–1748. http://dx.doi.org/10.3109/09638281003734334

LaRocca, N., Kalb, R., Kendall, P., & Scheinberg, L. (1982). The role of disease and demographic factors in the employment of patients with multiple sclerosis. *Archives of Neurology, 39,* 256. http://dx.doi.org/10.1001/archneur.1982.00510160062016

LaRocca, N., Kalb, R., Scheinberg, L., & Kendall, P. (1985). Factors associated with unemployment of patients with multiple sclerosis. *Journal of Chronic Diseases, 38,* 203–210. http://dx.doi.org/10.1016/0021-9681(85)90093-1

Lin, R. L., Shah, C. P., & Svoboda, T. J. (1995). The impact of unemployment on health: A review of the evidence. *African Journal of Medical Practice, 2,* 176–179.

Linn, M. W., Sandifer, R., & Stein, S. (1985). Effects of unemployment on mental and physical health. *American Journal of Public Health, 75,* 502–506. http://dx.doi.org/10.2105/AJPH.75.5.502

Lunde, H. M. B., Telstad, W., Grytten, N., Kyte, L., Aarseth, J., Myhr, K.-M., & Bø, L. (2014). Employment among patients with multiple sclerosis—a population study. *PLoS ONE, 9,* e103317. http://dx.doi.org/10.1371/journal.pone.0103317

Lundin, A., Lundberg, I., Hallsten, L., Ottosson, J., & Hemmingsson, T. (2010). Unemployment and mortality—A longitudinal prospective study on selection and causation in 49321 Swedish middle-aged men. *Journal of Epidemiology and Community Health, 64,* 22–28. http://dx.doi.org/10.1136/jech.2008.079269

Miller, A., & Dishon, S. (2006). Health-related quality of life in multiple sclerosis: The impact of disability, gender and employment status. *Quality of Life Research, 15,* 259–271. http://dx.doi.org/10.1007/s11136-005-0891-6

Miller, J., Schooler, C., Kohn, M. L., & Miller, K. A. (1979). Women and work: The psychological effects of occupational conditions. *American Journal of Sociology, 85,* 66–94. http://dx.doi.org/10.1086/226974

Moore, P., Harding, K. E., Clarkson, H., Pickersgill, T. P., Wardle, M., & Robertson, N. P. (2013). Demographic and clinical factors associated with changes in employment in multiple sclerosis. *Multiple Sclerosis Journal, 19,* 1647–1654.

Morales-Gonzáles, J. M., Benito-León, J., Rivera-Navarro, J., Mitchell, A. J., & the GEDMA Study Group. (2004). A systematic approach to analyse health-related quality of life in multiple sclerosis: The GEDMA study. *Multiple Sclerosis, 10,* 47–54. http://dx.doi.org/10.1191/1352458504ms967oa

Morrow, S. A., Drake, A., Zivadinov, R., Munschauer, F., Weinstock-Guttman, B., & Benedict, R. H. B. (2010). Predicting loss of employment over three years in multiple sclerosis: Clinically meaningful cognitive decline. *The Clinical Neuropsychologist, 24,* 1131–1145. http://dx.doi.org/10.1080/13854046.2010.511272

Morse, C. L., Schultheis, M. T., McKeever, J. D., & Leist, T. (2013). Multitasking in multiple sclerosis: Can it inform vocational functioning? *Archives of Physical Medicine and Rehabilitation, 94,* 2509–2514. http://dx.doi.org/10.1016/j.apmr.2013.06.033

O'Connor, R. J., Cano, S. J., Ramió i Torrentà, L., Thompson, A. J., & Playford, E. D. (2005). Factors influencing work retention for people with multiple sclerosis: Cross-sectional studies using qualitative and quantitative methods. *Journal of Neurology, 252,* 892–896. http://dx.doi.org/10.1007/s00415-005-0765-4

Pack, T. G., Szirony, G. M., Kushner, J. D., & Bellaw, J. R. (2014). Quality of life and employment in persons with multiple sclerosis. *Work, 49,* 281–287.

Pattani, S., Constantinovici, N., & Williams, S. (2004). Predictors of re-employment and quality of life in NHS staff one year after early retirement because of ill health: A national prospective study. *Occupational and Environmental Medicine, 61,* 572–576. http://dx.doi.org/10.1136/oem.2003.011817

Patti, F., Pozzilli, C., Montanari, E., Pappalardo, A., Piazza, L., Levi, A., . . . the Italian Study Group on Quality of Life in MS. (2007). Effects of education level and employment status on HRQoL in early relapsing-remitting multiple sclerosis. *Multiple Sclerosis, 13,* 783–791. http://dx.doi.org/10.1177/1352458506073511

Phillips, L. J., & Stuifbergen, A. K. (2006). Predicting continued employment in persons with multiple sclerosis. *Journal of Rehabilitation, 72,* 35–43.

Pompeii, L. A., Moon, S. D., & McCrory, D. C. (2005). Measures of physical and cognitive function and work status among individuals with multiple sclerosis: A review of the literature. *Journal of Occupational Rehabilitation, 15,* 69–84. http://dx.doi.org/10.1007/s10926-005-0875-y

Putzki, N., Fischer, J., Gottwald, K., Reifschneider, G., Ries, S., Siever, A., . . . Hartung, H. P. (2009). Quality of life in 1000 patients with early relapsing–remitting multiple sclerosis. *European Journal of Neurology, 16,* 713–720. http://dx.doi.org/10.1111/j.1468-1331.2009.02572.x

Raggi, A., Covelli, V., Schiavolin, S., Scaratti, C., Leonardi, M., & Willems, M. (2016). Work-related problems in multiple sclerosis: A literature review on its associates and determinants. *Disability and Rehabilitation, 38,* 936–944. http://dx.doi.org/10.3109/09638288.2015.1070295

Rätsep, T., Kallasmaa, T., Pulver, A., & Gross-Paju, K. (2000). Personality as a predictor of coping efforts in patients with multiple sclerosis. *Multiple Sclerosis, 6,* 397–402. http://dx.doi.org/10.1191/135245800701566386

Roberts, B. W., & Chapman, C. N. (2000). Change in dispositional well-being and its relation to role quality: A 30-year longitudinal study. *Journal of Research in Personality, 34,* 26–41. http://dx.doi.org/10.1006/jrpe.1999.2259

Rozin, R., Schiff, Y., Kahana, E., & Soffer, D. (1975). Vocational status of multiple sclerosis patients in Israel. *Archives of Physical Medicine and Rehabilitation, 56,* 300–304.

Scheinberg, L., Holland, N., Larocca, N., Laitin, P., Bennett, A., & Hall, H. (1981). Vocational disability and rehabilitation in multiple sclerosis. *International Journal of Rehabilitation Research, 4,* 61–63. http://dx.doi.org/10.1097/00004356-198103000-00008

Schuring, M., Mackenbach, J., Voorham, T., & Burdorf, A. (2011). The effect of re-employment on perceived health. *Journal of Epidemiology and Community Health, 65,* 639–644. http://dx.doi.org/10.1136/jech.2009.103838

Simmons, R. D., Tribe, K. L., & McDonald, E. A. (2010). Living with multiple sclerosis: Longitudinal changes in employment and the importance of symptom management. *Journal of Neurology, 257*, 926–936. http://dx.doi.org/10.1007/s00415-009-5441-7

Smith, M. M., & Arnett, P. A. (2005). Factors related to employment status changes in individuals with multiple sclerosis. *Multiple Sclerosis, 11*, 602–609. http://dx.doi.org/10.1191/1352458505ms1204oa

Solari, A., & Radice, D. (2001). Health status of people with multiple sclerosis: A community mail survey. *Neurological Sciences, 22*, 307–315. http://dx.doi.org/10.1007/s10072-001-8173-8

Strober, L. B. (2017). Personality in multiple sclerosis (MS): Impact on health, psychological well-being, coping, and overall quality of life. *Psychology, Health and Medicine, 22*, 152–161. http://dx.doi.org/10.1080/13548506.2016.1164321

Strober, L. B., & Arnett, P. A. (2015). Unemployment among women with multiple sclerosis: The role of coping and perceived stress and support in the workplace. *Psychology, Health & Medicine, 112*, 1–9. http://dx.doi.org/10.1080/13548506.2015.1093645

Strober, L. B., Chiaravalloti, N., Moore, N., & DeLuca, J. (2014). Unemployment in multiple sclerosis (MS): Utility of the MS Functional Composite and cognitive testing. *Multiple Sclerosis, 20*, 112–115. http://dx.doi.org/10.1177/1352458513488235

Strober, L. B., Christodoulou, C., Benedict, R. H. B., Westervelt, H. J., Melville, P., Scherl, W. F., . . . Krupp, L. B. (2012). Unemployment in multiple sclerosis: The contribution of personality and disease. *Multiple Sclerosis Journal, 18*, 647–653. http://dx.doi.org/10.1177/1352458511426735

Sumowski, J. F., Chiaravalloti, N., & DeLuca, J. (2009). Cognitive reserve protects against cognitive dysfunction in multiple sclerosis. *Journal of Clinical and Experimental Neuropsychology, 31*, 913–926. http://dx.doi.org/10.1080/13803390902740643

Uccelli, M. M., Specchia, C., Battaglia, M. A., & Miller, D. M. (2009). Factors that influence the employment status of people with multiple sclerosis: A multinational study. *Journal of Neurology, 256*, 1989–1996. http://dx.doi.org/10.1007/s00415-009-5225-0

van der Hiele, K., Middelkoop, H. A. M., Ruimschotel, R., Kamminga, N. G. A., & Visser, L. H. (2014). A pilot study on factors involved with work participation in the early stages of multiple sclerosis. *PloS One, 9*, e105673. http://dx.doi.org/10.1371/journal.pone.0105673

van der Hiele, K., van Gorp, D., Ruimschotel, R., Kamminga, N. G. A., Visser, L., & Middelkoop, H. (2015). Work participation and executive abilities in patients with relapsing-remitting multiple sclerosis. *PloS ONE, 10*, e0129228. http://dx.doi.org/10.1371/journal.pone.0129228

10

ECONOMIC IMPACT OF COGNITIVE IMPAIRMENT IN MULTIPLE SCLEROSIS

STEN FREDRIKSON

Multiple sclerosis (MS) is an inflammatory and degenerative disease of the central nervous system. The age at onset of MS is usually between 20 and 40 years of age. The global prevalence of MS is estimated to be around 2.5 million people, with a very uneven geographical distribution. The areas with the highest prevalence of MS are found in North America and Europe. In the United States, it has been estimated that there are approximately 400,000 persons with MS. Several recent studies from various countries have reported an increase in both incidence and prevalence of the disease. In prevalent areas, MS is a potentially disabling disease with a great impact on the life of the patient and the patient's family. The symptoms of MS are highly variable between different individuals and include sensory and motor disturbances, sometimes making the patient wheelchair bound, presenting problems with vision, bladder, coordination, and speech. During the latest

I would like to thank Gösta Bergendal, PhD (neuropsychologist), and Alice Fredrikson, MSc (economics), for carefully reviewing the manuscript based on their respective fields of expertise.

http://dx.doi.org/10.1037/0000097-011
Cognition and Behavior in Multiple Sclerosis, J. DeLuca and B. M. Sandroff (Editors)

three decades, so-called "invisible symptoms," including pain, depression, fatigue, and cognitive impairment, have been highlighted as important symptoms in MS.

Objective neuropsychological findings show cognitive dysfunction in 45 to 70% of the patients with MS. The most common cognitive symptoms include slowed information processing, impaired short-term memory, and attention deficits (for a review, see DeLuca, Yates, Beale, & Morrow, 2015). Longitudinal studies have shown decline in cognitive function over the disease course, e.g., information processing over 8 and 17 years of follow-up (Bergendal, Fredrikson, & Almkvist, 2007; Granberg et al., 2015). In a population-based study, approximately half of the persons with MS showed cognitive dysfunction at screening (Einarsson et al., 2006), a finding in line with results from studies in clinical settings. The concurrent occurrence of depression and fatigue may be confounders when evaluating the cognitive functions in a person with MS. Fatigue is one of the most debilitating symptoms in MS and may interfere with social activities (Dettmers & DeLuca, 2015). Fatigue is subjective and sometimes difficult to evaluate. Fatigue and anxiety (but not depression, as reported by others) have recently been found to be the strongest predictor of self-reported cognitive concerns (Beier, Amtmann, & Ehde, 2015). When looking at the complete picture, it is also of importance to evaluate the possible influence of comorbid diagnoses and medication on cognitive function. It is also of interest to note that accuracy to predict the neuropsychological test results based on the ordinary neurologist's examination is not better than chance (Romero, Shammi, & Feinstein, 2015). This finding should be considered when discussing how employers may interpret the cognitive function of their employed MS patients. Taken together, it is now well established that impaired cognitive functioning disrupts the societal and professional life in patients with MS (Benedict & Zivadinov, 2011).

A chronic and disabling disease with young adult onset (i.e., during the early and most productive years of life) will, of course, have societal consequences with health care costs as well as costs due to unemployment and early retirement. It has been reported that more than 90% of patients with MS have been working before diagnosis, while only 20% to 40% remain employed following their diagnosis. In a cross-sectional and longitudinal American study of more than 8,000 patients, based on registry data, almost 60% of the MS patients were unemployed (Julian, Vella, Vollmer, Hadjimichael, & Mohr, 2008). Several studies have shown a correlation between decreased physical function, as measured by Expanded Disability Status Scale (EDSS), and higher levels of unemployment. It has, however, also been reported that fatigue, cognitive dysfunction, and issues with employers contribute to why people stop working (for a review, see Pompeii, Moon, & McCrory, 2005).

Indeed, some early studies have shown that cognitive function differs between employed and unemployed (Beatty, Blanco, Wilbanks, Paul, & Hames, 1995; Rao et al., 1991), with cognitively impaired patients being less likely to be employed. Even self-perceived cognitive deficit has been associated with unemployment (Edgley, Sullivan, & Dehoux, 1991). In summary, although absence from work may be a multi-factorial process, in that it is difficult to exactly specify one single reason for inability to work at the individual level, impaired cognition might play an important role.

The present chapter provides an overview of the economic burden of MS as described in various countries and makes an attempt to evaluate to what extent cognitive dysfunction will contribute to the economic burden of MS. It is an "expensive" disease from a societal perspective, which often also influences the financial situation of the individual patient. The indirect costs (i.e., costs for sick leave and unemployment) usually dominate. The societal costs of MS will usually increase during the course of the disease as a consequence of increasing cognitive and physical disability. Because cognitive impairment is an important factor leading to unemployment, there is a logical link between impaired cognition and higher societal costs. A major challenge in evaluating cognitive impairment in MS is to exclude, or at least compensate for, the confounding factors like fatigue or depression.

ECONOMIC ASPECTS OF MS

The different types of studies in health economy are outlined in Exhibit 10.1 and Figure 10.1. There are several costs to consider when performing cost-of-illness studies in MS (see Exhibit 10.1). First, there are the direct medical costs including medication, in- and outpatient care, and medical and paraclinical consultations. Second, there are nonmedical direct costs, including devices, transportation, modifications of living environments, and informal care provided by family and friends. As a third component, there are indirect costs mainly due to productivity loss, including sick leave and early retirement. The fourth cost, an intangible cost, is an attempt to evaluate the cost of suffering and refers to the impact of MS on quality of life. The costs can then be looked at from three different perspectives: (a) at the individual level (what it means for the patient); (b) at the payer's (budgetary) perspective, including direct cost for medications; and (c) at the societal perspective, taking into account all costs, regardless of who pays. The latter approach is often most appropriate when evaluating the gross economic burden of a disease.

It should already be clear from the beginning, that the economic impact of cognitive impairment in MS has rarely been commented on as a specific part in the economic evaluations that have been published about MS. The evidence that cognition has an economic impact is mostly indirect.

Some early health economic studies in MS in the 1990s were cost-of-illness based. These studies were descriptive, and the aim was to show the total cost of MS to society. One early cost-of-illness study from the United States estimated the annual cost of MS to be $34,000 USD per person, giving

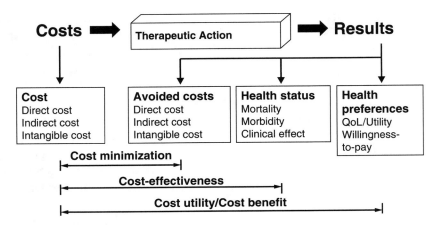

Figure 10.1. Structure of economic evaluation in health economy.

a conservative estimate of a national annual cost of at least $6.8 billion USD and a total lifetime cost per case of $2.2 million USD (Whetten-Goldstein, Sloan, Goldstein, & Kulas, 1998). In this study, indirect costs and costs of informal care dominated. Many of the cost-of-illness studies from the 1990s were based on data collected from patients before the broader use of disease-modifying therapies. Some of these early studies did show that costs increase with the severity of disease (Henriksson, Fredrikson, Masterman, & Jönsson, 2001), a finding that was later confirmed (Kobelt, Berg, Lindgren, Fredrikson, & Jönsson, 2006; see also Figure 10.2).

Other types of MS economic studies are the cost-effectiveness studies and cost-utility studies (see Exhibit 10.1 and Figure 10.1). The aim of these studies is to evaluate the cost-effectiveness of different interventions. A cost-effectiveness study is focused on a unidimensional outcome variable, e.g., "number of relapses avoided" after a specific intervention. The cost-utility study has an advantage over a cost-effectiveness study in that it enables the evaluation of the effect on the quality of life of the patient, combined with the time of the effect. In cost-utility studies, this combined outcome measure

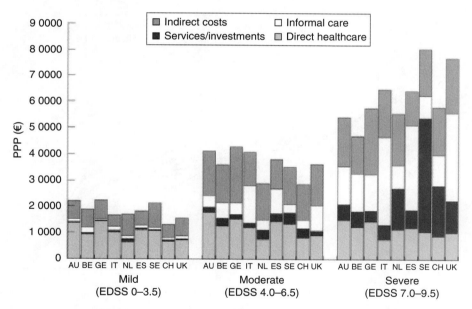

Figure 10.2. Total costs of MS increase at higher EDSS levels in several European countries. AU = Austria; BE = Belgium; CH = Switzerland; ES = Spain; GE = Germany; IT = Italy; NL = The Netherlands; SE = Sweden; UK = United Kingdom. From "Costs and Quality of Life of Patients With Multiple Sclerosis in Europe," by G. Kobelt, J. Berg, P. Lindgren, S. Fredrikson, and B. Jönsson, 2006, *Journal of Neurology, Neurosurgery, and Psychiatry, 77*, p. 922. Copyright 2006 by BMJ Publishing Group. Adapted with permission.

is called quality adjusted life years (QALY). Because it has been shown (see Figure 10.3) that the quality of life deteriorates dramatically over the disease course in MS (Kobelt et el., 2006), preservation of QALY is an important outcome measure after interventions.

During recent years, there have been several studies aimed at evaluating the total and individual cost of MS. A huge study examined the cost of brain disorders in Europe (adjusted to 2010 values) and reported the cost of MS, based on an estimation of approximately 540,000 patients in Europe, to be 14.6 billion euro (Gustavsson et al., 2011). This total cost is similar to that of epilepsy (13.8 billion euro), though epilepsy is a much more prevalent disorder (2.6 million people with epilepsy vs. 540,000 people with MS). The annual cost per subject was 26,974 euro for MS compared with 5,221 euro for epilepsy. Among the studied neurological diseases (MS, Parkinson's disease, stroke, traumatic brain injury, brain tumors, epilepsy, migraine), one of the highest costs per person has been found in MS (Andlin-Sobocki, Jönsson, Wittchen, & Olesen, 2005; Gustavsson et al., 2011). See Figure 10.4.

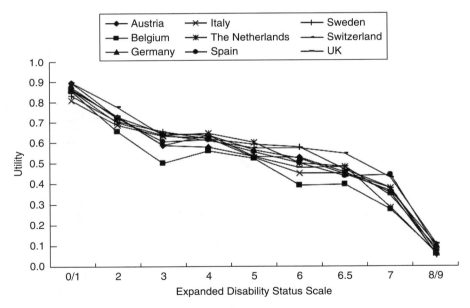

Figure 10.3. Utility scores, signifying the satisfaction accruing to a person from the consumption of a good or service. Calculated with the original EuroQol—five domains (EQ-5D) health status system in all countries. From "Costs and Quality of Life of Patients With Multiple Sclerosis in Europe," by G. Kobelt, J. Berg, P. Lindgren, S. Fredrikson, and B. Jönsson, 2006, *Journal of Neurology, Neurosurgery, and Psychiatry, 77*, p. 924. Copyright 2006 by BMJ Publishing Group. Adapted with permission.

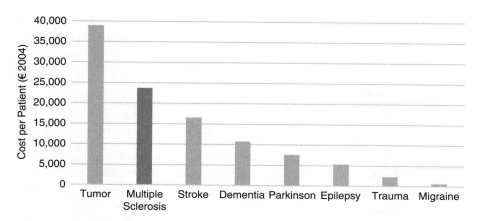

Figure 10.4. Cost per patient for some neurological disorders. From "Cost of Disorders of the Brain in Europe," by P. Andlin-Sobocki, B. Jönsson, H.-U. Wittchen, and J. Olesen, 2005, *European Journal of Neurology, 12*, Suppl. 1, p. 11. Copyright 2005 by John Wiley and Sons. Adapted with permission.

In another study based on more than 13,000 patients in nine European countries, the proportion of patients in early retirement due to MS ranged from 33% to 45%, while the proportion of patients still employed and working ranged between 26% to 42% (Kobelt et al., 2006). This study found that the single highest contributor to societal costs was productivity losses. A systematic review of the cost burden of MS in the United States found MS to be the second most costly chronic condition (after congestive heart failure) for average annual direct costs (Adelman, Rane, & Villa, 2013). The total mean costs (converted from "cost year" to U.S. dollars in 2011) for patients with MS ranged from $8,528 US to $54,244 US per patient per year. In the studies included in the systematic review, there was a wide range of indirect costs, up to $19,733 US per patient per year. Based on five studies in this review, direct costs comprised 64% to 91% and indirect costs comprised 9% to 36% (23% on average) of the total annual cost. This distribution with predominant direct costs is not a general finding in other (mainly European) studies.

A review aimed at identifying the relationship between EDSS and the cost of MS, written by American authors, found that both direct and indirect costs rise continuously with increasing EDSS, a rise that is qualitatively exponential (Patwardhan et al., 2005). The total costs are more similar in studies involving persons with MS with lower EDSS levels and vary significantly in studies involving those with higher EDSS levels. The significant variation is probably a result of the difference in the various national health care systems.

A recent review of the annual cost of MS in the United States reported the annual economic cost to be approximately $28 billion USD, with out-of-pocket expenditures for neurological disorders like MS exceeding expenditures for diabetes, stroke, mental illness, and heart disease (Ma, Chan, & Carruthers, 2014).

A systematic review of the economic burden of MS identified 29 cost-of-illness studies (Naci, Fleurence, Birt, & Duhig, 2010) from Europe, the United States, Canada, and Australia. A major finding among them was that there was a significant increase in costs associated with an increase in disease severity and disability measured by EDSS. Naci and colleagues (2010) found that indirect costs far outweighed the direct costs in later stages of the disease, mainly due to productivity losses, while direct costs (mainly disease-modifying drugs) contributed importantly during earlier stages of the disease. The review included studies from Austria, Australia, Belgium, Canada, France, Germany, Italy, the Netherlands, Poland, Spain, Sweden, Switzerland, the United Kingdom, and the United States. Differences in cultural norms played a significant role in the economic implications of MS when so many countries were reviewed.

In examining studies at the national level, one recent Italian study found that, in 2011, 0.8% of health care expenditure was referred to MS, corresponding to 2.5 billion euro (Ponzio et al., 2015). In another national study from Australia, the largest component (48%) of the societal cost of MS was indirect costs due to loss of productivity (Palmer, Colman, O'Leary, Taylor, & Simmons, 2013). Interestingly, this study found that the total costs of MS to Australian society increased with 58% between 2005 and 2010. When comparing results of health economy studies in MS over the years, it should be remembered that the prevalence of this disease is constantly changing (i.e., increasing), partly due to new diagnostic criteria, which include more benign and early cases of MS.

One part of the economic analysis that can be difficult to evaluate is the importance of intangible costs—the costs associated with disease-related changes in patient reported quality of life (hrQoL). The QALY is assigned a monetary value to calculate the intangible cost. Because it is known from studies in different countries that patients with MS report low hrQoL (see Figure 10.3), the intangible costs of this disease cannot be neglected. In a review of 13 identified studies from 10 countries, the intangible costs accounted for 17.5% to 47.8% of the total costs of MS, which is a substantial contribution to the overall economic burden of MS (Wundes, Brown, Bienen, & Coleman, 2010). The authors found that the largest increase in intangible costs occurred at the transition between mild and moderate disability (i.e., where disability is severe enough to prevent full daily activities). The hrQoL decreases with increasing EDSS, but it is not fully clear how cognitive impairment affects the intangible costs.

COGNITION AND EMPLOYMENT

A separate chapter in this book provides a detailed overview of cognition and employment. It has been described that employment rates in MS are affected up to 8 years before diagnosis and drop steadily after diagnosis, such that at 5 years postdiagnosis, only 50% are employed. Regarding overall employment status in patients with MS, the reported rate of unemployment varies between 22% and 80% (for a review, see Cadden & Arnett, 2015). Several MS symptoms may predict the future employment status, including cognition, fatigue, depression, and motor difficulties (for a review, see Cadden & Arnett, 2015). When comparing unemployed with employed MS patients, performance on tests of processing speed, working memory, and verbal fluency was worse in those who were unemployed (Morrow et al., 2010; Strober, Chiaravalloti, Moore, & DeLuca, 2014).

It is well-established in cross sectional studies that there is a correlation between neuropsychological test performance and vocational status in MS (Beatty et al., 1995; for a review, see Morrow et al., 2010; Rao et al., 1991). Fatigue, perceived cognitive dysfunction, and poor performance on neuropsychological tests have all been associated with employment problems in MS (for a review, see Julian et al., 2008). Unemployment (among females) with MS has recently been evaluated and found to be higher in patients who were older, had a longer disease duration and progressive course, reported greater fatigue, and performed worse on cognitive tests (Strober & Arnett, 2016). At an individual level, cognitive function, motor symptoms and fatigue have been found to be significantly associated with unemployment.

There are also several disease-specific factors that may contribute to inability to work. One recent study evaluated motor function, cognition, depression, and fatigue in employed versus unemployed persons with MS (the study population was 85% females; Cadden & Arnett, 2015). Briefly, it was found that only cognitive, motor, and fatigue composite scores were significantly associated with unemployed individuals (Cadden & Arnett, 2015).

What test can be used to evaluate cognition in relation to employment status? Symbol Digit Modalities Test (SDMT) has been suggested as a tool to access cognition and work disability (Benedict & Zivadinov, 2011; Krause, Kern, Horntrich, & Ziemssen, 2013). Others have found SDMT (but not PASAT) to be a significant predictor of employment status (Strober et al., 2014). One recent study established benchmark scores of SDMT that is associated with specific degree of impairment in work status (Benedict et al., 2016).

Decline in the SDMT and California Verbal Learning Test-Total Learning (CVLT2-TL) have been shown among patients employed at baseline to predict a clinical meaningful functional decline (Morrow et al., 2010). The factor of time on cognition (i.e., the correlation between disease duration and cognitive dysfunction) is not as clear as what has been shown about the correlation between EDSS and disease duration (Lynch, Parmenter, & Denney, 2005).

A vicious cycle has been described in the interplay between fatigue, cognition, and employment status—fatigue increased cognitive problems, leading to increased mental effort, and more fatigue—all symptoms that are invisible at the workplace that directly affect the ability to work (Johnson et al., 2004). Thus, memory and processing speed are influential on work capacity and these abilities should be considered (together with other symptoms) if or when making vocational suggestions.

It is obvious that the employment status will influence the financial status of most individuals with MS. The employment status and household income are closely related to the quality of life (Miller & Dishon, 2006).

DISCUSSION

As the text above indicates, specific evaluations of the economic impact of cognitive impairment are scarce. Data on such basic aspects as the extent to which cognitive rehabilitation can keep MS patients at work for additional years seem to be lacking.

MS is associated with high personal and societal costs due to its early onset (usually the third or fourth decade of life) and duration, which covers the most productive years in life. Cognitive impairment has been shown to cause unemployment, resulting in higher indirect costs. Indirect costs are the dominant driver of the economic burden from a societal perspective. Thus, cognitive impairment will cause economic burden not only to the affected individual, but also to society.

The study of cognition in MS has a short history (even though Charcot mentioned cognitive symptoms almost a century ago), and the history of health economy in MS is even shorter. In a study 25 years ago about work performance in persons with MS, cognition was not even mentioned among possible factors impeding work ability (Gulick, Yam, & Touw, 1989). The interplay among MS symptoms expressed as cognitive impairment and fatigue, work participation, and financial security of the individual patient and the societal costs is a complex matter. There is a clear need of further studies to delineate the specific economic impact of cognitive impairment. Future approaches to improve cognitive impairment may be of great economic value.

First of all, it must be understood that the effects of cognitive impairment on societal costs (including sick leave, early retirement, etc.) should be considered in the context of a specific health care insurance system. Despite variations in national health care systems, it is interesting to see the similarities between various health economy studies in MS.

Some findings seem to be clear regarding cognition in MS and the economic burden of the disease: (a) direct costs of disease-modifying treatments play, so far, a role mainly in earlier phases of the disease; (b) most studies show that indirect costs, mainly due to productivity loss, constitute the major economic burden of the disease, and dominate in later stages of the disease; (c) unemployment is common in patients diagnosed with MS; (d) unemployed patients with MS score worse on neuropsychological tests and perceive more cognitive deficits compared to employed MS patients; (e) cognitive dysfunction can occur at any disease stage in MS and, if it occurs early in the disease course, it may influence the ability to work when the patient is in the prime of life; (f) cognitive impairment can be expected to persist and deteriorate once apparent. Thus, cognition in MS has a major impact on the economic burden and societal costs of MS. However, the dollar/euro amount per year for the economic cost of cognitive impairment in MS has never been calculated.

Metacognition is self-perceived, cognitive functioning. It is not only objective cognitive impairment that may interfere with social activities, but also individuals who perceive themselves to be cognitively impaired may be less likely to participate in daily social activities and work. So that, metacognition, the perception of cognitive dysfunction, also may have economic consequences (Hughes et al., 2015). It does seem probable that the metacognition is more accurate in MS patients with mild cognitive impairment than in individuals with more advanced neuropsychological dysfunction. Thus, the costs of self-reported cognitive decline early in the disease can be expected to be lower than the costs of actual long-term cognitive impairment.

Because it is well known that MS mainly affects females, most studies of cognition and employment status have included a majority of females. Male patients with early evidence of cerebral gray matter atrophy have been reported to be most prone to cognitive impairment (Benedict & Zivadinov, 2011). Since the socioeconomic conditions differ between the sexes, further analysis of the economic burden of gender-specific cognitive decline will be of interest.

Can any measure be taken to reduce the impact of cognition on the economic burden of MS? This is, of course, a very important question. Because it is clear that cognitive impairment can occur early in the course of the disease in some patients with MS, an early intervention seems appropriate. Based on the cognitive reserve hypothesis, stating that a high level of cognitive functioning from onset may be protective to cognitive decline, it seems reasonable that early initiated cognition enhancement activities could be beneficial to prevent cognitive decline (and thus unemployment and higher societal costs). The saved economic burden from early intervention, of course, cannot yet be estimated, but considering the major role of cognitive impairment for unemployment, the potential savings can be expected to be of great importance.

CONCLUSIONS AND FUTURE DIRECTIONS

A question to be analyzed in future research is to what extent the evolution and use of new disease modifying therapies, connected with high direct costs, will influence the long term outcome on cognitive impairment and on indirect societal costs of sick leave and early retirement. Hopefully, and most likely, there will be new drugs introduced in the near future, with new modes of action including prevention of neurodegeneration. Some of these new drugs may also be used in later stages of the disease, which may increase direct costs in later (and progressive) phases of MS, while ultimately aiming to reduce indirect costs. An interesting study would be to evaluate the cost savings over time that could be achieved by a new drug aimed at preventing cognitive decline. Because unemployment due to cognitive decline occurs early, the savings may be important.

Another future challenge will be to evaluate whether the complex interactions of factors that, on an epidemiological study level, influence unemployment in MS (e.g., years of education, premorbid financial situation, degree of disability, cognitive dysfunction, occupational prestige, fatigue, desire to work, workplace conditions) can be adapted to the individual level for prediction of work capacity in a single MS patient and the corresponding economic burden. It will also be of great interest to develop paraclinical methods to measure cognition, such as imaging studies that can visualize cerebral degeneration and correlate the findings to cognitive symptoms. When this is possible, it will facilitate the possibility of objectively following the results of therapeutic interventions. Although today it may seem like science fiction to discuss a biochemical marker in blood that may predict or measure cognitive symptoms, such a marker, if found, would definitely be of great value in measuring the cost-effectiveness of different cognitive interventions.

Because cognitive dysfunction and fatigue have become more accepted as symptoms of substantial importance to the vocational and financial status of MS patients, and also of great importance for work ability and societal costs, it should be easy to motivate the treating neurologists to highlight these symptoms in the clinical evaluation. However, so far, this has not been widely adopted. A short, only minutes long, screening of cognitive status by using the SDMT could be feasible even in a busy clinical setting and may prove worthwhile in the long run. An early awareness and detection of cognitive impairment could initiate preventive measures aiming at avoiding unemployment and economic burden.

REFERENCES

Adelman, G., Rane, S. G., & Villa, K. F. (2013). The cost burden of multiple sclerosis in the United States: A systematic review of the literature. *Journal of Medical Economics*, *16*, 639–647. http://dx.doi.org/10.3111/13696998.2013.778268

Andlin-Sobocki, P., Jönsson, B., Wittchen, H.-U., & Olesen, J. (2005). Cost of disorders of the brain in Europe. *European Journal of Neurology*, *12* (Suppl. 1), 1–27. http://dx.doi.org/10.1111/j.1468-1331.2005.01202.x

Beatty, W. W., Blanco, C. R., Wilbanks, S. L., Paul, R. H., & Hames, K. A. (1995). Demographic, clinical and cognitive characteristics of multiple sclerosis patients who continue to work. *Neurorehabilitation and Neural Repair*, *9*, 167–173. http://dx.doi.org/10.1177/154596839500900306

Beier, M., Amtmann, D., & Ehde, D. M. (2015). Beyond depression: Predictors of self-reported cognitive function in adults living with MS. *Rehabilitation Psychology*, *60*, 254–262. http://dx.doi.org/10.1037/rep0000045

Benedict, R. H. B., Drake, A. S., Irwin, L. N., Frndak, S. E., Kunker, K. A., Khan, A. L., . . . Weinstock-Guttman, B. (2016). Benchmarks of meaningful impairment on the MSFC and BICAMS. *Multiple Sclerosis Journal*, *22*, 1874–1882. http://dx.doi.org/10.1177/1352458516633517

Benedict, R. H. B., & Zivadinov, R. (2011). Risk factors for and management of cognitive dysfunction in multiple sclerosis. *Nature Reviews. Neurology*, *7*, 332–342. http://dx.doi.org/10.1038/nrneurol.2011.61

Bergendal, G., Fredrikson, S., & Almkvist, O. (2007). Selective decline in information processing in subgroups of multiple sclerosis: An 8-year longitudinal study. *European Neurology*, *57*, 193–202. http://dx.doi.org/10.1159/000099158

Cadden, M., & Arnett, P. (2015). Factors associated with employment status in individuals with multiple sclerosis. *International Journal of MS Care*, *17*, 284–291. http://dx.doi.org/10.7224/1537-2073.2014-057

DeLuca, G. C., Yates, R. L., Beale, H., & Morrow, S. A. (2015). Cognitive impairment in multiple sclerosis: Clinical, radiologic and pathologic insights. *Brain Pathology*, *25*, 79–98. http://dx.doi.org/10.1111/bpa.12220

Dettmers, C., & DeLuca, J. (2015). Editorial: Fatigue in multiple sclerosis. *Frontiers in Neurology*, *6*, 266. http://dx.doi.org/10.3389/fneur.2015.00266

Edgley, K., Sullivan, M. J., & Dehoux, E. (1991). A survey of multiple sclerosis: II. Determinants of employment status. *Canadian Journal of Rehabilitation*, *4*, 127–132.

Einarsson, U., Gottberg, K., von Koch, L., Fredrikson, S., Ytterberg, C., Jin, Y. P., . . . Holmqvist, L. W. (2006). Cognitive and motor function in people with multiple sclerosis in Stockholm County. *Multiple Sclerosis Journal*, *12*, 340–353. http://dx.doi.org/10.1191/135248506ms1259oa

Granberg, T., Martola, J., Bergendal, G., Shams, S., Damangir, S., Aspelin, P., . . . Kristoffersen-Wiberg, M. (2015). Corpus callosum atrophy is strongly associated with cognitive impairment in multiple sclerosis: Results of a 17-year longitudinal study. *Multiple Sclerosis Journal*, *21*, 1151–1158. http://dx.doi.org/10.1177/1352458514560928

Gulick, E. E., Yam, M., & Touw, M. M. (1989). Work performance by persons with multiple sclerosis: Conditions that impede or enable the performance of work. *International Journal of Nursing Studies*, *26*, 301–311. http://dx.doi.org/10.1016/0020-7489(89)90017-5

Gustavsson, A., Svensson, M., Jacobi, F., Allgulander, C., Alonso, J., Beghi, E., . . . the CDBE2010 Study Group. (2011). Cost of disorders of the brain in Europe 2010. *European Neuropsychopharmacology*, *21*, 718–779. http://dx.doi.org/10.1016/j.euroneuro.2011.08.008

Henriksson, F., Fredrikson, S., Masterman, T., & Jönsson, B. (2001). Costs, quality of life and disease severity in multiple sclerosis: A cross-sectional study in Sweden. *European Journal of Neurology*, *8*, 27–35. http://dx.doi.org/10.1046/j.1468-1331.2001.00169.x

Hughes, A. J., Hartoonian, N., Parmenter, B., Haselkorn, J. K., Lovera, J. F., Bourdette, D., & Turner, A. P. (2015). Cognitive impairment and community integration outcomes in individuals living with multiple sclerosis. *Archives of Physical Medicine and Rehabilitation*, *96*, 1973–1979. http://dx.doi.org/10.1016/j.apmr.2015.07.003

Johnson, K. L., Yorkston, K. M., Klasner, E. R., Kuehn, C. M., Johnson, E., & Amtmann, D. (2004). The cost and benefits of employment: A qualitative study of experiences of persons with multiple sclerosis. *Archives of Physical Medicine and Rehabilitation*, *85*, 201–209.

Julian, L. J., Vella, L., Vollmer, T., Hadjimichael, O., & Mohr, D. C. (2008). Employment in multiple sclerosis. Exiting and re-entering the work force. *Journal of Neurology*, *255*, 1354–1360. http://dx.doi.org/10.1007/s00415-008-0910-y

Kobelt, G., Berg, J., Lindgren, P., Fredrikson, S., & Jönsson, B. (2006). Costs and quality of life of patients with multiple sclerosis in Europe. *Journal of Neurology, Neurosurgery, and Psychiatry*, *77*, 918–926. http://dx.doi.org/10.1136/jnnp.2006.090365

Krause, I., Kern, S., Horntrich, A., & Ziemssen, T. (2013). Employment status in multiple sclerosis: Impact of disease-specific and non-disease-specific factors. *Multiple Sclerosis Journal*, *19*, 1792–1799. http://dx.doi.org/10.1177/1352458513485655

Lynch, S. G., Parmenter, B. A., & Denney, D. R. (2005). The association between cognitive impairment and physical disability in multiple sclerosis. *Multiple Sclerosis Journal*, *11*, 469–476. http://dx.doi.org/10.1191/1352458505ms1182oa

Ma, V. Y., Chan, L., & Carruthers, K. J. (2014). Incidence, prevalence, costs, and impact on disability of common conditions requiring rehabilitation in the

United States: Stroke, spinal cord injury, traumatic brain injury, multiple sclerosis, osteoarthritis, rheumatoid arthritis, limb loss, and back pain. *Archives of Physical Medicine and Rehabilitation, 95,* 986–995.e1. http://dx.doi.org/10.1016/j.apmr.2013.10.032

Miller, A., & Dishon, S. (2006). Health-related quality of life in multiple sclerosis: The impact of disability, gender and employment status. *Quality of Life Research: An International Journal of Quality of Life Aspects of Treatment, Care & Rehabilitation, 15,* 259–271. http://dx.doi.org/10.1007/s11136-005-0891-6

Morrow, S. A., Drake, A., Zivadinov, R., Munschauer, F., Weinstock-Guttman, B., & Benedict, R. H. B. (2010). Predicting loss of employment over three years in multiple sclerosis: Clinically meaningful cognitive decline. *The Clinical Neuropsychologist, 24,* 1131–1145. http://dx.doi.org/10.1080/13854046.2010.511272

Naci, H., Fleurence, R., Birt, J., & Duhig, A. (2010). Economic burden of multiple sclerosis: A systematic review of the literature. *PharmacoEconomics, 28,* 363–379. http://dx.doi.org/10.2165/11532230-000000000-00000

Palmer, A. J., Colman, S., O'Leary, B., Taylor, B. V., & Simmons, R. D. (2013). The economic impact of multiple sclerosis in Australia in 2010. *Multiple Sclerosis Journal, 19,* 1640–1646. http://dx.doi.org/10.1177/1352458513488230

Patwardhan, M. B., Matchar, D. B., Samsa, G. P., McCrory, D. C., Williams, R. G., & Li, T. T. (2005). Cost of multiple sclerosis by level of disability: A review of literature. *Multiple Sclerosis Journal, 11,* 232–239. http://dx.doi.org/10.1191/1352458505ms1137oa

Pompeii, L. A., Moon, S. D., & McCrory, D. C. (2005). Measures of physical and cognitive function and work status among individuals with multiple sclerosis: A review of the literature. *Journal of Occupational Rehabilitation, 15,* 69–84.

Ponzio, M., Gerzeli, S., Brichetto, G., Bezzini, D., Mancardi, G. L., Zaratin, P., & Battaglia, M. A. (2015). Economic impact of multiple sclerosis in Italy: Focus on rehabilitation costs. *Neurological Sciences, 36,* 227–234. http://dx.doi.org/10.1007/s10072-014-1925-z

Rao, S. M., Leo, G. J., Ellington, L., Nauertz, T., Bernardin, L., & Unverzagt, F. (1991). Cognitive dysfunction in multiple sclerosis: II. Impact on employment and social functioning. *Neurology, 41,* 692–696. http://dx.doi.org/10.1212/WNL.41.5.692

Romero, K., Shammi, P., & Feinstein, A. (2015). Neurologists? accuracy in predicting cognitive impairment in multiple sclerosis. *Multiple Sclerosis and Related Disorders, 4,* 291—295. http://dx.doi.org/10.1016/j.msard.2015.05.009

Strober, L. B., & Arnett, P. A. (2016). Unemployment among women with multiple sclerosis: The role of coping and perceived stress and support in the workplace. *Psychology, Health & Medicine, 12,* 1–9. http://dx.doi.org/10.1080/13548506.2015.1093645

Strober, L. B., Chiaravalloti, N., Moore, N., & DeLuca, J. (2014). Unemployment in multiple sclerosis (MS): Utility of the MS functional composite and cognitive testing. *Multiple Sclerosis Journal, 20,* 112–115. http://dx.doi.org/10.1177/1352458513488235

Whetten-Goldstein, K., Sloan, F. A., Goldstein, L. B., & Kulas, E. D. (1998). A comprehensive assessment of the cost of multiple sclerosis in the United States. *Multiple Sclerosis Journal, 4,* 419–425. http://dx.doi.org/10.1177/135245859800400504

Wundes, A., Brown, T., Bienen, E. J., & Coleman, C. I. (2010). Contribution of intangible costs to the economic burden of multiple sclerosis. *Journal of Medical Economics, 13,* 626–632. http://dx.doi.org/10.3111/13696998.2010.525989

11

PEDIATRIC MULTIPLE SCLEROSIS AND COGNITION

NADINE AKBAR, CHRISTINE TILL, AND BRENDA BANWELL

There has been increased recognition of multiple sclerosis (MS) in children and adolescents, with approximately 5% of MS patients diagnosed prior to age 18 (Chitnis, Glanz, Jaffin, & Healy, 2009; Harding et al., 2013). The cognitive sequelae of pediatric-onset MS are particularly worrisome considering that the disease affects the primary acquisition of abilities required for adequate functioning in adulthood.

Given the relatively recent recognition and rarity of pediatric MS, studies on the cognitive sequelae of pediatric MS remain challenged by limited longitudinal follow-up data. Descriptions of the cognitive characteristics of pediatric MS have come from cohorts in Canada, Italy, and the United States (Amato et al., 2008; Julian et al., 2013; Till, Ghassemi, et al., 2011). Some studies report serial evaluations, which are especially crucial in terms of determining the extent, pattern, and risk factors for cognitive decline. Information regarding the impact of pediatric-onset MS on adulthood is

http://dx.doi.org/10.1037/0000097-012
Cognition and Behavior in Multiple Sclerosis, J. DeLuca and B. M. Sandroff (Editors)

limited to a few studies (Baruch et al., 2016; Krysko & O'Connor, 2016). This chapter reviews studies of cognition in pediatric MS, highlighting the nature, impact, and progression of cognitive deficits; the assessment tools utilized; and the relationships between cognitive functioning and disease-related characteristics, and neuroimaging. Potential therapeutic strategies, including cognitive rehabilitation, are also presented.

PREVALENCE OF COGNITIVE IMPAIRMENT IN PEDIATRIC MS

Prevalence of cognitive impairment in pediatric MS approximates 30%, although some variability exists (29%, 31%, 35%, and 35% reported by Till, Ghassemi, et al., 2011; Amato et al., 2008; MacAllister et al., 2005; and Julian et al., 2013, respectively). This is likely related, in part, to differences in study inclusion criteria (variable disease duration, disease severity, treatment exposures), by the definitions used for cognitive impairment, and by the controls used (normative data vs region-, age-, and sex-matched healthy participants).

CORE DEFICITS/DOMAINS AFFECTED

Pediatric MS is associated with deficits in the domains of memory, attention, and information processing speed, which overlaps with the cognitive profile in adult MS. In addition to those domains, and not common in adult MS, are deficits in language, visuomotor, and academic abilities (math, spelling). IQ is also more likely to be reduced in pediatric MS, with approximately 8% showing an IQ falling in the intellectual deficiency range (IQ score less than 70, see Amato et al., 2008) compared with 2% of the general population. Differences in the cognitive profiles between adult and pediatric MS likely reflect the co-occurrence of MS with the maturation of these abilities and/or due to the greater insult (lesion volume) to infratentorial regions in pediatric MS (Ghassemi et al., 2014). A review of more detailed studies, providing more insight into the nature of core deficits, is covered herein.

Memory

The prevalence of memory impairment ranges considerably across studies for both verbal and visual domains. In a United States study of 37 pediatric MS patients (MacAllister et al., 2005), impairment in immediate and delayed recall of visual information was found in 8% and 11% of patients, respectively. Impairment in delayed recall (but not immediate recall) of verbal information was slightly more common (19%), pointing to greater verbal compared with visual long-term memory deficits in pediatric MS. Higher rates of visual and verbal memory impairment were documented in a later Italian multicenter study, in which 63 pediatric MS patients were compared with 57 matched healthy controls (Amato et al., 2008). Deficits were observed among approximately half of the sample when required to recall both verbal (56%) and visual (53%) information immediately after presentation, whereas long-term recall was lower for verbal information (39%) relative to visuospatial information (18%), pointing again to greater verbal compared with visual long-term memory deficits in pediatric MS.

In a Canadian cohort of 32 pediatric MS patients and 26 age- and sex-matched healthy (Fuentes et al., 2012), verbal and nonverbal memory were evaluated using the Test of Memory and Learning, Second Edition (TOMAL–2). The TOMAL–2 subtests administered included the Word Selective Reminding, Memory for Stories, Abstract Verbal Memory, and Facial Memory tests. The only subtest that showed significant differences between groups was Memory for Stories with 9% of pediatric MS patients showing impaired performance 1.5 SD or more below norms. Rocca et al. (2016) found 10 (19%) out of 53 pediatric MS patients to be impaired (performance below the 5th percentile of healthy controls) on verbal memory, and the same percentage impaired on visual memory. In summary, the majority of studies document memory impairment occurring in approximately one fifth or fewer of pediatric patients with MS, with the exception of one study (Amato et al., 2008) where memory impairment was as found in roughly half of the sample for both visual and verbal information.

Executive Function

Deficits in executive functions are particularly vulnerable to disruption as these skills continue to mature throughout childhood and adolescence. In children and adolescents with MS, working memory (the cognitive system that temporarily stores information in the course of executing a goal) is one of the major executive functions affected (Amato et al., 2008; MacAllister et al., 2005; Till, Ho, et al., 2012). Approximately half of pediatric MS patients demonstrate difficulties with working memory and cognitive flexibility, as assessed by the Contingency Naming Test, Part B of the Trail Making Test (TMT-B), Modified Card Sorting Test, and the Tower of London (Amato et al., 2008; MacAllister, 2010; MacAllister et al., 2005), but not on the Wisconsin Card Sorting Task (Banwell & Anderson, 2005; Till, Ghassemi, et al., 2011), likely reflecting differences in specific task demands. This percentage is substantially higher than the reported prevalence of executive function deficits in adult-onset MS (e.g., approximately 17%, as reported by Drew, Tippett, Starkey, & Isler, 2008).

Deficits in at least one aspect of everyday executive function have also been reported by approximately half of parents of children and adolescents with MS, using the Behavior Rating Inventory of Executive Function (Till, Ho, et al., 2012). Using this subjective measure, organization of materials and working memory were the skills most frequently rated (30%) as being impaired by parents of pediatric MS patients. Given the reliance of working memory on efficient processing, it has been proposed that the observed difficulties in working memory may emerge or be exacerbated as a consequence of a primary processing speed deficit that frequently characterizes MS patients (Drew, Starkey, & Isler, 2009).

Information Processing Speed and Attention

Slowed performance relative to healthy controls has been demonstrated across numerous studies and measures of information processing speed, including Part A of the Trail Making Test (TMT-A; Till, Ghassemi, et al., 2011), the Symbol Digit Modalities Test (SDMT; Bethune et al., 2011; Till, Ghassemi, et al., 2011), and visual matching subtest from the Woodcock-Johnson III Test of Cognitive Abilities (Bethune et al., 2011; Till, Ghassemi, et al., 2011). Especially high rates of impairment have been found for the TMT-A (50% in Amato et al., 2008; 38% in Till, Deotto, et al., 2011; 32% in Julian et al., 2013; 30% in MacAllister et al., 2005) and SDMT (35% in Julian et al., 2013; 28% in Amato et al., 2008) across studies.

Todorow, DeSouza, Banwell, and Till (2014) performed a study evaluating selective attention in 15 pediatric-onset MS patients (age range, 13–21 years) with high average intellectual functioning compared with 15 age-matched controls. The task involved asking participants to detect a target stimulus presented among distractors. The pediatric-MS group had more difficulty ignoring task-irrelevant information compared with age-matched healthy controls. In a different analysis from the same cohort, evaluation of sustained attention (Till, Ghassemi, et al., 2011) found similar performance between pediatric MS patients and healthy controls on the Conners Continuous Performance Test—Fifth Edition, a task requiring participants to refrain from responding when a target stimulus appears. Further research is required to determine whether sustained attention is spared in pediatric MS.

Visuomotor Ability and Fine-Motor Coordination

Fine motor concerns have been reported in pediatric MS, similar to what is observed in adults with MS. Julian et al. (2013) showed that fine motor speed and coordination as measured by the grooved pegboard test was most frequently impaired (54%) among a battery of cognitive and motor tests. Fine motor difficulty on the nine-hole peg test, but not hand strength, was also reported in another study of adolescents with pediatric MS relative to controls (Squillace, Ray, & Milazzo, 2015). Taken together, these findings suggest that fine motor dexterity may be especially sensitive to deficits in pediatric MS and visible early in the course of disease (e.g., as in Julian et al., 2013). Especially high rates of impairment and worse performance relative to controls have also been demonstrated in pediatric MS patients using the Beery-Buktenica Developmental test of Visual Motor Integration (Beery VMI), a measure that also requires fine motor coordination. Impairment on this test, which requires participants to copy designs of increasing complexity, was found among 24% and 50% of pediatric MS patients in the study of Till, Ghassemi, et al. (2011) and Julian et al. (2013), respectively.

Language

Deficits in both expressive (Amato et al., 2008; MacAllister et al., 2005; Till, Ghassemi, et al., 2011) and receptive language (Amato et al., 2008; MacAllister et al., 2005) have been reported in pediatric MS. The study of Amato et al. (2008) reported an especially high rate of receptive language deficits (39%) using the Token Test. MacAllister and colleagues (2005) reported a lower rate of receptive language (14%) deficits, as well as naming deficits in 19% of 37 tested pediatric MS patients. Two studies which administered the Wechsler Abbreviated Scale of Intelligence (WASI) Vocabulary noted impairment in approximately 10% of 31 and 13% of 231 pediatric MS patients, respectively (Till et al.; Julian et al., 2013). Despite lower rates of impairment in language compared with other cognitive domains, it is notable that language deficits are much less commonly seen in adult MS (Rao, Leo, Bernardin, & Unverzagt, 1991), making this a relatively unique aspect of pediatric MS.

Social Cognition

Theory of mind (ToM), which refers to the ability to infer the mental state of others with respect to their knowledge, beliefs, and emotions, was recently investigated by Charvet, Cleary, et al. (2014). Three ToM tasks were administered to 28 pediatric-onset MS patients and 32 healthy controls measuring (a) facial emotion recognition, (b) identification of social faux pas, and (c) first- and second-order false beliefs. Relative to controls, the pediatric-onset MS group performed worse on the facial recognition and social faux pas test, and approached significance on the false beliefs task. Deficits in

ToM are also found in adults with MS, particularly in the recognition of negative facial emotions (Bora, Özakbaş, Velakoulis, & Walterfang, 2016; Cotter et al., 2016) and ability to recognize lies and sarcasm (Genova, Cagna, Chiaravalloti, DeLuca, & Lengenfelder, 2016). As social cognitive ability is an important component of adolescent and adult functioning, assessment of this domain in youth with MS should further be addressed.

Academic Performance

In a study of 31 youths with pediatric MS and 34 healthy controls, the pediatric MS group performed significantly worse than controls on the Calculation, Letter-Word Identification (measuring the ability to read words), and Spelling subtests of the WJ-III Tests of Achievement (Till, Deotto, et al., 2011), all measuring important abilities related to academic performance. Although the average range performance was demonstrated as a group by the pediatric MS patients on all of these subtests, deficits in written arithmetic ability were identified among 26% of patients, defined as performance at least 1 *SD* below the normative mean compared with 6% of the healthy controls. Difficulty with arithmetic is exacerbated by deficits in other cognitive abilities that are commonly affected in MS (e.g., processing speed, working memory, visual-spatial processing). Arithmetic difficulties, therefore, might become more pronounced as the disease progresses.

One of the most concerning aspects of pediatric MS is how the disease affects school performance. Approximately one-third of pediatric MS patients require a reduced class load, accommodations, and academic assistance due to fatigue and cognitive dysfunction (MacAllister et al., 2005). Examples of impact on school performance include increased time required to finish examinations, difficulty maintaining focus, frequently missing class (e.g., due to medical appointments, relapses, therapy side effects) which, in addition to cognitive dysfunction, can increase risk of grade retention or school dropout. Amato, Goretti, Ghezzi, Hakiki, et al. (2014) reported that school activities and achievements were negatively affected in 33% of 30 pediatric MS patients, as determined by requiring extra support teacher(s) (10%) and having to repeat a year in school (23%). All 33% of these patients were cognitively impaired. Disrupted participation in hobbies and sports was also demonstrated in 41% of patients, over half of whom (56%) were cognitively impaired. Finally, family and social relationships were negatively affected in 28% of patients (of note, of these patients, 73% were cognitively impaired). In summary, pediatric MS can have a very large impact on school performance and social functioning—one that is especially pronounced in patients with cognitive impairment.

LONGITUDINAL PROGRESSION OF DEFICITS

In the first longitudinal cognitive study in pediatric MS, MacAllister, Christodoulou, Milazzo, and Krupp (2007) evaluated changes in neuropsychological performance in a small cohort of 12 pediatric MS patients (mean age of onset = 12.5 years, mean disease duration = 22 months) evaluated at baseline and after a mean of 22 months (range, 11–30 months) follow-up. Decline was determined by comparing the frequency of tests failed by each participant at follow-up relative to a baseline evaluation. Failure on any one test was defined by performance ≥ 1.5 SD or more below age-matched means. Using this study's frequency-based approach, five patients (42%) were classified as demonstrating cognitive decline. Deterioration in performance was most pronounced for TMT-B and the Beery VMI. Younger age of disease onset was associated with greater decline in cognitive performance (change in mean composite z-score), perhaps reflecting a failure to acquire emerging cognitive skills.

Two- and 5-year follow-up data from the original cohort of Amato and colleagues (2008) have been published (Amato et al., 2010; Amato, Goretti, Viterbo, et al., 2014). After 2 years, 39 out of 56 (70%) pediatric MS patients were classified as cognitively impaired, compared with 19 out of 61 (31%) at baseline. Functions that were more prone to deterioration were those of verbal memory, complex attention, verbal fluency, and receptive language. However, at a longer-term follow-up (5 years post-baseline), only 18 out of 48 (38%) were cognitively impaired, mainly reflecting deterioration on measures of memory, yet improvement on tasks of attention/information processing speed and expressive language. Comparison of results across the 2- and 5-year follow-up assessments is limited based on use of different healthy control groups (used for defining cognitive impairment) at each time point. Also, the test version administered at 2-year follow-up was different from the version used at baseline and at 5 years, which may have had a small effect on explaining the marked deterioration in cognitive performance from baseline to 2 years. With respect to improvements observed, this could be due to the effects of disease-modifying treatments, which reduce disease activity over time, and may lead to stabilization of the negative impact of MS on cognitive development.

In one study that used the Reliable Change Index to determine individual changes on test scores over a 15-month interval (Till et al., 2013), improvements in cognitive functioning were reported among 18% of patients in the MS group as compared with 69% of participants in the control group. These results highlight a lack of maturational-expected improvements in the MS patients relative to age-matched healthy peers. Deterioration in functioning, defined as significant decline on three or more tests, was observed in seven of 28 patients (25%), as compared with only one of 26 controls (4%).

In contrast with the above results, a United States-based longitudinal study including 62 individuals with pediatric MS and five individuals with clinically isolated syndrome found that after a 1.6-year follow-up, most patients remained stable (Charvet, O'Donnell, et al., 2014). Only 6% of patients declined and 9% improved on two or more tasks. Differences in sample characteristics, assessment tools, and method of classifying change and accounting for practice effects may, in part, explain the differing results.

With respect to predictors of change, Hosseini, Flora, Banwell, and Till (2014) used growth curve modeling to demonstrate that older age of disease onset was associated with greater increases in TMT-B and SDMT scores over time. This suggests that older age of onset may help facilitate developmental increases in processing speed and prevent decline seen in patients with younger age of disease onset. Furthermore, patient-related factors, such as higher baseline IQ (Pastò et al., 2016) and higher parental education (Till et al., 2013), have been shown to relate to better cognitive outcomes in pediatric MS. The identification of any additional factors associated with resiliency to cognitive decline should be an area further pursued in pediatric MS.

ASSESSMENT TOOLS

Following initial studies reporting on the prevalence of cognitive dysfunction in pediatric MS, it became evident that a standardized cognitive battery was necessary for routine evaluation of children and adolescents with MS. To this aim, Portaccio et al. (2009) employed discriminant function analysis to determine the most sensitive measures from a comprehensive neuropsychological test battery that was used in a study of 61 pediatric MS patients and 58 healthy controls (Amato et al., 2008). Failure on any test was defined as performance below the 5th percentile of healthy controls. Using a cutoff of at least 4 tests failed, 41% of patients were classified as cognitively impaired. The most frequently affected cognitive domains were IQ (30% of patients impaired), verbal and spatial memory (23% were impaired on each of immediate recall measures of Selective Reminding Test and Spatial Recall Test), information processing speed (SDMT, TMT), and language (semantic verbal fluency, 18%, and token test, 18%). The tests with the highest discriminating ability were Wechsler Intelligence Scale for Children—Revised Vocabulary, SDMT, TMT-B, and Selective Reminding Test (Continuous Long-term Retrieval variable), which were thus selected for inclusion in the 30-minute Brief Neuropsychological Battery for Children (BNBC; Portaccio et al., 2009). Failure on at least one test of the BNBC yielded a sensitivity of 96% and specificity of 76% for detecting impairment, as defined on the full battery. The BNBC, however, requires further validation in independent samples to ensure the battery meets psychometric standards for reliability and validity.

In addition to the BNBC, the Brief International Cognitive Assessment for MS (BICAMS; Langdon et al., 2012) has been proposed for use in pediatric MS. Widely recognized and validated for use in adult MS, the BICAMS consists of the SDMT, learning trials from the California Verbal Learning Test Second Edition (CVLT-II), and the Brief Visuospatial Memory Test-Revised (BVMT-R). The CVLT-II can be replaced with the Rey Auditory Verbal Learning Test in order to permit use in children as young as 8 years. Despite no currently published validation studies of the BICAMS in pediatric MS, the BICAMS is still supported for use in this population (Krupp, Charvet, Porter, Amadiume, & Belman, 2014).

In 2011, Smerbeck et al. compared performance on a neuropsychological battery between 43 pediatric MS patients with 45 healthy controls, in order to determine which tests were most sensitive in distinguishing between groups. The battery included measures of intelligence (WASI), language (Expressive One Word Picture Vocabulary Test), visual memory (BVMT-R), and processing speed (SDMT). Patients had statistically significant worse performance on measures of visual memory (BVMT-R Total Learning and Delayed Recall) and processing speed (SDMT) than controls. This study did not include an evaluation of the sensitivity of the Beery-Buktenica Developmental Test of Visual-Motor Integration, which has shown one of the highest rates of impairment in pediatric MS (50% in Julian et al., 2013; 24% in Till, Ghassemi, et al., 2011). All of the aforementioned tasks with high sensitivity involve visual processing ability, suggesting that measures probing this ability should be incorporated into cognitive evaluations of individuals with pediatric MS.

In line with previous reports (Portaccio et al., 2009; Smerbeck et al., 2011), several recent studies have reported SDMT to be an effective screening measure for identifying cognitive impairment in pediatric MS. In the study of Charvet, Beekman, and colleagues (2014), 31 pediatric MS patients completed a neuropsychological evaluation within 1 year of completing the SDMT. Thirty-seven percent of patients demonstrated impairment on the SDMT. Impairment, however, was defined using liberal criteria of 1 or more SD below the normative mean values. Sensitivity and specificity of the SDMT for detecting cognitive impairment on the neuropsychological test battery were high at 77% and 81%, respectively. This study also found that older age at testing and increased disability (higher Expanded Disability Status Scale [EDSS] score) were predictors of poorer SDMT performance. Further support for the SDMT in pediatric MS comes from its strong correlation with white matter integrity of the corpus callosum (Bethune et al., 2011), as well as global brain MRI metrics (Till, Ghassemi, et al., 2011). Despite its promise as a screening instrument for cognitive impairment, the impact of other potential confounds for performance on the SDMT, including visual acuity, oral-motor planning, and practice effects, should be considered.

CLINICAL CORRELATES OF COGNITIVE DYSFUNCTION

In one of the first published reports of cognition in pediatric MS (Banwell & Anderson, 2005), deficits were almost exclusively found in patients with remote disease (mean time since first attack = 5.1 years), primarily in the areas of (a) executive function, particularly those tests requiring self-generated organizational strategies; (b) processing speed; and (c) working memory. Other studies have similarly reported that cognitive impairment is more likely in patients with longer disease duration and younger age of disease onset (Amato et al., 2008; MacAllister et al., 2005; Till, Ghassemi, et al., 2011). While longer disease duration provides a longer period of time for accrual of both local and global disease-related CNS insult, the fact that younger children are more likely to be impaired also implicates vulnerability of the developing neural networks to MS-related insult.

A significant association between physical disability, as assessed by the EDSS, and cognitive function has not been consistently demonstrated in either of the pediatric and adult MS populations. In pediatric MS, this lack of relationship is likely due to the limited amount of physical disability present in these patients.

Particularly as noted by parents (Till, Udler, et al., 2012), mood disturbance and behavioral problems are frequently reported in pediatric MS (Goretti et al., 2010; Weisbrot et al., 2014), perhaps reflecting reduced insight. With respect to the relationship between mood and cognitive function, higher anxiety and depression (as reported by the caregiver of pediatric MS patients) has been shown to have moderate to strong correlations (range, $r = .44$ to $r = .55$) with worse executive function, as measured by performance on the TMT and Digit Span task (Holland, Graves, Greenberg, & Harder, 2014), highlighting the difficulty in teasing apart these cognitive sequelae from mood-related symptomatology. Weisbrot and colleagues (2014) observed that pediatric MS patients with either a mood or anxiety disorder were more likely to be cognitively impaired when compared with pediatric MS patients with other psychiatric diagnosis (e.g., attention deficit hyperactivity disorder, oppositional defiant disorder) or no psychiatric diagnosis. Finally, the study of Charvet, Cersosimo, Schwarz, Belman, and

Krupp (2016) found that pediatric MS patients meeting criteria for cognitive impairment were more likely to have at least one behavioral and/or emotional problem in the clinically significant range (score 2% or less than age-normative database), as assessed using the Behavioral Assessment System for Children, Second Edition. The most frequently reported problems (based on both participant and parent reports) included those related to attention, somatization, and hyperactivity.

Fatigue is a common feature of MS. Approximately 50% of parents of pediatric MS patients describe their children as having fatigue (MacAllister et al., 2009). Both parent- and patient-reported fatigue correlates with cognitive impairment, particularly on measures of executive function, such as the TMT-A and TMT-B (Holland et al., 2014) and Tower of London (Goretti et al., 2012). Higher parent-reported cognitive fatigue has also been associated with impaired performance on tests of verbal memory (Selective Reminding Test), processing speed and attention (TMT-B), and language (Token Test).

In summary, given the associations between cognitive performance and fatigue, and mood and behavioral problems, it is important that these factors be accounted for in any study evaluating cognition in pediatric MS, as they may exert a confounding influence. These findings also highlight the importance of addressing issues related to behavioral problems and fatigue for the management of cognitive sequelae in pediatric MS.

NEUROIMAGING CORRELATES OF COGNITIVE FUNCTION IN PEDIATRIC MS

Over the past decade, there has been a rapid increase in the application of advanced magnetic resonance imaging (MRI) techniques to increase our understanding of the pathophysiology of cognitive impairment in pediatric MS, as well as the mechanisms contributing to its evolution. However, relative to adult MS, studies linking cognitive dysfunction to neuroimaging findings in pediatric MS are still very scarce. These studies have focused predominantly on the impact of white matter (WM) lesions, WM integrity and volume, and measures of axonal and neuronal damage, including abnormalities to gray matter (GM) and regional brain structure volume, such as the thalamus and cerebellum. In the following section, the structural and functional brain correlates of cognitive dysfunction in pediatric MS are reviewed.

Structural MRI Correlates

The frequency pattern of lesion distribution in pediatric-onset MS patients varies when compared with adult-onset MS. One major difference is the greater extent of infratentorial involvement in pediatric MS patients (Ghassemi et al., 2014; Waubant et al., 2009). Although the volume of supratentorial lesions has not been linked to performance on specific neuropsychological tests, global cognitive impairment is more common among pediatric MS patients who show a "posterior pattern" of pathology characterized by lesions in the right thalamus, middle and posterior corpus callosum, and bilateral parieto-occipital white matter relative to those without impairment (Rocca, Absinta, et al., 2014). Taking whole brain lesion burden into account, studies report a modest association between T_2 and T_1 lesion volume and neuropsychological test performance (Till, Ghassemi, et al., 2011). These lesion-based studies highlight the importance of a disconnection mechanism underlying the pathogenesis of cognitive impairment in pediatric MS. However, as with adult MS, lesion burden explains less variance in cognitive dysfunction than damage to normal appearing white matter and the involvement of GM.

Studies that evaluate white matter involvement using voxel-based morphology (for defining the regional location of WM abnormalities) and diffusion tensor imaging (which measures the extent of directionality in WM) lend further support to the notion of a disconnection syndrome in patients with pediatric-onset MS. In comparison with multiple MRI metrics, atrophy of the WM was the only MRI variable to distinguish between cognitively impaired and cognitively preserved patients with pediatric-onset MS (Rocca et al., 2015). Diffusion-weighted MRI abnormalities in the corpus callosum, particularly the genu and anterior body, was shown to predict reduced visual-perceptual speed (Bethune et al., 2011) and less efficient inhibition of irrelevant visual information on a global-local task (Todorow et al., 2014). Reduction in normal fiber alignment, as measured by fractional anisotropy, in the corpus callosum and in right frontal and parietal regions has also been shown to associate robustly with performance on a measure of calculation ability (Till, Deotto, et al., 2011), consistent with the important role of WM pathways underlying mathematical competence.

GM volume correlates negatively with cognitive performance in pediatric MS patients (Aubert-Broche et al., 2011; Kerbrat et al., 2012). Lower GM volume, which is found to occur in early stages of pediatric MS (Calabrese et al., 2012), correlated with reduced IQ and slower information processing speed (Till, Ghassemi, et al., 2011). The assessment of total GM volume did not differentiate cognitively impaired patients from cognitive-preserved patients in one pediatric MS study (Till, Ghassemi, et al., 2011), but did in another study when the topographic distribution of such damage was localized to specific structures, including the right precuneus and left middle temporal gyrus (Rocca, Absinta, et al., 2014).

Correlations between cognitive performance and deep GM structures were investigated in a sample of 35 pediatric-onset MS patients who underwent scanning on a 1.5T scanner. The thalamus, which was selected based on its active role in regulating information to cortical areas as well as its vulnerability to MS pathology (Mesaros et al., 2008), emerged as the most robust MRI predictor of global functional outcomes (Full Scale IQ, Cognitive Composite score), as well as measures of mental processing speed, visuomotor integration, and vocabulary (Till, Ghassemi, et al., 2011). In regression analyses, thalamic volume accounted for the largest amount of additional variance in predicting various neuropsychological outcomes and entered the models more frequently than any other MRI metric examined, including T_1- and T_2-lesion volume, corpus callosum area, normalized brain volume, and GM volume (Till, Deotto, et al., 2011). Relative to the global measures of brain volume analyzed in this study, only the regional structures (thalamic volume and corpus callosum area) differentiated pediatric MS patients identified as having cognitive impairment from those without (Till, Deotto, et al., 2011). In the same sample of patients, lower thalamic and frontal lobe volume were shown to predict executive dysfunction (Till, Ho, et al., 2012). Taken together, these findings indicate that the thalamus is crucially linked to a wide range of cognitive abilities in pediatric-onset MS.

Other studies have found the hippocampus and cerebellum to relate to poorer cognitive performance in pediatric MS. Fuentes et al. (2012) found that reduced performance on a verbal learning task was associated with reduced whole brain volume and hippocampal volume, even though the extent of hippocampal volume reduction was not as severe as the relative reduction in whole brain volume. Another study (Rocca et al., 2016) reported that cognitively impaired pediatric MS patients were shown to have reduced regional (head and body) right hippocampal volumes compared with cognitively preserved patients. Lower regional (head, body, or tail) hippocampal volumes were shown to correlate with worse attention and language performance, but not with measures of verbal or visuospatial memory. Regarding the cerebellum, Weier et al. (2016) found that cerebellar posterior lobe volume and infratentorial lesion volume explained additional variance (above sex and cerebral measures) in the WASI Vocabulary test and SDMT performance, despite no statistical differences in cerebellar volume between patients and controls. These findings suggest the cerebellum may contribute to abnormalities in cognitive function in pediatric MS, consistent with associations found in adult-onset MS (Cerasa et al., 2012; Weier et al., 2014).

Functional MRI Correlates

In one functional MRI (fMRI) study conducted in 35 pediatric-onset MS patients and 16 controls (Rocca, Absinta, et al., 2014), results showed decreased resting-state functional connectivity of the precuneus in cognitively impaired patients whereas cognitively preserved patients showed higher resting-state of the anterior cingulate cortex, both with other areas of the default-mode network, consistent with the idea of a functional reorganization process to delay functional decline. Another study from this group (Rocca, Valsasina, et al., 2014) observed that increased resting-state functional connectivity of the medial frontal gyrus (implicating the attention network) negatively correlated with T_2 lesion volume and was more pronounced in cognitively preserved MS patients, suggesting a possible mechanism that may serve to counteract the impact of structural damage. A study from a separate research group, consisting of solely cognitively preserved patients (Akbar, Till, et al., 2016), found that higher functional connectivity of the left frontal medial cortex with the bilateral anterior cingulate cortex and right precuneus was associated with lower overall performance on a neuropsychological test battery. This study suggests that in patients who are cognitively intact, reduced cognitive performance may be associated with the recruitment of greater neural resources while at rest. Overall, these mixed findings could be due to differences in sample characteristics, cognitive measures, and/or use of different resting-state fMRI analytic techniques.

Using an fMRI-version of the SDMT, Akbar, Banwell, et al. (2016) measured activation patterns and behavioral performance/task speed in 20 pediatric-onset MS patients (age range, 13–24; mean age = 19) and 16 age- and sex-matched healthy controls. Despite equal performance across both groups, the pediatric MS group demonstrated lower activation of the right middle frontal gyrus compared with the healthy control group, which could be due to structural damage or incomplete development of frontally mediated attentional networks. Greater activation, particularly of occipital regions, was associated with faster response time, suggesting this to be a mechanism for maintenance of intact processing speed performance. Further studies are needed to understand changes in other cognitive-relevant networks, to examine how changes in regional and global brain growth and/or connectivity in pediatric MS patients differs as a function of MS disease activity during key epochs of brain maturation, and how these functional changes contribute to the evolution of cognitive impairment.

THE IMPACT OF PEDIATRIC MS ON ADULT LIFE

Processing speed deficits in adulthood have been shown to be prominent in individuals diagnosed with pediatric-onset MS. Krysko and O'Connor (2016) reported that 53% of the 34 adults (age range, 18–30; mean age = 21; mean disease duration = 6.3 years) with pediatric-onset MS that they studied were impaired on the SDMT, as defined by a z-score equal to or less than

1.5 SD below age- and sex-matched normative data. Recently, Baruch et al. (2016) sought to determine whether childhood and adolescent onset of MS exerts more negative effects on cognition in comparison to disease-onset in adulthood. To do this, these authors compared SDMT performance in two groups of adult MS patients: 51 with pediatric-onset MS and 550 with adult-onset disease (mean age of pediatric-onset MS group = 32.7; mean disease duration = 17.2 years). Using normative z-scores, the pediatric-onset MS group demonstrated poorer SDMT performance compared with the adult-onset group, after adjusting for age at testing and disease duration. This suggests that the co-occurrence of pediatric MS during the development of pathways underlying processing speed exerts a more negative impact than if MS onset occurred during adulthood, purportedly when these pathways would have already been developed.

MANAGEMENT OF COGNITIVE DEFICITS

Management of cognitive deficits in pediatric MS should involve the prevention of cognitive decline, management of existing deficits, as well as identifying and treating factors, such as fatigue and depression, that may negatively impact cognitive performance. Currently, cognitive deficits in pediatric MS are generally managed on a case-by-case basis, primarily involving academic accommodations according to areas of deficit. For example, children with attention deficits may be placed in a distraction-free area during class, children with reduced processing speed may get more time to finish exams, or children with memory deficits may be taught compensatory strategies, such as using a day planner which may help improve academic and daily functioning.

What is now beginning to emerge is research on the potential role of cognitive rehabilitation in pediatric MS. In the study of Hubacher and colleagues (2015), five patients received computerized working memory training for 4 weeks, four times per week, for 45 minutes each session (Hubacher et al., 2015). The training tool (BrainStim) consisted of three modules targeting both verbal and visuospatial working memory, in which participants have to remember spatial routes, the location of cards, or numbers presented on the screen. Two patients showed positive changes on tests of working memory and alertness following training. These patients also demonstrated increased and more widespread brain activation, as well as increases in functional connectivity during a working memory fMRI task. Thus, increased activation could be underlying the observed treatment effect. It was noted, however, that the two patients showing positive treatment response were those with longer time since last relapse and higher general intelligence at baseline.

This small study shows some promise for cognitive rehabilitation but, clearly, larger studies are required.

As in adult MS, cognitive rehabilitation interventions in pediatric MS could involve the use of other computer-assisted rehabilitation programs, such as the Attention Processing Training program (Amato, Goretti, Viterbo, et al., 2014). Teaching of specific memory and behavioral strategies (e.g., Chiaravalloti, Moore, Nikelshpur, & DeLuca, 2013; Hanssen, Beiske, Landrø, Hofoss, & Hessen, 2016), as commonly done with adult MS patients, or completion of home-based written and computer-based materials (e.g., Gich et al., 2015) have received less attention in pediatric-onset MS patients. Further research in pediatric MS should also evaluate the influence of other types of behavioral interventions, such as exercise and meditation, based on literature in preadolescent children of the general population (Hillman, Erickson, & Kramer, 2008). In addition, the effect of disease-modifying agents on cognition have yet to be investigated and should be a further area of inquiry.

CONCLUSIONS AND FUTURE DIRECTIONS

The impact of pediatric-onset MS on long-term adult outcomes remains to be fully appreciated. Vocational (e.g., ability to work part-time or full-time) and social outcomes, such as relationships and parenthood, and quality of life should all be considered. In addition, further characterization of the neuropsychological profile in relation to risk and protective factors as well as brain related changes are needed to aid in early identification and for the management of pediatric MS. In particular, the role of "cognitive reserve" as a potential moderator of cognitive decline should be investigated. Although difficult to determine in pediatric populations, cognitive reserve could be quantified by such measures as performance on premorbid standardized test measures, socioeconomic status, parental education, and parental occupation level. Standardization and validation of measures for assessment of functional impairment, as well as detection of early changes, will also help advance the field and promote much needed multi-center comparisons and collaborative research. Finally, it is imperative to appreciate the impact of MS onset during childhood on developing neural networks and to determine whether neuro-rehabilitation strategies can mitigate the impact of this serious disease.

REFERENCES

Akbar, N., Banwell, B., Sled, J. G., Binns, M. A., Doesburg, S. M., Rypma, B., . . . Till, C. (2016). Brain activation patterns and cognitive processing speed in patients with pediatric-onset multiple sclerosis. *Journal of Clinical and Experi-*

mental Neuropsychology, 38, 393–403. http://dx.doi.org/10.1080/13803395.2015.1119255

Akbar, N., Till, C., Sled, J. G., Binns, M. A., Doesburg, S. M., Aubert-Broche, B., . . . Banwell, B. (2016). Altered resting-state functional connectivity in cognitively preserved pediatric-onset MS patients and relationship to structural damage and cognitive performance. *Multiple Sclerosis Journal, 22,* 792–800. http://dx.doi.org/10.1177/1352458515602336

Amato, M. P., Goretti, B., Ghezzi, A., Hakiki, B., Niccolai, C., Lori, S., . . . Trojano, M. (2014). Neuropsychological features in childhood and juvenile multiple sclerosis: Five-year follow-up. *Neurology, 83,* 1432–1438. http://dx.doi.org/10.1212/WNL.0000000000000885

Amato, M. P., Goretti, B., Ghezzi, A., Lori, S., Zipoli, V., Moiola, L., . . . Trojano, M. (2010). Cognitive and psychosocial features in childhood and juvenile MS: Two-year follow-up. *Neurology, 75,* 1134–1140. http://dx.doi.org/10.1212/WNL.0b013e3181f4d821

Amato, M. P., Goretti, B., Ghezzi, A., Lori, S., Zipoli, V., Portaccio, E., . . . Trojano, M. (2008). Cognitive and psychosocial features of childhood and juvenile MS. *Neurology, 70,* 1891–1897. http://dx.doi.org/10.1212/01.wnl.0000312276.23177.fa

Amato, M. P., Goretti, B., Viterbo, R. G., Portaccio, E., Niccolai, C., Hakiki, B., . . . Trojano, M. (2014). Computer-assisted rehabilitation of attention in patients with multiple sclerosis: Results of a randomized, double-blind trial. *Multiple Sclerosis Journal, 20,* 91–98. http://dx.doi.org/10.1177/1352458513501571

Aubert-Broche, B., Fonov, V., Ghassemi, R., Narayanan, S., Arnold, D. L., Banwell, B., . . . Collins, D. L. (2011). Regional brain atrophy in children with multiple sclerosis. *NeuroImage, 58,* 409–415. http://dx.doi.org/10.1016/j.neuroimage.2011.03.025

Banwell, B. L., & Anderson, P. E. (2005). The cognitive burden of multiple sclerosis in children. *Neurology, 64,* 891–894. http://dx.doi.org/10.1212/01.WNL.0000152896.35341.51

Baruch, N. F., O'Donnell, E. H., Glanz, B. I., Benedict, R. H. B., Musallam, A. J., Healy, B. C., . . . Chitnis, T. (2016). Cognitive and patient-reported outcomes in adults with pediatric-onset multiple sclerosis. *Multiple Sclerosis Journal, 22,* 354–361. http://dx.doi.org/10.1177/1352458515588781

Bethune, A., Tipu, V., Sled, J. G., Narayanan, S., Arnold, D. L., Mabbott, D., . . . Banwell, B. (2011). Diffusion tensor imaging and cognitive speed in children with multiple sclerosis. *Journal of the Neurological Sciences, 309,* 68–74. http://dx.doi.org/10.1016/j.jns.2011.07.019

Bora, E., Özakbaş, S., Velakoulis, D., & Walterfang, M. (2016). Social cognition in multiple sclerosis: A meta-analysis. *Neuropsychology Review, 26,* 160–172. http://dx.doi.org/10.1007/s11065-016-9320-6

Calabrese, M., Seppi, D., Romualdi, C., Rinaldi, F., Alessio, S., Perini, P., & Gallo, P. (2012). Gray matter pathology in MS: A 3-year longitudinal study in a pediatric population. *AJNR. American Journal of Neuroradiology, 33,* 1507–1511. http://dx.doi.org/10.3174/ajnr.A3011

Cerasa, A., Passamonti, L., Valentino, P., Nisticò, R., Pirritano, D., Gioia, M. C., . . . Quattrone, A. (2012). Cerebellar-parietal dysfunctions in multiple sclerosis patients with cerebellar signs. *Experimental Neurology, 237,* 418–426. http://dx.doi.org/10.1016/j.expneurol.2012.07.020

Charvet, L. E., Beekman, R., Amadiume, N., Belman, A. L., & Krupp, L. B. (2014). The Symbol Digit Modalities Test is an effective cognitive screen in pediatric onset multiple sclerosis (MS). *Journal of the Neurological Sciences, 341,* 79–84. http://dx.doi.org/10.1016/j.jns.2014.04.006

Charvet, L. E., Cersosimo, B., Schwarz, C., Belman, A., & Krupp, L. B. (2016). Behavioral symptoms in pediatric multiple sclerosis: Relation to fatigue and cognitive impairment. *Journal of Child Neurology, 31,* 1062–1067. http://dx.doi.org/10.1177/0883073816636227

Charvet, L. E., Cleary, R. E., Vazquez, K., Belman, A. L., & Krupp, L. B. (2014). Social cognition in pediatric-onset multiple sclerosis (MS). *Multiple Sclerosis Journal, 20,* 1478–1484. http://dx.doi.org/10.1177/1352458514526942

Charvet, L. E., O'Donnell, E. H., Belman, A. L., Chitnis, T., Ness, J. M., Parrish, J., . . . Krupp, L. B. (2014). Longitudinal evaluation of cognitive functioning in pediatric multiple sclerosis: Report from the U.S. Pediatric Multiple Sclerosis Network. *Multiple Sclerosis Journal, 20,* 1502–1510. http://dx.doi.org/10.1177/1352458514527862

Chiaravalloti, N. D., Moore, N. B., Nikelshpur, O. M., & DeLuca, J. (2013). An RCT to treat learning impairment in multiple sclerosis: The MEMREHAB trial. *Neurology, 81,* 2066–2072. http://dx.doi.org/10.1212/01.wnl.0000437295.97946.a8

Chitnis, T., Glanz, B., Jaffin, S., & Healy, B. (2009). Demographics of pediatric-onset multiple sclerosis in an MS center population from the Northeastern United States. *Multiple Sclerosis Journal, 15,* 627–631. http://dx.doi.org/10.1177/1352458508101933

Cotter, J., Firth, J., Enzinger, C., Kontopantelis, E., Yung, A. R., Elliott, R., & Drake, R. J. (2016). Social cognition in multiple sclerosis: A systematic review and meta-analysis. *Neurology, 87,* 1727–1736. http://dx.doi.org/10.1212/WNL.0000000000003236

Drew, M., Tippett, L. J., Starkey, N. J., & Isler, R. B. (2008). Executive dysfunction and cognitive impairment in a large community-based sample with multiple sclerosis from New Zealand: A descriptive study. *Archives of Clinical Neuropsychology, 23,* 1–19. http://dx.doi.org/10.1016/j.acn.2007.09.005

Drew, M. A., Starkey, N. J., & Isler, R. B. (2009). Examining the link between information processing speed and executive functioning in multiple sclerosis. *Archives of Clinical Neuropsychology, 24,* 47–58. http://dx.doi.org/10.1093/arclin/acp007

Fuentes, A., Collins, D. L., Garcia-Lorenzo, D., Sled, J. G., Narayanan, S., Arnold, D. L., . . . Till, C. (2012). Memory performance and normalized regional brain volumes in patients with pediatric-onset multiple sclerosis. *Journal of the International Neuropsychological Society, 18,* 471–480. http://dx.doi.org/10.1017/S1355617711001913

Genova, H. M., Cagna, C. J., Chiaravalloti, N. D., DeLuca, J., & Lengenfelder, J. (2016). Dynamic assessment of social cognition in individuals with multiple sclerosis: A pilot study. *Journal of the International Neuropsychological Society, 22,* 83–88. http://dx.doi.org/10.1017/S1355617715001137

Ghassemi, R., Narayanan, S., Banwell, B., Sled, J. G., Shroff, M., & Arnold, D. L. (2014). Quantitative determination of regional lesion volume and distribution in children and adults with relapsing-remitting multiple sclerosis. *PLoS One, 9,* e85741. http://dx.doi.org/10.1371/journal.pone.0085741

Gich, J., Freixanet, J., García, R., Vilanova, J. C., Genís, D., Silva, Y., . . . Ramió-Torrentà, L. (2015). A randomized, controlled, single-blind, 6-month pilot study to evaluate the efficacy of MS-Line! A cognitive rehabilitation programme for patients with multiple sclerosis. *Multiple Sclerosis Journal, 21,* 1332–1343. http://dx.doi.org/10.1177/1352458515572405

Goretti, B., Ghezzi, A., Portaccio, E., Lori, S., Zipoli, V., Razzolini, L., . . . Amato, M. P. (2010). Psychosocial issue in children and adolescents with multiple sclerosis. *Neurological Sciences, 31,* 467–470. http://dx.doi.org/10.1007/s10072-010-0281-x

Goretti, B., Portaccio, E., Ghezzi, A., Lori, S., Moiola, L., Falautano, M., . . . Amato, M. P. (2012). Fatigue and its relationships with cognitive functioning and depression in paediatric multiple sclerosis. *Multiple Sclerosis Journal, 18,* 329–334. http://dx.doi.org/10.1177/1352458511420846

Hanssen, K. T., Beiske, A. G., Landrø, N. I., Hofoss, D., & Hessen, E. (2016). Cognitive rehabilitation in multiple sclerosis: A randomized controlled trial. *Acta Neurologica Scandinavica, 133,* 30–40. http://dx.doi.org/10.1111/ane.12420

Harding, K. E., Liang, K., Cossburn, M. D., Ingram, G., Hirst, C. L., Pickersgill, T. P., . . . Robertson, N. P. (2013). Long-term outcome of paediatric-onset multiple sclerosis: A population-based study. *Journal of Neurology, Neurosurgery, and Psychiatry, 84,* 141–147. http://dx.doi.org/10.1136/jnnp-2012-303996

Hillman, C. H., Erickson, K. I., & Kramer, A. F. (2008). Be smart, exercise your heart: Exercise effects on brain and cognition. *Nature Reviews Neuroscience, 9,* 58–65. http://dx.doi.org/10.1038/nrn2298

Holland, A. A., Graves, D., Greenberg, B. M., & Harder, L. L. (2014). Fatigue, emotional functioning, and executive dysfunction in pediatric multiple sclerosis. *Child Neuropsychology, 20,* 71–85. http://dx.doi.org/10.1080/09297049.2012.748888

Hosseini, B., Flora, D. B., Banwell, B. L., & Till, C. (2014). Age of onset as a moderator of cognitive decline in pediatric-onset multiple sclerosis. *Journal of the International Neuropsychological Society, 20,* 796–804. http://dx.doi.org/10.1017/S1355617714000642

Hubacher, M., DeLuca, J., Weber, P., Steinlin, M., Kappos, L., Opwis, K., & Penner, I.-K. (2015). Cognitive rehabilitation of working memory in juvenile multiple sclerosis-effects on cognitive functioning, functional MRI and network related connectivity. *Restorative Neurology and Neuroscience, 33,* 713–725. http://dx.doi.org/10.3233/RNN-150497

Julian, L., Serafin, D., Charvet, L. E., Ackerson, J., Benedict, R. H. B., Braaten, E., . . . Krupp, L. B. (2013). Cognitive impairment occurs in children and adolescents with multiple sclerosis: Results from a United States network. *Journal of Child Neurology, 28,* 102–107. http://dx.doi.org/10.1177/0883073812464816

Kerbrat, A., Aubert-Broche, B., Fonov, V., Narayanan, S., Sled, J. G., Arnold, D. A., . . . Collins, D. L. (2012). Reduced head and brain size for age and disproportionately smaller thalami in child-onset MS. *Neurology, 78,* 194–201. http://dx.doi.org/10.1212/WNL.0b013e318240799a

Krupp, L. B., Charvet, L. E., Porter, M., Amadiume, N., & Belman, A. (2014, September). *Application of the Brief International Cognitive Assessment for Multiple Sclerosis (BICAMS) to pediatric-onset MS.* Poster presented at the 2014 Joint ACTRIMS-ECTRIMS Meeting, Boston, MA.

Krysko, K. M., & O'Connor, P. (2016). Quality of life, cognition and mood in adults with pediatric multiple sclerosis. *The Canadian Journal of Neurological Sciences, 43,* 368–374. http://dx.doi.org/10.1017/cjn.2015.354

Langdon, D. W., Amato, M. P., Boringa, J., Brochet, B., Foley, F., Fredrikson, S., . . . Benedict, R. H. B. (2012). Recommendations for a Brief International Cognitive Assessment for Multiple Sclerosis (BICAMS). *Multiple Sclerosis Journal, 18,* 891–898. http://dx.doi.org/10.1177/1352458511431076

MacAllister, W. S. (2010). Multiple sclerosis in children and adolescents: Neurocognitive disorders. In D. Riva & C. Njiokiktjien (Eds.), *Brain lesion localization and developmental functions. Basal ganglia, connecting systems, cerebellum, mirror neurons* (pp. 81–88). France: John Libbey Eurotext.

MacAllister, W. S., Belman, A. L., Milazzo, M., Weisbrot, D. M., Christodoulou, C., Scherl, W. F., . . . Krupp, L. B. (2005). Cognitive functioning in children and adolescents with multiple sclerosis. *Neurology, 64,* 1422–1425. http://dx.doi.org/10.1212/01.WNL.0000158474.24191.BC

MacAllister, W. S., Christodoulou, C., Milazzo, M., & Krupp, L. B. (2007). Longitudinal neuropsychological assessment in pediatric multiple sclerosis. *Developmental Neuropsychology, 32,* 625–644. http://dx.doi.org/10.1080/87565640701375872

MacAllister, W. S., Christodoulou, C., Troxell, R., Milazzo, M., Block, P., Preston, T. E., . . . Krupp, L. B. (2009). Fatigue and quality of life in pediatric multiple sclerosis. *Multiple Sclerosis Journal, 15,* 1502–1508. http://dx.doi.org/10.1177/1352458509345902

Mesaros, S., Rocca, M. A., Absinta, M., Ghezzi, A., Milani, N., Moiola, L., . . . Filippi, M. (2008). Evidence of thalamic gray matter loss in pediatric multiple sclerosis. *Neurology, 70,* 1107–1112. http://dx.doi.org/10.1212/01.wnl.0000291010.54692.85

Pastò, L., Portaccio, E., Goretti, B., Ghezzi, A., Lori, S., & Hakiki, B., . . . Amato, M. P. (2016). The cognitive reserve theory in the setting of pediatric-onset multiple sclerosis. *Multiple Sclerosis Journal, 22,* 1741–1749.

Portaccio, E., Goretti, B., Lori, S., Zipoli, V., Centorrino, S., Ghezzi, A., . . . Amato, M. P. (2009). The brief neuropsychological battery for children: A screening tool for cognitive impairment in childhood and juvenile multiple sclerosis. *Multiple Sclerosis Journal, 15,* 620–626. http://dx.doi.org/10.1177/1352458508101950

Rao, S. M., Leo, G. J., Bernardin, L., & Unverzagt, F. (1991). Cognitive dysfunction in multiple sclerosis. I. Frequency, patterns, and prediction. *Neurology, 41,* 685–691. http://dx.doi.org/10.1212/WNL.41.5.685

Rocca, M. A., Absinta, M., Amato, M. P., Moiola, L., Ghezzi, A., Veggiotti, P., . . . Filippi, M. (2014). Posterior brain damage and cognitive impairment in pediatric multiple sclerosis. *Neurology, 82,* 1314–1321. http://dx.doi.org/10.1212/WNL.0000000000000309

Rocca, M. A., De Meo, E., Amato, M. P., Copetti, M., Moiola, L., Ghezzi, A., . . . Filippi, M. (2015). Cognitive impairment in paediatric multiple sclerosis patients is not related to cortical lesions. *Multiple Sclerosis Journal, 21,* 956–959. http://dx.doi.org/10.1177/1352458514557303

Rocca, M. A., Morelli, M. E., Amato, M. P., Moiola, L., Ghezzi, A., Veggiotti, P., . . . Filippi, M. (2016). Regional hippocampal involvement and cognitive impairment in pediatric multiple sclerosis. *Multiple Sclerosis Journal, 22,* 628–640. http://dx.doi.org/10.1177/1352458515598569

Rocca, M. A., Valsasina, P., Absinta, M., Moiola, L., Ghezzi, A., Veggiotti, P., . . . Filippi, M. (2014). Intranetwork and internetwork functional connectivity abnormalities in pediatric multiple sclerosis. *Human Brain Mapping, 35*(8), 4180–4192. http://dx.doi.org/10.1002/hbm.22469

Smerbeck, A. M., Parrish, J., Serafin, D., Yeh, E. A., Weinstock-Guttman, B., Hoogs, M., . . . Benedict, R. H. B. (2011). Visual-cognitive processing deficits in pediatric multiple sclerosis. *Multiple Sclerosis Journal, 17,* 449–456. http://dx.doi.org/10.1177/1352458510391689

Squillace, M., Ray, S., & Milazzo, M. (2015). Changes in gross grasp strength and fine motor skills in adolescents with pediatric multiple sclerosis. *Occupational Therapy in Health Care, 29,* 77–85. http://dx.doi.org/10.3109/07380577.2014.967441

Till, C., Deotto, A., Tipu, V., Sled, J. G., Bethune, A., Narayanan, S., . . . Banwell, B. L. (2011). White matter integrity and math performance in pediatric multiple sclerosis: A diffusion tensor imaging study. *NeuroReport, 22,* 1005–1009. http://dx.doi.org/10.1097/WNR.0b013e32834dc301

Till, C., Ghassemi, R., Aubert-Broche, B., Kerbrat, A., Collins, D. L., Narayanan, S., . . . Banwell, B. L. (2011). MRI correlates of cognitive impairment in childhood-onset multiple sclerosis. *Neuropsychology, 25,* 319–332. http://dx.doi.org/10.1037/a0022051

Till, C., Ho, C., Dudani, A., García-Lorenzo, D., Collins, D. L., & Banwell, B. L. (2012). Magnetic resonance imaging predictors of executive functioning in patients with pediatric-onset multiple sclerosis. *Archives of Clinical Neuropsychology, 27*, 495–509. http://dx.doi.org/10.1093/arclin/acs058

Till, C., Racine, N., Araujo, D., Narayanan, S., Collins, D. L., Aubert-Broche, B., . . . Banwell, B. (2013). Changes in cognitive performance over a 1-year period in children and adolescents with multiple sclerosis. *Neuropsychology, 27*, 210–219. http://dx.doi.org/10.1037/a0031665

Till, C., Udler, E., Ghassemi, R., Narayanan, S., Arnold, D. L., & Banwell, B. L. (2012). Factors associated with emotional and behavioral outcomes in adolescents with multiple sclerosis. *Multiple Sclerosis Journal, 18*, 1170–1180. http://dx.doi.org/10.1177/1352458511433918

Todorow, M., DeSouza, J. F., Banwell, B. L., & Till, C. (2014). Interhemispheric cooperation in global-local visual processing in pediatric multiple sclerosis. *Journal of Clinical and Experimental Neuropsychology, 36*, 111–126. http://dx.doi.org/10.1080/13803395.2013.867013

Waubant, E., Chabas, D., Okuda, D. T., Glenn, O., Mowry, E., Henry, R. G., . . . Pelletier, D. (2009). Difference in disease burden and activity in pediatric patients on brain magnetic resonance imaging at time of multiple sclerosis onset vs adults. *Archives of Neurology, 66*(8), 967–971. http://dx.doi.org/10.1001/archneurol.2009.135

Weier, K., Penner, I. K., Magon, S., Amann, M., Naegelin, Y., Andelova, M., . . . Sprenger, T. (2014). Cerebellar abnormalities contribute to disability including cognitive impairment in multiple sclerosis. *PLoS One, 9*, e86916. http://dx.doi.org/10.1371/journal.pone.0086916

Weier, K., Till, C., Fonov, V., Yeh, E. A., Arnold, D. L., Banwell, B., & Collins, D. L. (2016). Contribution of the cerebellum to cognitive performance in children and adolescents with multiple sclerosis. *Multiple Sclerosis Journal, 22*, 599–607. http://dx.doi.org/10.1177/1352458515595132

Weisbrot, D., Charvet, L., Serafin, D., Milazzo, M., Preston, T., Cleary, R., . . . Krupp, L. (2014). Psychiatric diagnoses and cognitive impairment in pediatric multiple sclerosis. *Multiple Sclerosis Journal, 20*, 588–593. http://dx.doi.org/10.1177/1352458513504249

12

PHARMACOLOGICAL TREATMENT FOR COGNITIVE IMPAIRMENT IN MULTIPLE SCLEROSIS

MARIA PIA AMATO AND BENEDETTA GORETTI

Cognitive impairment in multiple sclerosis (MS) affects from 40% up to 70% or more of patients, sometimes from the early stages of the disease. It presents a considerable burden to patients and to society, due to the negative impact on maintaining employment, social and daily living activities, and the capacity to benefit from in-patient rehabilitation (Amato et al., 2013). Therefore, interventions to ameliorate or reduce cognitive impairment, through pharmacological and/or rehabilitation approaches, may significantly benefit patient function and quality of life.

In this chapter, we provide an updated overview of available evidence of pharmacological approaches for ameliorating cognitive impairment, based either on disease-modifying treatments (DMTs) or symptomatic treatments.

http://dx.doi.org/10.1037/0000097-013
Cognition and Behavior in Multiple Sclerosis, J. DeLuca and B. M. Sandroff (Editors)

DISEASE-MODIFYING TREATMENTS

Since the approval of immunomodulatory-injected therapies in the early 1990s, a considerable body of evidence has accumulated on the impact of DMTs on relapse rate, disability progression, and magnetic resonance parameters in MS. In principle, DMTs also have the potential to positively influence the cognitive outcomes, by acting on some key pathogenic mechanisms of MS-related cognitive impairment. In particular, all the approved DMTs reduce the accumulation of T2 and T1 lesions in the brain, and some of them also reduce the progression of brain atrophy. Moreover, the decrease of the ongoing inflammatory activity may also contribute to better cognitive performance. Finally, based on preclinical data, some of the new DMTs may also exert a direct neuroprotective/neurotrophic effect, for instance, through the delivery of neurotrophic factors or activation of anti-oxidative stress pathways (Gold, Wolinksy, Amato, & Comi, 2010). However, evidence in the field remains extremely limited. Interpretation of available data is complicated by issues largely related to methodological problems of study design and execution (Amato et al., 2013).

In the majority of randomized controlled trials on DMTs, cognition has been only a secondary or even a tertiary, explorative outcome. In most cases, the Paced Auditory Serial Addition Test (PASAT), a test of information processing speed and complex attention, has been included as the only measure of cognition in the context of the Multiple Sclerosis Functional Composite (MSFC; Rudick et al., 1997). Moreover, the inclusion criteria have not taken into account the patients' cognitive status at entry into the trial and the studies have not been powered based on cognitive parameters. As for postmarketing, observational studies on DMTs, the vast majority are nonrandomized, have included small sample of patients with different clinical characteristics, and used heterogeneous cognitive assessment tools and outcome measures.

Most of the DMT studies have shown at least some positive effects on cognition. However, all of the above limitations have meant that cognitive results available to date can only be interpreted with caution.

Interferons Beta

Interferons (IFNs) are a group of signaling proteins made and released by host cells in response to the presence of several pathogens, such as viruses, bacteria, parasites, and tumor cells (Gold et al., 2010). The bulk of the evidence for the effects of DMTs on cognitive outcomes in MS has been collected with the IFN b-1a and IFN b-1b. They act through similar immunomodulating effects, including inhibitory effects on proliferation of leukocytes and antigen presentation. Furthermore, they may modulate the profile of cytokine production toward an anti-inflammatory phenotype and can reduce T-cell migration into the central nervous system (CNS; Gold et al., 2010). They are given subcutaneously or intramuscularly in relapsing-remitting (RR) MS. IFN b-1b is also approved in Europe for secondary progressive (SP) MS.

With IFN bs, overall, available evidence suggests some modest, positive effect on cognition (Amato et al., 2013). One of the earliest trials (Pliskin et al., 1996) explored the effects of low-dose IFN b-1b (50 mg, $n = 8$), high dose IFN b-1b (250 mg, $n = 9$) and placebo ($n = 13$) on cognition in a small group of 30 RR MS patients from one center. A focused neuropsychological battery was administered to the patients between the second and fourth years, whereas baseline cognitive performance was not assessed. High-dose IFN b-1b treatment was associated with better performance on only one test measuring delayed visual recall. This finding was significantly related to reduced MRI lesion burden.

The most rigorous and extensive study explored the effects of intramuscular IFN b-1a on cognition in the context of a multicenter, 2-year, phase III randomized clinical trial (Fischer et al., 2000). Both a comprehensive and a brief neuropsychological battery were administered to 166 RR MS patients. After 2 years, adjusting for baseline performance, IFN b-1a showed a significant beneficial effect on tests of information processing speed, learning and memory, as well as a positive trend on tests of visuospatial abilities and problem solving. Moreover, the brief battery revealed improved cognitive performance in both arms, possibly due to "practice effects," which was significantly more pronounced in the treatment arm. Finally, the treatment arm also exhibited a significantly increased time to sustained deterioration in the performance on the PASAT. In interpreting the study's results, a few caveats should be considered. The analysis of results after 2 years included only 60% of the baseline group of patients (i.e., 40% attrition). Moreover, it is difficult to generalize the trial results to everyday practice, because the neuropsychological assessment in the trial was particularly extensive—taking nearly 3 hours. The effect of IFNB-1b on cognition in patients with clinically isolated syndromes (CIS) has been assessed in the phase III, BENEFIT trial (Kappos et al., 2006) and its extension at 3 (Kappos et al., 2007) and 5 years (Kappos et al., 2009). In the original 2-year trial, patients with a first clinical demyelinating event (CIS) were randomized to receive IFN b-1b immediately after the clinical event (i.e., early treatment group) or at the end of the trial (i.e., delayed treatment group). The mean MSFC score improved over the 5 years in most patients belonging to either treatment group. This improvement was largely driven by improvement in the PASAT, whose scores were in the normal range in the vast majority of the subjects at baseline. Improvement on the PASAT was significantly more pronounced in the early treatment group compared with the delayed treatment group after 5 years, suggesting an effect of early treatment in maintaining an intact cognitive functioning (Penner et al. 2012).

No cognitive data have been published from the IFN b trials in subjects with secondary and primary progressive (PP) MS (e.g., Montalban et al., 2009).

As for postmarketing observational studies involving interferons and cognition in MS, the current chapter will focus only on the largest ones (i.e., studies that have included at least one hundred patients). As compared to clinical trials, these observational studies reflect therapeutic choices in everyday clinical practice. Due to the lack of randomization, they are prone to several sources of bias, such as heterogeneous demographic and clinical characteristics of the subjects, different assessment tools and cognitive outcomes, so that their results are difficult to compare and should be interpreted with caution. The effects IFN b-1a on cognitive function in early, mildly disabled RR MS patients were addressed in the Italian multicenter, postmarketing Cognitive Impairment in Multiple Sclerosis (COGIMUS) study (Patti et al., 2010). This prospective cohort study included early RR MS patients treated with IFN b-1a s.c. 22 or 44 mcg in everyday clinical practice. The patients were assessed through the Brief Repeatable Neuropsychological Battery (BRNB) and the Stroop test at baseline and at 12-month intervals for 3 years for a total of four cognitive assessments. At baseline there were no differences between the two groups in demographic and clinical characteristics or in the proportions of patients impaired on more than three tests. Data on cognitive function at baseline and 3 years were available for 318 patients of the original cohort (72.1 %; 22 mcg, $n = 153$; 44 mcg, $n = 165$) and showed a 32% risk reduction of developing impairment in three or more tests for patients on high dose compared with those on the lower dose. The authors suggested that higher and more frequent doses of the drug can be more effective than lower doses in terms of the cognitive outcome of the subjects, although, due to the above-mentioned limitations of observational studies, the results should be interpreted with caution.

Glatiramer Acetate

Glatiramer acetate (GA) is a polypeptide-based therapy approved for the treatment of RR MS. Most investigations have attributed the immunomodulatory effect of GAs to its capability to alter T-cell differentiation, promoting development of Th2-polarized GA-reactive CD4(+) T-cells, which may dampen inflammation within the CNS. GA also exerts immunomodulatory activity on antigen presenting cells, which participate in innate immune responses (Gold et al., 2010). The effect of GA on cognition was also evaluated as part of a phase III trial (Weinstein et al., 1999) on RRMS where patients were randomized to receive GA (20 mg sc daily) or placebo. Two hundred forty-eight patients were tested at baseline and after 1 to 2 years using the BRNB. At baseline, neuropsychological test performance was similar in both arms, with mean scores falling within the range of normal performance with the exception of a verbal fluency test. Both arms showed a significant improvement in cognitive performance because of "practice effects." No differences were detected between the treatment groups for any of the neuropsychological tests. Both the low level of baseline cognitive abnormalities and the short-term observation period may explain the absence of an effect of GA on cognitive function. A subgroup of 153 patients (65%) was reexamined 10 years after inclusion into the clinical trial (Schwid, Goodman, Weinstein, McDermott, & Johnson, 2007). Only attention tests and the PASAT showed a significant decline in patients who originally received either GA or placebo. There were no differences in cognitive performance between patients originally in the placebo arm or the GA arm, again suggesting the absence of an effect of GA on cognitive function. However, the high rate of patients not included in the long-term evaluation and the substantial stability of cognitive functioning in these subjects render it difficult to draw any firm conclusions about the effect of GA on cognition. Finally, although the MSFC was included in a phase III trial of GA in PP MS, no cognitive data have been published (Wolinsky et al., 2007).

Natalizumab

Natalizumab is a humanized monoclonal antibody that binds to the α_4 subunit of $\alpha_4\beta_1$ and $\alpha_4\beta_7$ integrins of activated leukocytes and blocks their binding to their endothelial receptors (VCAM-1 and mucosal addressin cell adhesion molecule 1, respectively), thereby preventing their passage across the blood-brain barrier and attenuating inflammation in the CNS (Gold et al., 2010). In natalizumab Phase III clinical trials of RR MS patients— the Natalizumab Safety and Efficacy in Relapsing Remitting Multiple Sclerosis (AFFIRM) trial (Polman et al., 2006) and Safety and Efficacy of Natalizumab in Combination with Interferon Beta-1a in Patients with Relapsing Remitting Multiple Sclerosis (SENTINEL) trial (Rudick et al., 2006)—the PASAT was the only cognitive tool used. In the AFFIRM trial, RR MS patients were randomly assigned to receive either natalizumab (at the standard dose of 300 mg) or placebo by intravenous infusion every 4 weeks for up to 116 weeks. In the SENTINEL trial, patients were randomly assigned to receive 300 mg of natalizumab or placebo intravenously every 4 weeks in addition to interferon beta-1a at a dose of 30 μg intramuscularly once weekly for up to 116 weeks. The PASAT data suggested a positive effect on cognition in the arm treated with natalizumab in both studies.

The impact of natalizumab on cognitive functioning was also investigated in a few observational studies. In an uncontrolled, observational study

(Iaffaldano et al., 2012), cognitive performance was examined by the BRNB and the Stroop test calculating a Cognitive Impairment Index (CII) every 12 months. In two arms, 100 patients and 53 patients completed 1- and 2-year-natalizumab treatment, respectively, at the standard dose of 300 mg iv every four weeks. After 1 year of treatment, the percentage of cognitively impaired patients decreased from 29% to 19%, and the mean baseline values of the CII and fatigue scores were significantly reduced. These effects were confirmed in the patients treated for up to 2 years. In a prospective, uncontrolled study in 333 patients, after 12 months of natalizumab treatment, 69% to 88% of patients reported an improvement in patient-reported outcomes measures, including quality of life, fatigue, and cognition (Stephenson et al., 2012). Reduction of self-reported fatigue was also reported in the large TYNERGY study (Svenningsson et al., 2013).

In the above studies, the nonrandomized study design, together with the absence of a control group and/or of objective measures of cognitive performance, limits the validity of conclusions.

Other DMTs

Fingolimod is an oral sphingosine-1-phosphate receptor modulator marketed for the treatment of RR MS. The drug acts by preventing lymphocyte egress from lymph nodes, thus leading to a reduced infiltration of potentially autoaggressive lymphocytes into the CNS. Preclinical findings also suggest that fingolimod may promote neuroprotective and reparative processes within the CNS through modulation of sphingosine-1-phosphate receptors expressed on neural cells (Gold et al., 2010). In the Safety and Efficacy of Fingolimod in Patients with Relapsing-Remitting Multiple Sclerosis (FREEDOMS) trial, a 24-month, randomized controlled trial of oral fingolimod (0.5 mg/day or 1.25 mg/day) was compared with placebo in patients with RR MS; a significant effect on the MSFC was observed in both active groups compared with the placebo group (Cohen et al., 2010), although no data for the PASAT have been published.

Similarly, trials on newer oral and biologic DMTs recently introduced in the market for RR MS patients have included the PASAT in the context of the MSFC, although no cognitive results have been published thus far. Postmarketing studies of these newer drugs are underway.

Conclusions and Future Directions

The effect of DMTs on cognition has not been adequately studied and methodological limitations render it difficult to draw any firm conclusions. Further, some of the studies with DMTs have shown weak, positive effects on cognition. It is hypothesized that early treatment may be the most effective way to help preserve intact cognitive functioning and delay the development of cognitive impairment. There is consensus among the experts that future trials should assess cognition more systematically to shed some light on the potential effect of DMTs on the patient cognitive outcome (Amato et al., 2013).

SYMPTOMATIC DRUGS

Studies on symptomatic drugs in MS have focused on improving performance in specific, impaired cognitive domains and have used specific inclusion criteria relative to baseline cognitive performance. Most of the studies have focused on information processing, speed and complex attention, or episodic memory and share a few methodological shortcomings, in particular, small sample sizes, study design (often crossover rather than parallel-group), heterogeneity of cognitive measures (impaired cognition was often not an inclusion criterion), and outcomes (see Table 12.1).

Antifatigue Drugs

Due to frequent association between fatigue and cognitive impairment in MS patients and the hypothesis of a shared pathophysiologic basis, it has been speculated that drugs used for the symptomatic management of fatigue in MS may also be beneficial for cognitive functioning (Tur, 2016).

Amantadine and Pemoline

Amantadine may increase dopaminergic, noradrenergic, and serotoninergic transmissions, inhibit monoaminoxidase A, and block N-methyl-D-aspartic acid (NMDA) receptors (Tur, 2016). Further, it could enhance endorphin system activity. Pemoline is a central nervous system (CNS) stimulant: animal studies indicate that it may act through dopaminergic mechanisms (Tur). Geisler and colleagues (1996) studied the effects of 6 weeks treatment with amantadine, pemoline, or placebo on cognitive functioning in MS, evaluating 45 patients with MS and severe fatigue. All patients underwent comprehensive neuropsychological testing. Primary outcome measures were tests of attention, memory, and motor speed. All three treatment groups improved on tests of attention, verbal memory, and motor speed, probably due to "practice effects," and there were no significant differences in cognitive performance between amantadine, pemoline, and placebo patients (Geisler et al., 1996).

TABLE 12.1
Summary of Studies on Symptomatic Treatments for Cognitive Dysfunction in Multiple Sclerosis

Authors	Drug	Number treated	Design	Duration	Cognitive results
Antifatigue drugs					
Geisler et al., 1996	Amantadine, pemoline	16	DB, PC, RCT	6 weeks	−
Möller et al., 2011	Modafinil	62	DB, PC, RCT	8 weeks	−
Lange et al., 2009	Modafinil	8	DB, PC, RCT	8 weeks	+
Stankoff et al., 2005	Modafinil	59	DB, PC, RCT	5 weeks	−
Wilken et al., 2008	Modafinil	23	Randomized, evaluator blind	4 months	+
Bruce et al., 2012	Armodafinil	16	DB, PC, CO	1 week	+
Ford-Johnson et al., 2016	Modafinil	16	DB, CO	5 weeks	+
Alzheimer's drugs					
Shaygannejad et al., 2008	Rivastigmine	30	DB, PC, RCT	12 weeks	−
Parry et al., 2003	Rivastigmine	10	OLT	4–6 weeks	+
Cader et al., 2009	Rivastigmine	15	CO, SB	4–6 weeks	−
Krupp et al., 2004	Donepezil	35	DB, PC, RCT	24 weeks	+
Krupp et al., 2011	Donepezil	61	DB, PC, RCT	24 weeks	−
Lovera et al., 2010	Memantina	58	DB, PC, RCT	16 weeks	−
Villoslada et al., 2009	Memantina	19	DB, PC, CO	12 months	−

		Stimulants			
Benedict et al., 2008	l-amphetamine	19	Counterbalanced, within-subject	4x single doses	+
Morrow et al., 2009	l-amphetamine	108	DB, PC, RCT	4 weeks	–
Sumowski et al., 2011 (re-analysis of Morrow et al., 2009)	l-amphetamine	108	DB, PC, RCT	4 weeks	+
Harel et al., 2009	Methylphenidate	14	DB, PC, RCT	Single dose	+
Lovera et al., 2007	Ginkgo biloba	20	DB, PC, RCT	12 weeks	–
Lovera et al., 2010	Ginkgo biloba	61	DB, PC, RCT	12 weeks	–
Johnson et al., 2006	Ginkgo biloba	12	DB, PC, PG	4 weeks	+ variable responses
		Potassium channel blockers			
Magnin et al., 2015	Fampridine	50	OLT	4 weeks	+
Pavsic et al., 2015	Fampridine	30	OLT	4 weeks	–
Jensen et al., 2014	Fampridine	108	OLT	26–28 days	+

Note. + = positive results, – = negative results; DB = double blind, PC = placebo controlled, RCT = randomized controlled trial, CO = crossover, SB = single blind, OLT = open-label trial, PG = parallel group.

Modafinil

Modafinil (and its R-isomer, armodafinil) is a wakefulness-promoting agent used for treatment of a few sleep disorders. The drug acts as a selective, relatively weak, atypical dopamine reuptake inhibitor. However, it appears that other additional mechanisms may also be at play (Mignot, 2012). Overall, there is no consistent evidence to date that modafinil can help improve cognitive impairments in MS, based on multiple randomized trials providing inconsistent findings. A double-blind, placebo-controlled randomized trial involving 121 patients with MS and fatigue (Möller et al., 2011) found that modafinil had no significant effects on fatigue or cognitive dysfunction. In this study, there was a significant improvement on the SDMT with modafinil, but not in the PASAT, which actually improved significantly in the placebo group. In a double-blind, placebo-controlled randomized trial of 21 patients with MS, published by Lange, Volkmer, Heesen, and Liepert (2009), a total of 18 patients were tested using the D2 Alertness Test, which measures focusing of attention. Although modafinil-treated patients showed relative improvement on the D2 test and subjectively reported less fatigue, another larger study involving 115 patients did not replicate the benefit on fatigue (Stankoff et al., 2005). Another study with modafinil suggested a positive treatment effect on other neuropsychological tests, but this study was not placebo-controlled (Wilken et al., 2008).

Bruce et al. (2012) conducted a small double-blind, placebo-controlled, crossover study testing the efficacy of armodafinil in reducing cognitive problems in 23 MS patients. After correcting for multiple comparisons, the patients had significantly improved delayed memory on a list-learning task after they took armodafinil, but no improvement on measures of executive function, visual memory, processing speed, or self-reported fatigue. More recently, Ford-Johnson et al. (2016) assessed the efficacy of modafinil for the treatment of new learning and memory deficits, as well as fatigue, in persons with MS. Sixteen patients with a diagnosis of MS and documented new learning impairment completed the study. In a 5-week randomized, double-blind, crossover design, participants received either a single daily oral dose of modafinil (200 mg) or placebo for 2 weeks. A 1-week washout period was included between study arms. No effect of modafinil was noted on learning and memory performance. However, participants taking 200 mg of modafinil showed improvement in one of the two working memory measures administered, as compared with those on placebo. Treatment with modafinil did not have any beneficial effect in reducing self-reported fatigue.

Acetylcholinesterase Inhibitors

Acetylcholinesterase inhibitors used in Alzheimer's disease have been tested for improving cognition in other neurological disorders, including

MS. In MS, it is hypothesized that disruption of cholinergic pathways and impaired axonal transport of acetylcholine may reduce cholinergic drive that might underlie, at least in part, cognitive dysfunction. (Amato et al., 2013). Moreover, neuroimaging studies have shown hippocampal atrophy and altered connectivity in MS subjects, which have been associated with patients' memory impairments (Sicotte et al., 2008).

Rivastigmine

Parry, Scott, Palace, Smith, and Matthews (2003) suggested that rivastigmine, a central cholinesterase inhibitor, is able to perform an acute modulation of potentially adaptive functional changes in cognitive processing. They studied 10 patients with MS and 11 healthy controls using a functional MRI (fMRI) counting Stroop task. All the MS patients and four controls took the drug. Each subject was studied on 2 separate days: once with administration of rivastigmine (3 mg orally) and once with administration of placebo 150 min before fMRI scanning. In five of the 10 MS patients there was a relative normalization of the abnormal Stroop-associated pattern of brain activation, although no change in brain activation was found in any of four healthy controls taking the drug.

In a single investigator-blind, crossover treatment design, Cader, Palace, and Matthews (2009) studied 15 patients with MS taking rivastigmine (4.5 mg by mouth twice daily) and domperidone, a *peripherally selective dopamine D_2 receptor* antagonist (10 mg by mouth once a day) or domperidone alone. Both a Stroop task and an N-back task were used to assess changes in brain activity using fMRI. Subjects were required to attend the imaging center on three separate occasions, 4 to 6 weeks apart, in a crossover design. Patients were imaged twice: (1) 4 weeks after randomization to treatment with either domperidone and rivastigmine or domperidone alone, and (2) after the alternative treatment that had been administered for approximately 4 weeks. Administration of rivastigmine significantly increased fMRI activation in the right inferior frontal gyrus for the Stroop task. Incremental fMRI activation with progressively greater N-back task difficulty was enhanced by rivastigmine in prefrontal and parietal cortical regions. Functional connectivity analysis also showed increased connectivity in a few brain regions associated with the performance on the N-back task. However, there were no statistically significant changes in the neuropsychological task performance with rivastigmine in this small study (Cader et al., 2009).

In a 3-month single-center, double-blind, placebo-controlled clinical trial, Shaygannejad, Janghorbani, Ashtari, Zanjani, and Zakizade (2008) enrolled 60 MS patients with cognitive impairment. Patients were randomly allocated to receive a 12-week treatment course of either rivastigmine (1.5 mg once a day increment over 4 weeks increased to 3 mg twice daily) or placebo. Response to treatment was assessed by the Wechsler Memory Scale (WMS) at baseline and 12 weeks after the start of therapy. A slight, but significant memory improvement occurred in both groups, possibly due to "practice effects." The average WMS general memory score at the end of trial did not change between rivastigmine and placebo group (Shaygannejad et al., 2008).

Taken as a whole the above results do not support a clear role of rivastigmine in improving MS-related cognitive dysfunction.

Donepezil

Donepezil binds and reversibly inactivates the cholinesterases, thus inhibiting hydrolysis of acetylcholine (Krupp et al., 2004). The pivotal study on donepezil published by Krupp et al. (2004) was a randomized, double-blind, placebo-controlled, single-center clinical trial of 69 patients with MS, who were selected for initial memory difficulties and randomly assigned to receive a 24-week treatment course of either donepezil (10 mg daily) or placebo. Subjects underwent neuropsychological assessment at weeks 0 and 24, consisting primarily of a modified version of the Brief Repeatable Battery. The Selective Reminding Test (SRT) was chosen as the primary outcome measure. Donepezil improved memory performance on the SRT, when compared with placebo. Moreover, patients in the donepezil group were significantly more likely to self-report memory improvement than those receiving placebo. The drug was generally well-tolerated, with the exception that unusual/abnormal dreams occurred more frequently in the donepezil-treated group. A subsequent double-blind, parallel-group, placebo-controlled, multicenter randomized trial was performed by the same group of researchers (Krupp et al., 2011). The study investigated the effects of 10 mg daily of donepezil ($n = 61$) versus 10 mg of placebo ($n = 59$) in 120 cognitively impaired MS patients. After 24 weeks, there were no improvements in memory performance on SRT in the donepezil group. Post hoc analyses, however, revealed significant memory improvements in the subgroup of patients exhibiting more severe degrees of cognitive dysfunction (Krupp et al., 2011).

Conflicting data from donepezil studies may be interpreted in different ways, including a real lack of effect of the drug in MS patients, the inclusion in the trial of patients with memory defects that were too mild—as suggested by post hoc analyses—or even a different pathogenesis of memory defects in MS subjects. These defects might derive primarily either from information processing speed problems, which are not sensitive to donepezil effects, or be mainly secondary to hippocampal involvement, where, in hypothesis, donepezil might exert its beneficial effects.

Memantine

Memantine acts on activated NMDA receptors by binding to a site located in the channel of the receptor. A multicenter, double-blind, placebo-controlled clinical trial in MS patients with cognitive impairment ($n = 126$: RR, PP, and SP) was conducted by Lovera et al. (2010). Fifty-eight MS patients treated with memantine at 20 mg daily and 68 controls were tested. The primary outcome was the change from baseline to exit on the PASAT and the California Verbal Learning Test-II (CVLT-II) Long Delay Free Recall. The first results showed that patients in the memantine group showed no improvements in performance on PASAT and CVLT-II. Subjects on memantine had no serious adverse events (AEs), but had more fatigue and neurological AEs, as well as less cognitive improvement and greater neuropsychiatric symptoms than subjects on placebo as reported by family members (Lovera et al.). Villoslada, Arrondo, Sepulcre, Alegre, and Artieda (2009) conducted a 1-year, randomized, double-blind, crossover trial to compare memantine (30 mg/day) against a placebo in 60 patients with MS and cognitive impairment. Using the BRNB, the primary endpoint was improvement of verbal memory. Seven of the nine patients in the memantine group reported some transient worsening of neurological impairment during the trial. However, one patient who had exhibited deteriorating cognitive performance during the treatment did not recover to the baseline level. Concerns about safety of memantine discourage its use for treating cognitive impairment in MS (Villoslada et al.).

Stimulants

In MS patients, slowed mental processing often coexists with impairments in various aspects of complex information processing, as well as attention capacity. It is, therefore, reasonable to consider CNS stimulants for MS patients.

L-Amphetamine Sulphate

L-amphetamine sulphate, or 1-methyl-2-phenylethylamine sulphate (2:1), is a synthetic sympathomimetic amine. The L-isomer of amphetamine is a psychostimulant that acts by stimulating dopamine release and dopamine-reuptake inhibition. It seems to be less potent in facilitating dopamine transmission than the D-isomer, but it does produce equivalent increases in norepinephrine in the hippocampus and cortex (Benedict et al., 2008). In a pilot double-blind, placebo-controlled study involving 19 MS patients (Benedict et al.), single 45 mg doses of L-amphetamine sulphate in MS were associated with improved performance on neuropsychological tests measuring information processing speed. In a subsequent larger-scale study, Morrow and colleagues (2009) tested 151 clinically definite MS patients randomized to L-amphetamine or to placebo in a 6-week, double-blind, parallel-group, dose-titration trial. The initial 5 mg dose of L-amphetamine was progressively increased up to 30 mg, and this dose was maintained for 14 days. The trial results did not confirm any significant improvement on the SDMT or subjective ratings of cognition. However, in a reanalysis of the study results focusing on memory function, there was a significant effect of L-amphetamine sulphate on auditory/verbal and visual/spatial memory in the cognitively impaired MS patients (Sumowski et al., 2011), suggesting that the drug may act by improving hippocampal function. In the above studies, L-amphetamine proved to be well tolerated, although tolerability in the long-term remains questionable.

Methylphenidate

Methylphenidate is a CNS stimulant of the *phenethylamine* and *piperidine classes* that is used in the treatment of attention-deficit/hyperactivity disorder and narcolepsy (Markowitz, Straughn, & Patrick, 2003). Harel, Appleboim, Lavie, and Achiron (2009) studied 26 MS patients with impaired attention in a double-blind, placebo-controlled trial. The patients were randomized to receive a single dose of 10 mg methylphenidate or placebo. Attention was assessed using PASAT-3" and PASAT-2" at baseline and one hour after drug/placebo administration. Methylphenidate significantly improved performance of both PASAT-3" and PASAT-2" tests, by 22.8% and 25.6%, respectively, while no significant changes were observed in placebo-treated patients.

Ginkgo Biloba

Ginkgo biloba is an herbal extract tested to enhance cognitive function in patients with Alzheimer's disease or other dementias. This drug has been tested in two small MS trials. The first one reported improvements in fatigue, symptom severity, and functional performance (Johnson et al., 2006); however, no specific cognitive outcomes were reported. The second study, a 12-week, randomized, double-blind, placebo-controlled trial of 38 patients with MS, did not find significant benefits of ginkgo biloba treatment compared with placebo on any cognitive test (Lovera et al., 2007).

Potassium Channel Blockers

Fampridine

Fampridine (4-aminopyridine) is a potassium-channel blocker approved by FDA for improving gait performance disability in MS (Goodman et al., 2010). Due to its mechanism of action, however, a few studies have explored the impact of the drug on other motor and cognitive parameters. Fifty MS patients were included in a prospective, monocentric, open-label trial (Magnin et al., 2015). Assessments of verbal phonological and semantic fluencies were repeated twice (within 1 week) before fampridine treatment and twice after fampridine treatment. Gait velocity and fatigue (visual analogical scale) were also assessed. Verbal fluencies were significantly improved after fampridine treatment. Gait responders and gait nonresponders did not present significant differences in verbal fluency performance and fatigue score. The authors suggested that fampridine may have a favorable effect on phonological fluency, even in the gait nonresponder patients. Pavsic, Pelicon, Ledinek, and Sega (2015) conducted a nonrandomized study including 30 patients with different types of MS, treated with 10 mg of fampridine twice daily. The response rate in terms of gait performance was 56.7%. After 28 days of treatment, significant improvement among responders occurred in total MSFC score; however, there was no statistically significant improvement of PASAT. Jensen, Ravnborg, Mamoei, Dalgas, and Stenager (2014) performed another open-label study of 108 MS patients treated with fampridine 10 mg BID. After 26 to 28 days of treatment, results showed significant improvements on quantitative tests of upper and lower limb functions, as well as the SDMT, measuring information processing speed and working memory on visual scanning.

Conclusions and Future Directions

Overall, to date, due to sparse investigations, limitations of the study design, and conflicting study findings, there are no robust data supporting the use of any of the above described symptomatic drugs for improving MS-related cognitive impairments. In a few cases, positive results in the pilot trial have not been confirmed in larger-scale studies. Pharmacological treatment of comorbidities that can contribute to poor cognitive performance, such as depression, may also provide cognitive benefits. However, with the possible exception of fatigue, this area has been poorly addressed thus far. There are still many unanswered questions regarding the use of cognitive enhancer agents, including the effects of their long-term use in a chronic disease such as MS. A possible effect of agents used to enhance cognition in MS could be due to their capability of counteracting the side effects of other drugs (e.g., benzodiazepines, baclophen, alpha lytic) used to treat symptoms other than cognitive impairment. On the whole, the research in this field must be considered preliminary. It is premature to currently recommend the clinical use of these classes of medications, and their off-label prescription in clinical practice is limited to a few selected cases.

REFERENCES

Amato, M. P., Langdon, D., Montalban, X., Benedict, R. H. B., DeLuca, J., Krupp, L. B., . . . Comi, G. (2013). Treatment of cognitive impairment in multiple sclerosis: Position paper. *Journal of Neurology, 260,* 1452–1468. http://dx.doi.org/10.1007/s00415-012-6678-0

Benedict, R. H. B., Munschauer, F., Zarevics, P., Erlanger, D., Rowe, V., Feaster, T., & Carpenter, R. L. (2008). Effects of l-amphetamine sulfate on cognitive function in multiple sclerosis patients. *Journal of Neurology, 255,* 848–852. http://dx.doi.org/10.1007/s00415-008-0760-7

Bruce, J., Hancock, L., Roberg, B., Brown, A., Henkelman, E., & Lynch, S. (2012). Impact of armodafinil on cognition in multiple sclerosis: A randomized, double-blind crossover pilot study. *Cognitive and Behavioral Neurology, 25,* 107–114. http://dx.doi.org/10.1097/WNN.0b013e31826df7fd

Cader, S., Palace, J., & Matthews, P. M. (2009). Cholinergic agonism alters cognitive processing and enhances brain functional connectivity in patients with multiple sclerosis. *Journal of Psychopharmacology, 23,* 686–696. http://dx.doi.org/10.1177/0269881108093271

Cohen, J. A., Barkhof, F., Comi, G., Hartung, H.-P., Khatri, B. O., Montalban, X., . . . Kappos, L. (2010). Oral fingolimod or intramuscular interferon for relapsing multiple sclerosis. *The New England Journal of Medicine, 362,* 402–415. http://dx.doi.org/10.1056/NEJMoa0907839

Fischer, J. S., Priore, R. L., Jacobs, L. D., Cookfair, D. L., Rudick, R. A., Herndon, R. M., . . . Kooijmans-Coutinho, M. F. (2000). Neuropsychological effects of interferon beta-1a in relapsing multiple sclerosis. *Annals of Neurology, 48,* 885–892. http://dx.doi.org/10.1002/1531-8249(200012)48:6<885::AID-ANA9>3.0.CO;2-1

Ford-Johnson, L., DeLuca, J., Zhang, J., Elovic, E., Lengenfelder, J., & Chiaravalloti, N. D. (2016). Cognitive effects of modafinil in patients with multiple sclerosis: A clinical trial. *Rehabilitation Psychology, 61,* 82–91. http://dx.doi.org/10.1037/a0039919

Geisler, M. W., Sliwinski, M., Coyle, P. K., Masur, D. M., Doscher, C., & Krupp, L. B. (1996). The effects of amantadine and pemoline on cognitive functioning in multiple sclerosis. *Archives of Neurology, 53,* 185–188. http://dx.doi.org/10.1001/archneur.1996.00550020101021

Gold, R., Wolinsky, J. S., Amato, M. P., & Comi, G. (2010). Evolving expectations around early management of multiple sclerosis. *Therapeutic Advances in Neurological Disorders, 3,* 351–367. http://dx.doi.org/10.1177/1756285610385608

Goodman, A. D., Brown, T. R., Edwards, K. R., Krupp, L. B., Schapiro, R. T., Cohen, R., . . . Blight, A. R. (2010). A Phase 3 trial of extended release oral dalfampridine in multiple sclerosis. *Annals of Neurology, 68,* 494–502. http://dx.doi.org/10.1002/ana.22240

Harel, Y., Appleboim, N., Lavie, M., & Achiron, A. (2009). Single dose of methylphenidate improves cognitive performance in multiple sclerosis patients with impaired attention process. *Journal of the Neurological Sciences, 276,* 38–40. http://dx.doi.org/10.1016/j.jns.2008.08.025

Iaffaldano, P., Viterbo, R. G., Paolicelli, D., Lucchese, G., Portaccio, E., Goretti, B., . . . Trojano, M. (2012). Impact of natalizumab on cognitive performances and fatigue in relapsing multiple sclerosis: A prospective, open-label, two years observational study. *PLoS One, 7,* e35843. http://dx.doi.org/10.1371/journal.pone.0035843

Jensen, H. B., Ravnborg, M., Mamoei, S., Dalgas, U., & Stenager, E. (2014). Changes in cognition, arm function and lower body function after slow-release Fampridine treatment. *Multiple Sclerosis Journal, 20,* 1872–1880. http://dx.doi.org/10.1177/1352458514533844

Johnson, S. K., Diamond, B. J., Rausch, S., Kaufman, M., Shiflett, S. C., & Graves, L. (2006). The effect of ginkgo biloba on functional measures in multiple sclerosis: A pilot randomized controlled trial. *EXPLORE: The Journal of Science and Healing, 2,* 19–24. http://dx.doi.org/10.1016/j.explore.2005.10.007

Kappos, L., Freedman, M. S., Polman, C. H., Edan, G., Hartung, H.-P., Miller, D. H., . . . Sandbrink, R. (2007). Effect of early versus delayed interferon beta-1b treatment on disability after a first clinical event suggestive of multiple sclerosis: A 3-year follow-up analysis of the BENEFIT study. *The Lancet, 370,* 389–397. http://dx.doi.org/10.1016/S0140-6736(07)61194-5

Kappos, L., Freedman, M. S., Polman, C. H., Edan, G., Hartung, H.-P., Miller, D. H., . . . Pohl, C. (2009). Long-term effect of early treatment with interferon beta-1b after a first clinical event suggestive of multiple sclerosis: 5-year active treatment extension of the phase 3 BENEFIT trial. *The Lancet Neurology, 8,* 987–997. http://dx.doi.org/10.1016/S1474-4422(09)70237-6

Kappos, L., Polman, C. H., Freedman, M. S., Edan, G., Hartung, H. P., Miller, D. H., . . . Sandbrink, R. (2006). Treatment with interferon beta-1b delays conversion to clinically definite and McDonald MS in patients with clinically isolated syndromes. *Neurology, 67,* 1242–1249. http://dx.doi.org/10.1212/01.wnl.0000237641.33768.8d

Krupp, L. B., Christodoulou, C., Melville, P., Scherl, W. F., MacAllister, W. S., & Elkins, L. E. (2004). Donepezil improved memory in multiple sclerosis in a randomized clinical trial. *Neurology, 63,* 1579–1585. http://dx.doi.org/10.1212/01.WNL.0000142989.09633.5A

Krupp, L. B., Christodoulou, C., Melville, P., Scherl, W. F., Pai, L.-Y., Muenz, L. R., . . . Wishart, H. (2011). Multicenter randomized clinical trial of donepezil for memory impairment in multiple sclerosis. *Neurology, 76,* 1500–1507. http://dx.doi.org/10.1212/WNL.0b013e318218107a

Lange, R., Volkmer, M., Heesen, C., & Liepert, J. (2009). Modafinil effects in multiple sclerosis patients with fatigue. *Journal of Neurology, 256,* 645–650. http://dx.doi.org/10.1007/s00415-009-0152-7

Lovera, J., Bagert, B., Smoot, K., Morris, C. D., Frank, R., Bogardus, K., . . . Bourdette, D. (2007). Ginkgo biloba for the improvement of cognitive performance in multiple sclerosis: A randomized, placebo-controlled trial. *Multiple Sclerosis Journal, 13*, 376–385. http://dx.doi.org/10.1177/1352458506071213

Lovera, J. F., Frohman, E., Brown, T. R., Bandari, D., Nguyen, L., Yadav, V., . . . Bourdette, D. (2010). Memantine for cognitive impairment in multiple sclerosis: A randomized placebo-controlled trial. *Multiple Sclerosis Journal, 16*, 715–723. http://dx.doi.org/10.1177/1352458510367662

Magnin, E., Sagawa, Y., Jr., Chamard, L., Berger, E., Moulin, T., & Decavel, P. (2015). Verbal fluencies and fampridine treatment in multiple sclerosis. *European Neurology, 74*, 243–250. http://dx.doi.org/10.1159/000442348

Markowitz, J. S., Straughn, A. B., & Patrick, K. S. (2003). Advances in the pharmacotherapy of attention-deficit-hyperactivity disorder: Focus on methylphenidate formulations. *Pharmacotherapy, 23*, 1281–1299. http://dx.doi.org/10.1592/phco.23.12.1281.32697

Mignot, E. J. M. (2012). A practical guide to the therapy of narcolepsy and hypersomnia syndromes. *Neurotherapeutics, 9*, 739–752. http://dx.doi.org/10.1007/s13311-012-0150-9

Möller, F., Poettgen, J., Broemel, F., Neuhaus, A., Daumer, M., & Heesen, C. (2011). HAGIL (Hamburg Vigil Study): A randomized placebo-controlled double-blind study with modafinil for treatment of fatigue in patients with multiple sclerosis. *Multiple Sclerosis Journal, 17*, 1002–1009. http://dx.doi.org/10.1177/1352458511402410

Montalban, X., Sastre-Garriga, J., Filippi, M., Khaleeli, Z., Téllez, N., Vellinga, M. M., . . . Thompson, A. J. (2009). Primary progressive multiple sclerosis diagnostic criteria: A reappraisal. *Multiple Sclerosis Journal, 15*, 1459–1465. http://dx.doi.org/10.1177/1352458509348422

Morrow, S. A., Kaushik, T., Zarevics, P., Erlanger, D., Bear, M. F., Munschauer, F. E., & Benedict, R. H. B. (2009). The effects of L-amphetamine sulfate on cognition in MS patients: Results of a randomized controlled trial. *Journal of Neurology, 256*, 1095–1102. http://dx.doi.org/10.1007/s00415-009-5074-x

Parry, A. M. M., Scott, R. B., Palace, J., Smith, S., & Matthews, P. M. (2003). Potentially adaptive functional changes in cognitive processing for patients with multiple sclerosis and their acute modulation by rivastigmine. *Brain, 126*, 2750–2760. http://dx.doi.org/10.1093/brain/awg284

Patti, F., Amato, M. P., Bastianello, S., Caniatti, L., Di Monte, E., Ferrazza, P., . . . COGIMUS Study Group. (2010). Effects of immunomodulatory treatment with subcutaneous interferon beta-1a on cognitive decline in mildly disabled patients with relapsing-remitting multiple sclerosis. *Multiple Sclerosis Journal, 16*, 68–77. http://dx.doi.org/10.1177/1352458509350309

Pavsic, K., Pelicon, K., Horvat Ledinek, A., & Sega, S. (2015). Short-term impact of fampridine on motor and cognitive functions, mood and quality of life among multiple sclerosis patients. *Clinical Neurology and Neurosurgery, 139*, 35–40. http://dx.doi.org/10.1016/j.clineuro.2015.08.023

Penner, I.-K., Stemper, B., Calabrese, P., Freedman, M. S., Polman, C. H., Edan, G., . . . Sandbrink, R. (2012). Effects of interferon beta-1b on cognitive performance in patients with a first event suggestive of multiple sclerosis. *Multiple Sclerosis Journal, 18,* 1466–1471. http://dx.doi.org/10.1177/1352458512442438

Pliskin, N. H., Hamer, D. P., Goldstein, D. S., Towle, V. L., Reder, A. T., Noronha, A., & Arnason, B. G. W. (1996). Improved delayed visual reproduction test performance in multiple sclerosis patients receiving interferon beta-1b. *Neurology, 47,* 1463–1468. http://dx.doi.org/10.1212/WNL.47.6.1463

Polman, C. H., O'Connor, P. W., Havrdova, E., Hutchinson, M., Kappos, L., Miller, D. H., . . . Sandrock, A. W. (2006). A randomized, placebo-controlled trial of natalizumab for relapsing multiple sclerosis. *The New England Journal of Medicine, 354,* 899–910. http://dx.doi.org/10.1056/NEJMoa044397

Rudick, R., Antel, J., Confavreux, C., Cutter, G., Ellison, G., Fischer, J., . . . Willoughby, E. (1997). Recommendations from the national multiple sclerosis society clinical outcomes assessment task force. *Annals of Neurology, 42,* 379–382. http://dx.doi.org/10.1002/ana.410420318

Rudick, R. A., Stuart, W. H., Calabresi, P. A., Confavreux, C., Galetta, S. L., Radue, E.-W., . . . Sandrock, A. W. (2006). Natalizumab plus interferon beta-1a for relapsing multiple sclerosis. *The New England Journal of Medicine, 354,* 911–923. http://dx.doi.org/10.1056/NEJMoa044396

Schwid, S. R., Goodman, A. D., Weinstein, A., McDermott, M. P., & Johnson, K. P. (2007). Cognitive function in relapsing multiple sclerosis: Minimal changes in a 10-year clinical trial. *Journal of the Neurological Sciences, 255,* 57–63. http://dx.doi.org/10.1016/j.jns.2007.01.070

Shaygannejad, V., Janghorbani, M., Ashtari, F., Zanjani, H. A., & Zakizade, N. (2008). Effects of rivastigmine on memory and cognition in multiple sclerosis. *The Canadian Journal of Neurological Sciences, 35,* 476–481. http://dx.doi.org/10.1017/S0317167100009148

Sicotte, N. L., Kern, K. C., Giesser, B. S., Arshanapalli, A., Schultz, A., Montag, M., . . . Bookheimer, S. Y. (2008). Regional hippocampal atrophy in multiple sclerosis. *Brain, 131,* 1134–1141. http://dx.doi.org/10.1093/brain/awn030

Stankoff, B., Waubant, E., Confavreux, C., Edan, G., Debouverie, M., Rumbach, L., . . . French Modafinil Study Group. (2005). Modafinil for fatigue in MS: A randomized placebo-controlled double-blind study. *Neurology, 64,* 1139–1143. http://dx.doi.org/10.1212/01.WNL.0000158272.27070.6A

Stephenson, J. J., Kern, D. M., Agarwal, S. S., Zeidman, R., Rajagopalan, K., Kamat, S. A., & Foley, J. (2012). Impact of natalizumab on patient-reported outcomes in multiple sclerosis: A longitudinal study. *Health and Quality of Life Outcomes, 10,* 155. http://dx.doi.org/10.1186/1477-7525-10-155

Sumowski, J. F., Chiaravalloti, N., Erlanger, D., Kaushik, T., Benedict, R. H. B., & DeLuca, J. (2011). L-amphetamine improves memory in MS patients with objective memory impairment. *Multiple Sclerosis Journal, 17,* 1141–1145. http://dx.doi.org/10.1177/1352458511404585

Svenningsson, A., Falk, E., Celius, E. G., Fuchs, S., Schreiber, K., Berkö, S., . . . Penner, I.-K. (2013). Natalizumab treatment reduces fatigue in multiple sclerosis. Results from the TYNERGY trial; a study in the real life setting. *PLoS One, 8*, e58643. http://dx.doi.org/10.1371/journal.pone.0058643

Tur, C. (2016). Fatigue management in multiple sclerosis. *Current Treatment Options in Neurology, 18*, 26. http://dx.doi.org/10.1007/s11940-016-0411-8

Villoslada, P., Arrondo, G., Sepulcre, J., Alegre, M., & Artieda, J. (2009). Memantine induces reversible neurologic impairment in patients with MS. *Neurology, 72*, 1630–1633. http://dx.doi.org/10.1212/01.wnl.0000342388.73185.80

Weinstein, A., Schwid, S. I. L., Schiffer, R. B., McDermott, M. P., Giang, D. W., & Goodman, A. D. (1999). Neuropsychologic status in multiple sclerosis after treatment with glatiramer. *Archives of Neurology, 56*, 319–324. http://dx.doi.org/10.1001/archneur.56.3.319

Wilken, J. A., Sullivan, C., Wallin, M., Rogers, C., Kane, R. L., Rossman, H., . . . Quig, M. E. (2008). Treatment of multiple sclerosis-related cognitive problems with adjunctive modafinil: Rationale and preliminary supportive data. *International Journal of MS Care, 10*, 1–10. http://dx.doi.org/10.7224/1537-2073-10.1.1

Wolinsky, J. S., Narayana, P. A., O'Connor, P., Coyle, P. K., Ford, C., Johnson, K., . . . Ladkani, D. (2007). Glatiramer acetate in primary progressive multiple sclerosis: Results of a multinational, multicenter, double-blind, placebo-controlled trial. *Annals of Neurology, 61*, 14–24. http://dx.doi.org/10.1002/ana.21079

13

COGNITIVE REHABILITATION IN MULTIPLE SCLEROSIS

NANCY D. CHIARAVALLOTI AND JOHN DeLUCA

Cognitive and behavioral rehabilitation are designed to enhance a person's capacity to process and interpret information and to improve his or her ability to function in all aspects of family and community life (National Institutes of Health, 1998). Given the clear and consistent documentation of cognitive deficits and their impact on the lives of persons with multiple sclerosis (MS; e.g., Chiaravalloti & DeLuca, 2008), the need for effective cognitive rehabilitation is clear. Although the focus on designing and testing effective cognitive rehabilitation programs for persons with MS is a relatively recent phenomenon as compared with other rehabilitation populations, the growth in research studies addressing this need over the past decade has been substantial.

Cognitive rehabilitation studies conducted in the MS population have focused on various aspects of cognitive functioning, including attentional deficits (Plohmann, Kappos, & Ammann, et al., 1998), communication skills

http://dx.doi.org/10.1037/0000097-014
Cognition and Behavior in Multiple Sclerosis, J. DeLuca and B. M. Sandroff (Editors)

(Foley et al., 1994), and memory functioning (Allen, Goldstein, Heyman, & Rondinelli, 1998; Jønsson, Korfitzen, Heltberg, Ravnborg, & Byskov-Ottosen, 1993). Many more recent studies have focused on multimodal treatment paradigms designed to target several aspects of cognition either simultaneously or consecutively (Filippi et al., 2012; Gich et al., 2015; Mattioli, Stampatori, Scarpazza, Parrinello, & Capra, 2012; Mattioli, Stampatori, Zanotti, Parrinello, & Capra, 2010; Parisi, Rocca, Mattioli, et al., 2014).

O'Brien, Chiaravalloti, Goverover, and DeLuca (2008) completed the first systematic review to specifically address cognitive rehabilitation in MS and found only 16 studies conducted on the topic of cognitive rehabilitation within MS at the time. Learning and memory studies constituted the majority ($n = 6$), with a few focused on attention and unspecified or multiple skills. Only one practice guideline and one practice option could be recommended at that time largely due to a lack of methodological rigor. Mitolo, Venneri, Wilkinson, and Sharrack (2015) conducted a more recent systematic review; they identified 33 publications and noted that while earlier articles focused on memory and skill acquisition, more recent studies targeted the constructs of executive function (EF), attention, and processing speed (PS; see Figure 13.1). Findings, however, did not support new practice guidelines, and the authors concluded that there was a lack of evidence for the effectiveness of cognitive rehabilitation in improving subjective cognitive deficits, such as mood, quality of life (QOL), fatigue, or self-efficacy. Das Nair, Martin,

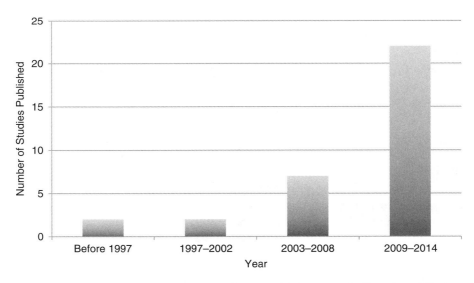

Figure 13.1. Cognitive rehabilitation studies in multiple sclerosis. Data from Mitolo, Venneri, Wilkinson, and Sharrack, 2015.

and Lincoln (2016) conducted a more recent Cochrane Review on memory rehabilitation and noted evidence to support memory rehabilitation as having a positive impact on memory abilities and QOL. Das Nair and colleagues highlighted the need for large-scale randomized clinical trials (RCTs) to provide rigorous data supporting effective treatments and the need for ecologically valid outcome assessments.

COGNITIVE REHABILITATION FOR LEARNING AND MEMORY

By far, the domain of learning and memory has received the most attention in the MS-related cognitive rehabilitation literature. Programs consist of computer-assisted technology, and paper and pencil approaches that focus on skills to improve function.

Many studies examining the effectiveness of structured training programs have shown promising results (see Table 13.1). Several studies have been conducted on the modified Story Memory Technique (mSMT), beginning with a pilot double-blind, placebo-controlled randomized clinical trial in 28 persons with mixed subtypes of MS (Chiaravalloti, DeLuca, Moore, & Ricker, 2005). The intervention group was taught the mSMT, which used context and imagery to improve learning and, therefore, recall. The placebo-control group met with equal frequency and duration and performed traditional memory exercises but did not receive training in context and imagery. Treated participants who had moderate to severe learning impairments showed significant improvement in learning abilities at immediate follow-up, with no change noted in the control group (see Figure 13.2). Self-report for memory function also was significantly better for participants in the experimental versus control group posttreatment. In a larger clinical trial on the mSMT (Chiaravalloti, Moore, Nikelshpur, & DeLuca, 2013), the treatment group ($n = 35$) showed significantly improved learning on the California Verbal Learning Test learning slope posttreatment relative to the placebo group ($n = 34$). Similar results were noted on objective measures of everyday memory, self-reported general contentment, and family report of apathy and executive dysfunction (see Figure 13.3). Posttreatment improvement in the treatment group was maintained on the list learning and self-report measures 6 months later. The efficacy of the mSMT has been further validated with neuroimaging data. Chiaravalloti, Wylie, Leavitt, and DeLuca (2012) examined 16 individuals with clinically definite MS randomly assigned to treatment ($n = 8$) or placebo-control ($n = 8$) groups, and matched for age, education, and disease characteristics. No baseline activation differences on functional magnetic resonance imaging (fMRI) were seen between groups.

TABLE 13.1

Studies Addressing Learning and Memory Dysfunction in MS

Reference	Treatment protocol or technique based?	Treatment ingredient	Results
Basso, Ghormley, Lowery, Combs, & Bornstein (2008)	Technique based	Self-generation	Treatment > control
Carr, das Nair, Schwartz, & Lincoln (2014)	Treatment protocol	ReMiND program	Mixed
Chiaravalloti, DeLuca, Moore, & Ricker (2005)	Treatment protocol	mSMT: Context and imagery	Treatment > control
Chiaravalloti, Moore, Nikelshpur, & DeLuca (2013)	Treatment protocol	mSMT: Context and imagery	Treatment > control
das Nair & Lincoln (2012)	Treatment protocol	ReMiND program	Mixed
Ernst et al. (2013)	Treatment protocol	Mental visual imagery	Treatment > control
Ernst, Blanc, De Seze, & Manning (2015)	Treatment protocol	Mental visual imagery	Treatment > control
Gentry (2008)	Compensation	Learning to use a PDA	Treatment gains were demonstrated
Goverover, Basso, Wood, Chiaravalloti, & DeLuca (2011)	Technique based	Self-generation in combination with spaced learning	Treatment > control
Goverover, Chiaravalloti, & DeLuca (2008)	Technique based	Self-generation	Treatment > control
Goverover, Chiaravalloti, & DeLuca (2014)	Technique based	Self-generation	Treatment > control
Goverover, Hillary, Chiaravalloti, Arango-Lasprilla, & DeLuca (2009)	Technique based	Spaced learning trials	Treatment > control
Moore, Peterson, O'Shea, McIntosh, & Thaut (2008)	Technique based	Spoken or sung version of the RAVLT	Treatment = control
Sumowski, Chiaravalloti, & DeLuca (2010)	Technique based	Spaced learning trials in combination with self-testing	Treatment > control
Thaut, Peterson, McIntosh, & Hoemberg (2014)	Technique based	Spoken or sung version of the RAVLT	Sung version better than spoken

Note. MS = multiple sclerosis; mSMT = modified Story Memory Technique; RAVLT = Rey Auditory Verbal Learning Test.

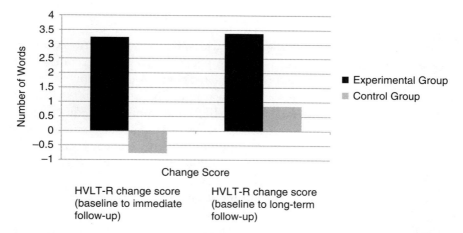

Figure 13.2. Improvements on the Hopkins Verbal Learning Test—Revised (HVLT–R) from before to after treatment with the modified Story Memory Technique (mSMT) as compared with a placebo control group ($p < .05$). Data from Chiaravalloti, DeLuca, Moore, and Ricker (2005).

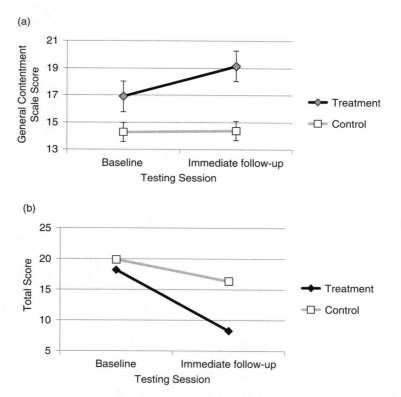

Figure 13.3. Improvements in (a) self-reported general contentment and (b) family report of executive dysfunction in daily life as reflected in the Frontal Systems Behavior Scale total score (including subscales assessing apathy, disinhibition, and executive dysfunction) in 35 participants undergoing treatment with the modified Story Memory Technique as compared with the placebo control group ($n = 34$). Both $p < .05$. Data from Chiaravalloti, Moore, Nikelshpur, and DeLuca (2013).

After treatment, greater activation was evident in the treatment group during performance of a memory task within a widespread cortical network involving frontal, parietal, precuneus, and parahippocampal regions. In contrast, the placebo-control group showed no significant changes in cerebral activation at follow-up. A significant association was found between increased activation in the right middle frontal gyrus (MFG) and improved memory performance posttreatment in the treatment group only. The authors concluded that the observed increases in MFG activation likely reflect increased use of strategies taught during treatment when learning new information. This group (Leavitt, Wylie, Girgis, DeLuca, & Chiaravalloti, 2014) also showed increased connectivity between left hippocampus and cortical regions specifically involved in memory for visual imagery, as well as among critical hubs of the default mode network (DMN) after treatment. Increased connectivity also was noted from the right hippocampus to left postcentral gyrus, precentral gyrus, MFG, and cingulate gyrus. These changes were not observed in the placebo control group, providing evidence for efficacy of a behavioral intervention to impact the integrity of neural networks subserving memory functions in persons with MS. Dobryakova, Wylie, DeLuca, and Chiaravalloti (2014) examined functional brain activity 6 months after mSMT treatment and showed that in addition to the maintenance of the behavioral improvement, the increases in patterns of cerebral activation during learning immediately after treatment were maintained 6 months posttraining.

Mendozzi et al. (1998) similarly examined the efficacy of the memory modules of RehaCom, a computer-assisted cognitive retraining program, in 60 persons with relapsing-remitting MS (RRMS) or secondary progressive MS (SPMS). There were three groups in the study: a no treatment control group, a nonspecific training group that received attention-only RehaCom modules, and a specific training group with RehaCom that included both memory and attention modules. Participants met for 15 biweekly sessions that were approximately 45 minutes in length. The specific training group significantly improved on four memory outcome measures, the nonspecific group improved on one, and the control group showed no improvement. The researchers concluded that the specific memory training was superior to both the nonspecific and the no-training conditions. Although RehaCom has been used extensively in MS, few studies have examined the efficacy of the memory modules in this population.

Group memory rehabilitation may be most practical in regard to insurance reimbursement. Carr, das Nair, Schwartz, and Lincoln (2014) conducted an RCT in 48 people with MS, reporting poor memory randomized to a group memory rehabilitation program or a wait-list control, for ten 1.5-hour sessions over 10 weeks. Although there were no significant effects of treatment relative to the control group at immediate or 4-month follow-up, the intervention group reported significantly better mood than controls at the 8-month follow-up. Das Nair and Lincoln (2012) compared the effectiveness of two group memory rehabilitation programs (i.e., compensation or restitution group treatment) with a self-help group control group in a single-blind randomized controlled trial. The compensation and restitution groups each used significantly more internal memory aids than the self-help group posttreatment. There were no significant differences between the groups on measures of mood, adjustment, and activities of daily living.

In addition to examining the efficacy of structured treatment protocols, studies have sought to evaluate the efficacy of well-known techniques from cognitive psychology in patients with MS (see Table 13.1). Such techniques have been well validated in healthy controls (HC), but only recently tested in memory-impaired MS participants. Research on these techniques is essential in that techniques noted to improve learning and memory in MS may be effectively developed into future treatment protocols. Chiaravalloti and DeLuca (2002) examined the memory benefit of self-generated learning compared with didactic presentation in MS and HC subjects. Self-generated learning resulted in significantly enhanced learning and memory in both groups. Basso, Ghormley, Lowery, Combs, and Bornstein (2008) extended this work by examining self-generated learning in MS patients with and without memory impairment, as well as HC. Participants learned word pairs that either were self-generated or didactically presented. All groups remembered more self-generated versus didactic words, and severity of memory impairment did not play a role in the degree of benefit. O'Brien, Chiaravalloti, Arango-Lasprilla, Lengenfelder, and DeLuca (2007) further noted that cognitively impaired persons with MS demonstrated a significant benefit from self-generation. Individuals with impairments in multiple cognitive domains recalled fewer words overall compared with those with no or one impaired cognitive domain; however, even those with impairments in multiple cognitive domains demonstrated a large effect size in recall of generated versus provided words.

Goverover, Chiaravalloti, and DeLuca (2008) examined a self-generation strategy to improve learning and performance of everyday functional tasks in persons with MS. Twenty participants with MS and 18 HC completed two meal preparation tasks and two financial management tasks. One task in each area was presented in a provided condition in which all instructions were provided to and read by the participants, and the other was presented in a generated condition in which participants were asked to generate the to-be-remembered information. Both persons with MS and HC showed enhanced memory performance for items learned in the generated condition as compared with the provided condition, demonstrating that self-generated learning can significantly improve activities of daily living for persons with MS. This group further examined the role of task meaningfulness and degree of cognitive impairment in the effectiveness of self-generated learning (Goverover et al., 2014). Thirty-five persons with MS with moderate to severe learning and memory impairments, and 35 persons with little to no impairment learned functional everyday tasks and laboratory tasks, each in two learning conditions (i.e., provided and generated). Self-generated learning was more effective in recall of the functional tasks compared with the laboratory tasks across participants, showing that self-generation may be influenced by variables, such as task meaningfulness. Taken together, self-generated learning has been shown to be a powerful technique in improving learning and memory in persons with MS.

Goverover, Hillary, Chiaravalloti, Arango-Lasprilla, and DeLuca (2009) examined a second technique from cognitive psychology to improve learning and memory: spaced learning. This technique compared *spaced learning trials*, when trials are distributed over time, versus *massed learning trials*, when learning trials are consecutive, on the acquisition of everyday functional tasks. Twenty participants with MS and 18 HC completed two route learning tasks and two paragraph reading tasks, with one task in each area presented in the "spaced" condition and the second task presented in the "massed" condition. Results showed that the spaced condition significantly enhanced memory performance relative to the massed condition—but for verbal stimuli only.

Goverover, Basso, Wood, Chiaravalloti, and DeLuca (2011) examined the potential benefit of combining memory-enhancing strategies to improve new learning. Twenty MS participants and 18 HC were presented with three tasks (i.e., learning names, appointments, object locations), each in three learning conditions (i.e., massed, spaced learning, combination of spaced- and generated learning). Combined spaced learning and self-generation yielded significantly better recall than spaced learning alone. In turn, spaced learning resulted in better recall than the massed condition.

A third cognitively enhancing technique demonstrating efficacy in persons with MS is retrieval practice (also called the testing effect), in which retesting previously learned information improves subsequent recall more than additional restudy trials. Sumowski, Chiaravalloti, and DeLuca (2010) had 32 persons with MS and 16 HC learn 48 verbal paired associates in three learning conditions: massed restudy, spaced restudy, and spaced testing. Spaced testing was superior to the other two conditions in both MS and HC. A second study by this group showed that the benefit of spaced testing was maintained 1 week later, resulting in a 25-fold improvement over massed learning (Sumowski et al., 2013). These studies showed that retrieval practice significantly improves memory more than additional restudy trials.

A final behavioral phenomenon from cognitive psychology, the repetition effect was tested in 64 participants with mixed MS subtypes and 20 HC on verbal list learning (Chiaravalloti et al., 2003). The results showed that persons with MS who required more repetition of the list to reach a learning criterion recalled fewer words at follow-up testing than persons who needed fewer repetitions to learn the list. Chiaravalloti et al. (2003) concluded that simple repetition alone does not necessarily improve learning and memory, and that interventions that improve the quality of encoding would more beneficial, such as increased organization. The greater the degree of cognitive impairment the less likely MS subjects benefited from simple repetition to enhance new learning.

Two studies examined the cognitive rehabilitation of autobiographical memory. In their first study, Ernst et al. (2013) utilized a program to treat deficits in autobiographical memory in 10 participants with MS. Persons with MS who completed a treatment program consisting of mental visual imagery focused on autobiographical memory showed significant improvement in memory and self-reported improvements in daily life functioning. In a second study by the same group, Ernst, Blanc, De Seze, and Manning (2015) examined 40 patients with a deficit in autobiographical memory randomized to three groups: an experimental group ($n = 17$) that completed the same mental visual imagery program as just described, a verbal control group ($n = 10$) that completed a sham verbal program, and a stability group ($n = 13$) that received no intervention. Improvement in autobiographical memory and executive control was observed in only in the experimental group, with self-reported transfer to daily life.

Taken together, these studies clearly showed that learning and memory dysfunction in MS is highly amenable to cognitive rehabilitation.

COGNITIVE REHABILITATION FOR ATTENTION, PROCESSING SPEED, AND/OR WORKING MEMORY

Similar to learning and memory research, substantial work has established the efficacy of interventions for attentional deficits in persons with MS. Early studies focused on non-computer-mediated retraining programs—with limited success. For example, Lincoln et al. (2002) randomized 240 MS participants to a control group, an assessment-only group, or a treatment group. Interventions included diaries, calendars, notebooks, lists, and visual mnemonics, and could last up to 6 months. No change in subjectively reported cognitive impairment (or mood or QOL) was observed.

Programs targeting attention transitioned to be largely computer-mediated treatment protocols, including Attention Process Training, Fresh Minder, BrainStim, and RehaCom, with many positive findings. Plohmann, Kappos, and Brunnschweiler (1994) enrolled MS participants into a computer-aided cognitive rehabilitation program consisting of sixteen 45- to 60-minute training sessions, four times a week, in a wait-list crossover design. Although cognitive improvement was reported, no aggregate data were provided nor were statistical analyses conducted. In a second study by this group (Plohmann, Kappos, Ammann, et al., 1998), 22 participants with mixed MS subtypes completed twelve 40-minute sessions over 3 weeks using a computer-assisted rehabilitation program targeting four types of attention: selective, divided, sustained, and vigilance. Significant improvement was seen in MS participants who received specific training in alertness and divided attention. Participants also showed self-reported improvements in cognitive functioning in everyday life and QOL, with treatment effects sustained for 9 weeks.

Amato et al. (2014) tested a home-based computerized program for retraining attentional deficits based on attention process training. RRMS subjects who failed more than two tests of attention were randomized to specific (i.e., treatment; $n = 55$) or nonspecific computerized training ($n = 33$). A benefit of the specific training was observed on the Paced Auditory Serial Addition Test (PASAT) but not on self-report measures. Pusswald, Mildner, Zebenholzer, Auff, and Lehrner (2014) examined the efficacy of Fresh Minder 2 plus psychosocial counseling in 40 patients with MS: 20 assigned to a treatment group and 20 to a no contact control group. A significant treatment effect was noted in attention and mental fatigue (simple and cued reaction time) in the treatment group only. Vogt et al. (2009) investigated the effects of BrainStim, a treatment program based on Baddeley's working memory (WM) model (Baddeley & Hitch, 1974), in 45 MS outpatients allocated to two different training groups (i.e., high and low intensity) and a no-training control group. Results showed significantly improved fatigue, WM, and mental speed in the treatment groups only. Hubacher et al. (2015) also examined BrainStim in 10 participants with MS (i.e., six treatment, four control). Despite the limited statistical analyses due to the small sample size, two different patterns of change after cognitive rehabilitation were identified: (a) decreased brain activation associated with increased PS and (b) a reorganization process associated with improved PS and WM. The authors thus cautioned against the use of traditional group statistics in analyzing imaging data related to treatment efficacy and emphasized individual differences to ensure a complete understanding of the data and response patterns.

Although PS deficits represent the most common cognitive deficits in persons with MS and have shown detrimental impact on daily life functioning, the examination of treatment for PS deficits in MS is in its infancy. Hancock, Bruce, Bruce, and Lynch (2015) conducted a pilot study examining the effect of computerized cognitive training consisting of Posit Science's Sweep Seeker and Road Tour, focusing on PS, and Master Gardener and the Brain Twister n-back task, addressing WM. Seventy-one participants who self-reported cognitive problems were randomized into an active or a sham training group; training occurred 6 days per week for 6 weeks in 30-minute intervals. This study suffered from substantial attrition, with the final N being 30. The active training group improved significantly on the PASAT following treatment, with other trends noted.

Rosti-Otajärvi, Mäntynen, Koivisto, Huhtala, and Hämäläinen (2013a) randomized 102 patients with RRMS with subjective and objective attentional deficits into an intervention or a no treatment control group. The intervention group received strategy-oriented neuropsychological rehabilitation once per week for 13 weeks in 60-minute sessions. After 3 and 6 months, no treatment effect was observed on cognitive test variables (Mäntynen et al., 2014). The intervention group, however, did report fewer depressive symptoms, less psychological burden from the disease, and reduced cognitive fatigue symptoms at 6 months and at 1-year posttreatment.

Research in cognitive rehabilitation has recently been applying neuroimaging procedures as a primary outcome to evaluate the impact of the treatment on brain structure and function. In an early study, Sastre-Garriga et al. (2011) investigated a cognitive rehabilitation program in 15 MS patients with cognitive impairment and five HC. The cognitive rehabilitation program was composed of 15 computer-aided drills and practice sessions, and five non-computer-aided cognitive stimulation group sessions (over 5 weeks). Increased brain activity on fMRI was observed after rehabilitation in several cerebellar areas in persons with MS as compared with healthy subjects. Patients also showed significant improvement on the backward version of the Digit Span Test and on a composite score of neuropsychological outcomes.

RehaCom is a computer mediated cognitive rehabilitation protocol that consists of multiple modules that address several cognitive domains. Several researchers have examined the efficacy of RehaCom for remediating attentional processes in patients with MS. For example, Cerasa et al. (2013) enrolled 23 MS patients in a double-blind RCT. After treatment, the RehaCom group showed improved performance in attention with a large effect size compared with an active control group. This increased performance was associated with increased activity on fMRI in the posterior cerebellar lobule and in the superior parietal lobule. These results demonstrated that intensive cognitive rehabilitation impacts neural plasticity and improves cognition.

COGNITIVE REHABILITATION
FOR EXECUTIVE DYSFUNCTION

Although the majority of studies have focused on the most commonly impaired aspects of cognition in MS, memory and attention, a handful of studies has investigated the cognitive rehabilitation of the less often cognitively impaired domain of EF. Lincoln, Dent, and Harding (2003) included EF as one of three domains targeted in their cognitive rehabilitation intervention and found no significant changes posttreatment. Birnboim and Miller (2004) examined 10 persons with mixed MS subtypes seen for twenty-four 1-hour weekly sessions over 6 months. Treatment used a metacognitive therapeutic approach emphasizing learning of metacognitive aspects of cognition in three phases (i.e., understanding, practice, transfer). Patients with RRMS showed a 36% improvement on a strategic application test compared with an approximately 16% improvement in persons with SPMS. Significant improvements also were reported on neuropsychological tests, including the Rey Auditory Verbal Learning Test delayed subtest, digit symbol coding, and a fluency task. Fink et al. (2010) compared a treatment group ($n = 11$) with a placebo control group ($n = 14$) and an untreated group ($n = 15$). Treatment group participants engaged in textbook exercises for executive functioning four times per week for 25- to 30-minute sessions, and received weekly feedback from a psychologist. Significantly greater improvements were seen in EF and verbal learning in the treatment group compared with the two other groups. Baseline brain atrophy (i.e., parenchymal fraction) was related to improvements in set shifting posttreatment. The authors concluded that cognitive intervention may indeed be beneficial in treating executive dysfunction and that baseline brain atrophy has some predictive value in determining treatment outcome.

Although EF impairments remain understudied in MS, these preliminary studies showed that cognitive interventions have shown some degree of efficacy.

MULTIMODAL TREATMENT PROGRAMS

Although RehaCom can be used to specifically target attentional abilities, many authors (e.g., Filippi et al., 2012; Parisi, Rocca, Mattioli, et al., 2014) have evaluated its impact on multiple cognitive processes simultaneously, namely, attention, information processing, and EF. In an early study, Solari et al. (2004) examined the remediation of attention and memory in 82 participants with mixed subtypes of MS. RehaCom was not supported as efficacious for improving attention (or memory) in MS. In contrast, Mattioli et al. (2010) enrolled 20 patients with impairment in PS and EF in a double-blind study in which the treatment group received intensive computer-assisted cognitive rehabilitation of attention, information processing, and EF for 3 months using RehaCom compared with a no treatment control. The treatment group significantly improved on tests of attention, PS, and EF, and showed reduced depression. The long-term maintenance was observed by Mattioli et al. (2012), showing statistically significant improvement in attention, PS, and EF 9 months following treatment in the RehaCom subjects only. In addition, treated patients showed decreased depression and improved QOL. Reliable change indices demonstrated the clinical significance of this improvement.

Neuroimaging data has provided substantial support of RehaCom in treating attention, PS, and EF in persons with MS. Twenty patients with RRMS and cognitive deficits at baseline were randomly assigned to a treatment group ($n = 10$) or to a no treatment control group ($n = 10$). Filippi et al. (2012) reported that the treatment group showed improved performance on tests of attention, PS, and EF from baseline to follow-up. Similarly, changes on fMRI were noted in the posterior cingulate cortex (PCC)/precuneus and dorsolateral prefrontal cortex (PFC) during the Stroop task, and modified activity of the anterior cingulum, PCC and/or precuneus, left dorsolateral PFC, and right inferior parietal lobule at rest in the treatment group compared with the control group. These changes on fMRI were correlated with cognitive improvement. The authors concluded that rehabilitation of attention, PS, and EF in RRMS may be impacted through enhanced recruitment of brain networks subserving the trained functions.

Using the same participants as Filippi et al. (2012), Parisi, Rocca, Valsasina, et al. (2014) examined how resting state functional connectivity (RSFC) of the anterior cingulate cortex (ACC) correlates with cognitive rehabilitation in RRMS patients. At the two study time points, ACC activity was correlated with the bilateral middle and inferior frontal gyrus, basal ganglia, PCC, cerebellum, precuneus, middle temporal gyrus, and inferior parietal lobule (IPL). At follow-up, compared with baseline, the treatment group showed increased functional connectivity (FC) of the ACC with the right MFG and right IPL, whereas the control group showed decreased FC of the ACC with the right cerebellar and right inferior temporal gyrus. Significant correlations were found between improvement in PASAT performance and RSFC of the ACC with the right MFG and right IPL. The authors concluded that cognitive rehabilitation correlates with changes in RSFC of brain regions subserving functions targeted by the training.

Parisi, Rocca, Mattioli, et al. (2014) further examined the long-term efficacy of 12 weeks of RehaCom in the same group of participants. The authors examined RSFC and neuropsychological performance before treatment, after 12 weeks of rehabilitation, and at 6-month follow-up. Participants who completed RehaCom treatment continued to show improvements on tests of attention, EF, depression, and QOL at 6-month follow-up. Neuro-psychological performance was significantly correlated with changes in RSFC in cognitive-related networks and the anterior cingulum. RSFC changes in the DMN from baseline to the 12-week follow-up predicted cognitive performance and less severe depression, whereas RSFC changes within the executive network from baseline to the 12-week follow-up predicted better QOL.

Bonavita et al. (2015) similarly examined changes in FC following treatment with RehaCom in 18 cognitively impaired RRMS patients, with 14 cognitively impaired RRMS patients completing a control condition (reading a newspaper twice per week for 30 minutes, then explaining the contents a neurology resident). Significant posttreatment improvement was noted on tests of PS, WM, and visual memory. A significant increase of the FC of the DMN was noted in the PCC and bilateral inferior parietal cortex. After cognitive rehabilitation, a significant negative correlation between Stroop Color–Word Interference Test and FC in the PCC was observed. The authors concluded that cognitive rehabilitation may induce adaptive cortical reorganization, resulting in improved cognitive performance.

Several treatment protocols have been developed to treat multiple aspects of cognition but each have been examined by one study to date, with promising results. Examples of such treatment programs include MS-Line! (Gich et al., 2015), designed for home use, and Dr Kawashima's Brain Training (DKBT; Nintendo, Japan), adapted into an 8-week, home-based cognitive rehabilitation program for attention, PS, and WM (De Giglio et al., 2015). Solari et al. (2004) examined an 8-week, 16-session, computer-aided intervention for memory and attention. Brissart, Leroy, and Debouverie (2010) examined ProCogSEP, a 13-session cognitive intervention addressing several cognitive domains, including verbal memory, visual memory, WM, associative memory, and EF. Memory, Attention, and Problem Solving Skills for Persons With Multiple Sclerosis is yet another 8-week computer-assisted cognitive rehabilitation intervention that includes eight weekly group sessions focused on using cognitive compensatory strategies, as well as home-based training (Stuifbergen et al., 2012). Janssen, Boster, Lee, Patterson, and Prakash (2015) similarly examined an 8-week, hybrid-variable priority training program in eliciting broad cognitive transfer effects. Hanssen, Beiske, Landrø, Hofoss, and Hessen (2016) conducted an RCT in which the intervention group participated in cognitive group sessions and individual sessions focusing on goal attainment scaling (GAS) goals for coping with cognitive challenges, with some success. This group also tested a 4-week, inpatient cognitive rehabilitation program in which patients were guided through the process of formulating GAS goals for coping with cognitive challenges in everyday life (Hanssen, Šaltytė Benth, Beiske, Landrø, & Hessen, 2015). The Sclerosi Multipla Intensive Cognitive Training (SMICT) trial (Mattioli et al., 2014) applied specific intensive cognitive training for attention/PS, EF, and memory over 1 year, noting improvement in memory and attention/PS posttraining. Two-year follow-up data on these initially enrolled participants showed some support for maintenance of cognitive improvement (Mattioli, Bellomi, Stampatori, Provinciali, et al., 2016). Although each of these studies has noted some degree of improvement following treatment, replication is necessary, and transfer to other cognitive domains and generalization to daily life require examination.

Rilo et al. (2016) examined a group-based multimodal treatment program, REHACOP, with 21 MS patients randomized to treatment and 21 to a wait-list control. REHACOP treatment consisted of 3 months of group treatment focused on attention, PS, learning and memory, language, executive functioning, and social cognition. The REHACOP group showed improvements in several areas, including PS, WM, verbal memory, and EF, all with medium to large effect sizes. This study demonstrated the need for future research examining this multimodal group treatment program to effectively treat cognitive deficits in persons with MS.

HOME-BASE COGNITIVE
REHABILITATION PROGRAMS

Home-based cognitive rehabilitation has been studied as an alternative to frequent clinic visits. As described earlier, Amato et al. (2014) tested a home-based computerized program for retraining attentional deficits based on attention process training, with noted benefit on the PASAT but not on self-report measures. Shatil, Metzer, Horvitz, and Miller (2010) examined training on a personalized, home-based, computerized cognitive training program (three times a week for 12 weeks). MS participants were assigned to a training group ($n = 59$) or no treatment control group ($n = 48$). The training group showed a significant improvement compared with the control group in general memory, and visual and verbal WM. Cognitive training also was associated with increased naming speed, speed of information recall, focused attention, and visuomotor vigilance. Hildebrandt et al. (2007) tested a home-based computer treatment with 42 patients with RRMS randomized to a treatment group or a control group. Improvements were noted on tasks assessing verbal learning, long delay verbal memory, and WM. Training had no effect on neurological status, QOL, or fatigue. This study also showed a relationship between lower brain atrophy (i.e., brain parenchymal fraction, ventricular fraction) and benefit from treatment on tasks of WM and learning but not delayed recall.

De Giglio et al. (2015) examined an 8-week, home-based cognitive rehabilitation program, based on the video game DKBT, in 35 individuals with MS with cognitive impairment randomized to a treatment group or a wait-list control group. The authors reported a significant improvement on PS and QOL. De Giglio et al. (2016) further tested the use of this video game-based cognitive rehabilitation as compared with a wait-list control group in 24 individuals with MS with cognitive impairment. They observed a significant improvement on the PASAT and the Stroop after 8 weeks of cognitive rehabilitation. The intervention group showed increased FC in the cingulum, precuneus, and bilateral parietal cortex and a lower FC in the cerebellum and in left PFC posttreatment as compared with the wait-list control group. FC changes in these regions also correlated with cognitive improvement.

Charvet et al. (2015) sought to develop a protocol for remotely supervised cognitive remediation. Twenty individuals with MS were randomized to an active cognitive remediation program using the Lumosity software (Lumos Labs, 2015) or an ordinary computer games control group. Participants were given laptop computers to take home, with a targeted training frequency of 30 hours total (5 days per week for 12 weeks). Compliance reached 80% of the target as determined via monitoring software installed on the laptops. Significant improvement was noted in the active training group on both the cognitive measures and motor tasks compared with the control group. Remote training was thus deemed feasible by the authors.

Taken together, these studies indicated that home-based cognitive rehabilitation may be an effective alternative to clinic-based treatment to facilitate ease of treatment delivery.

NONSPECIFIC COGNITIVE
REHABILITATION INTERVENTIONS

A small group of studies has attempted to improve cognition without focusing on any single or combination of specific skills. Improved psychological symptoms are commonly seen following such interventions, with changes in objectively evaluated cognitive processes being less common. For example, Mendoza, Pittenger, and Weinstein (2001) assigned certified nursing assistants to participants and observed decreased depression. Jønsson et al. (1993) utilized (a) cognitive training, which consisted of teaching compensation, substitution, and direct training; and (b) neuropsychotherapy, which consisted of individualized goal-directed treatment that aimed to help participants accept their present cognitive and behavioral levels of functioning, noting treatment effects on visual–spatial memory and visuomotor speed, and improvement in depression on short-term follow-up, sustained at 6 months following treatment. Brenk, Laun, and Haase (2008) evaluated a 6-week, nonspecific, home-based cognitive training protocol showing significant improvement attention, visuoconstructive and figural long-term memory, depression, and QOL. Lincoln et al. (2003) utilized psychoeducation and diaries that were reviewed, and strategies and/or assistive devices (e.g., diaries, calendars, alarms, lists, notes) were discussed and given (with training) to participants, noting more than 50% of patients reported fewer problems postintervention. Thus, although work examining nonspecific cognitive training generally does not involve methodologically rigorous RCTs, some promising results have been noted.

Factors Influencing Treatment Efficacy

Although the efficacy of cognitive rehabilitation is often examined in regard to the specific cognitive construct targeted by the treatment, it is important to recognize that cognitive deficits, and thus improvement following cognitive rehabilitation, present within a constellation of other cognitive, psychological, and physical symptomatology. Although many studies overlook the complex nature of these systems, a handful of studies have highlighted the influence of factors other than the targeted deficit on treatment efficacy. Rosti-Otajärvi, Mäntynen, Koivisto, Huhtala, and Hämäläinen (2013b) examined patient-related factors impacting the outcome of cognitive rehabilitation in 98 patients with RRMS receiving multimodal neuropsychological intervention consisting of attention retraining, teaching compensatory strategies, psychoeducation, psychological support, and homework assignments. Sessions were conducted once a week in 60-minute sessions across 13 weeks. Patient factors, such as baseline level of cognitive functioning and gender-impacted cognitive rehabilitation outcomes, were such that those with more severe attentional deficits at baseline showed greater benefit than those with milder deficits, and men reported a greater decrease in perceived cognitive deficits compared with women. In contrast, illness-related factors, such as duration and severity of the disease, did not impact cognitive rehabilitation outcome. Intervention-related factors, such as dosage and therapist characteristics, similarly did not impact benefit.

Rosti-Otajärvi, Mäntynen, Koivisto, Huhtala, and Hämäläinen (2014) similarly evaluated the effects of baseline patient-related (i.e., cognitive, mood and fatigue symptoms, cognitive status, demographic factors) and illness-related factors (i.e., duration and severity of the disease) on the patient–therapist alliance, as well as the effects of the alliance on cognitive rehabilitation outcome in 56 patients with RRMS. Patients received a multimodal cognitive intervention (i.e., attention retraining, learning strategies, psychoeducation, psychological support, homework assignments) conducted once a week for 13 weeks; sessions lasted for 60 minutes each. None of the baseline factors was related to the alliance. Better patient-evaluated alliance was associated with a more prominent decrease in fatigue symptoms and greater achievement of rehabilitation goals. Better therapist-evaluated alliance was associated with greater benefit from the intervention as evaluated by therapists and thus may be related to positive neuropsychological rehabilitation outcome in MS.

Specific cognitive impairments also may have an influence on other cognitive functions and benefit from cognitive rehabilitation. Chiaravalloti and DeLuca (2015) conducted a post hoc analysis on the MEMREHAB trial, investigating the role of deficits in PS on the impact of the mSMT to improve learning and memory in persons with MS. Results showed that in addition to displaying impaired learning and memory, participants with an additional deficit in PS ability benefited less from treatment with the mSMT, whereas participants with intact PS abilities showed significantly greater benefit from mSMT treatment. These findings highlighted the complex cognitive symptoms that occur in MS and their relationships with one another.

Alternative Approaches to Improving Cognition

Several studies have additionally sought to improve cognitive abilities via alternative treatment modalities. For example, Shevil and Finlayson (2010) tested a 5-week, group-based community program addressing strategies to self-manage the cognitive changes associated with MS. Actual neuropsychological test performance was not examined, but significant improvements were seen posttreatment in the person's understanding of cognitive impairments and their impact on daily life, including increased self-efficacy. Gentry (2008) evaluated the effects of an occupational therapy training protocol using PDAs as assistive technology for people with MS-related cognitive impairment and showing that functional performance increased significantly with PDA use, maintained at an 8-week follow-up. No effect was observed on cognitive testing. Pöttgen, Lau, Penner, Heesen, and Moritz (2015) developed and tested a cognitive-behavioral group intervention based on metacognition, Metacognitive Training in MS, in 11 patients with MS, noting improved self-efficacy, fatigue, and mood posttreatment. The authors also found significant improvements on the Test Battery for Attention Performance (TAP) phasic alertness and selective attention measures posttreatment. A trend was additionally seen on the TAP tonic alertness score and the Symbol Digit Modalities Test.

Several studies examined the use of music as a mnemonic device to improve learning and memory performance. Moore, Peterson, O'Shea, McIntosh, and Thaut (2008) examined the utility of music mnemonics as a compensatory learning strategy in persons with MS. Some benefit, albeit nonsignificant, was observed from learning information through music; such improvements were greatest in participants with the least cognitive impairment. Thaut, Peterson, McIntosh, and Hoemberg (2014) further examined the impact of music mnemonics on verbal memory by measuring brain activity via electroencephalogram (EEG) during music-assisted learning. The music condition resulted in better word memory, better word order memory, and stronger bilateral frontal alpha activity on EEG than the spoken condition.

In addition, several recent studies have examined the impact of a structured exercise regimen on cognitive functioning in persons with MS, with promising results (e.g., Leavitt, Cirnigliaro, et al., 2014; Motl, Sandroff, & DeLuca, 2016). Such approaches are discussed in a later chapter.

Rather than applying traditional cognitive rehabilitation, several authors have successfully addressed deficits in PS in persons with MS by manipulating the time allotment for cognitive processing of the stimulus. Leavitt, Lengenfelder, Moore, Chiaravalloti, and DeLuca (2011) had 53 individuals with MS and 36 HC complete a computerized cognitive task that manipulated cognitive load and the interval between presentation of stimuli. Individuals with MS with PS deficits showed improved accuracy on the task when provided with more time to complete the task. This is consistent with Lengenfelder et al. (2006), who showed that persons with MS were able to perform equivalent to HCs when provided with additional time to complete the task. Arnett (2004) similarly performed a PS manipulation of a learning task and showed similar results. Participants with MS were able to learn more information when the information was presented at a slower rate. These studies have highlighted the importance of PS in carrying out cognitive tasks accurately. These findings point to the need to develop effective treatments for PS deficits in persons with MS, which is likely to not only improve PS but also other aspects of cognition reliant on PS for effective completion.

Multiple authors have supplemented traditional cognitive therapy with other treatment modalities in an attempt to maximize the treatment effect. Mattioli and colleagues, for example, examined the adjunctive benefit of transcranial direct current stimulation (tDCS) and cognitive therapy consisting of modified PASAT tasks utilizing months and words, which have been proven to be effective in both traumatic brain injury and MS (Mattioli, Bellomi, Stampatori, Capra, & Miniussi, 2016). tDCS applied in conjunction with cognitive training resulted in significantly greater improvement on tests of PS and EF after treatment and 6 months later compared with cognitive training alone. Similarly, Martínez-González and Piqueras (2015) examined the long-term effectiveness of a combined cognitive behavioral therapy and neuropsychological intervention in one woman with MS for 1 year. Posttreatment increases in attention, verbal memory, and nonverbal executive functioning were noted. Mäntynen et al. (2014) examined the effects of strategy-oriented neuropsychological rehabilitation once per week for 13 weeks, consisting of computer-based attention and WM retraining, psychoeducation, strategy learning, and psychological support. A positive impact was observed in self-perceived cognitive deficits, but there were no treatment effects noted in cognitive performance. From these studies, one can conclude that the additive effect of cognitive rehabilitation and additional therapeutic modalities might maximize patient benefit.

CONCLUSIONS AND FUTURE DIRECTIONS

Given the devastating effects of cognitive impairment on social functioning, occupational functioning, and everyday life activities, the amelioration of cognitive deficits is paramount. As such, efforts to improve cognitive abilities in MS may result in significant improvements in everyday functioning and overall QOL, and the overall cost of the disease to society at large. The past decade has seen a tremendous increase in the quantity of research addressing cognitive deficits in MS, and the quality of such research has similarly improved.

Moving forward, future research should continue to pursue efforts to effectively treat cognitive deficits in individuals with MS as these deficits have a substantial impact on a person's ability to function effectively in daily life, maintain fulfilling social relationships, and maintain meaningful employment (e.g., Goverover, Genova, Hillary, & DeLuca, 2007). Efforts to overcome barriers to the practical application of cognitive rehabilitation in the clinical realm would be most beneficial, including the application of telerehabilitation to cognitive rehabilitation in MS to minimize the need for travel to clinical centers for repeated sessions. The development of effective group interventions would effectively address difficulty with third-party payment for cognitive rehabilitation services seen at the level of individual therapy. More RCTs are needed to identify effective interventions for cognitive deficits in persons with MS at the most rigorous level of scientific evidence. Following the identification of effective interventions, research addressing the specific questions of which patients are most likely to benefit from treatment, at what point in the disease process the treatment is most effective, and what is the optimal dosage for maximal benefit is needed. Also, studying the benefits of cognitive rehabilitation on everyday functional activity should be a major goal of future research. Finally, the paucity of research focused on cognitive rehabilitation in progressive forms of MS has become more evident in recent years and is needed in future studies.

Although much work has been accomplished in establishing the efficacy of cognitive rehabilitation programs in MS in recent years, many questions remain unaddressed. Future research is necessary to address these many remaining issues and identify treatment that will maximize cognitive functioning, and thus everyday life functioning and overall QOL in persons diagnosed with MS.

REFERENCES

Allen, D. N., Goldstein, G., Heyman, R. A., & Rondinelli, T. (1998). Teaching memory strategies to persons with multiple sclerosis. *Journal of Rehabilitation Research and Development, 35*, 405–410.

Amato, M. P., Goretti, B., Viterbo, R. G., Portaccio, E., Niccolai, C., Hakiki, B., . . . Trojano, M. (2014). Computer-assisted rehabilitation of attention in patients with multiple sclerosis: Results of a randomized, double-blind trial. *Multiple Sclerosis Journal, 20*, 91–98. http://dx.doi.org/10.1177/1352458513501571

Arnett, P. A. (2004). Speed of presentation influences story recall in college students and persons with multiple sclerosis. *Archives of Clinical Neuropsychology, 19*, 507–523. http://dx.doi.org/10.1016/j.acn.2003.07.006

Baddeley, A. D., & Hitch, G. J. (1974). Working memory. In G. H. Bower (Ed.), *Psychology of Learning and Motivation Series: Advances in Research and Theory* (Vol. 8, pp. 47–89). London, England: Academic Press.

Basso, M. R., Ghormley, C., Lowery, N., Combs, D., & Bornstein, R. A. (2008). Self-generated learning in people with multiple sclerosis: An extension of Chiaravalloti and DeLuca (2002). *Journal of Clinical and Experimental Neuropsychology, 30*, 63–69. http://dx.doi.org/10.1080/13803390601186957

Birnboim, S., & Miller, A. (2004). Cognitive rehabilitation for multiple sclerosis patients with executive dysfunction. *Journal of Cognitive Rehabilitation, 22*, 11–18.

Bonavita, S., Sacco, R., Della Corte, M., Esposito, S., Sparaco, M., d'Ambrosio, A., . . . Tedeschi, G. (2015). Computer-aided cognitive rehabilitation improves cognitive performances and induces brain functional connectivity changes in relapsing remitting multiple sclerosis patients: An exploratory study. *Journal of Neurology, 262*, 91–100. http://dx.doi.org/10.1007/s00415-014-7528-z

Brenk, A., Laun, K., & Haase, C. G. (2008). Short-term cognitive training improves mental efficiency and mood in patients with multiple sclerosis. *European Neurology, 60*, 304–309. http://dx.doi.org/10.1159/000157885

Brissart, H., Leroy, M., & Debouverie, M. (2010). Première évaluation d'un programme de remédiation cognitive chez des patients atteints de sclérose en plaques: PROCOG-SEP [First evaluation of a cognitive remediation program in patients with multiple sclerosis: PROCOG-SEP]. *Revue Neurologique, 166*, 406–411. http://dx.doi.org/10.1016/j.neurol.2009.06.008

Carr, S. E., das Nair, R., Schwartz, A. F., & Lincoln, N. B. (2014). Group memory rehabilitation for people with multiple sclerosis: A feasibility randomized controlled trial. *Clinical Rehabilitation, 28*, 552–561. http://dx.doi.org/10.1177/0269215513512336

Cerasa, A., Gioia, M. C., Valentino, P., Nisticò, R., Chiriaco, C., Pirritano, D., ... Quattrone, A. (2013). Computer-assisted cognitive rehabilitation of attention deficits for multiple sclerosis: A randomized trial with fMRI correlates. *Neurorehabilitation and Neural Repair, 27*, 284–295. http://dx.doi.org/10.1177/1545968312465194

Charvet, L. E., Kasschau, M., Datta, A., Knotkova, H., Stevens, M. C., Alonzo, A., ... Bikson, M. (2015). Remotely-supervised transcranial direct current stimulation (tDCS) for clinical trials: Guidelines for technology and protocols. *Frontiers in Systems Neuroscience, 9*, 26. http://dx.doi.org/10.3389/fnsys.2015.00026

Chiaravalloti, N. D., & DeLuca, J. (2002). Self-generation as a means of maximizing learning in multiple sclerosis: An application of the generation effect. *Archives of Physical Medicine and Rehabilitation, 83*(8), 1070–1079. http://dx.doi.org/10.1053/apmr.2002.33729

Chiaravalloti, N. D., & DeLuca, J. (2008). Cognitive impairment in multiple sclerosis. *Lancet Neurology, 7*, 1139–1151. http://dx.doi.org/10.1016/S1474-4422(08)70259-X

Chiaravalloti, N. D., & DeLuca, J. (2015). The influence of cognitive dysfunction on benefit from learning and memory rehabilitation in MS: A sub-analysis of the MEMREHAB trial. *Multiple Sclerosis Journal, 21*, 1575–1582. http://dx.doi.org/10.1177/1352458514567726

Chiaravalloti, N. D., DeLuca, J., Moore, N. B., & Ricker, J. H. (2005). Treating learning impairments improves memory performance in multiple sclerosis: A randomized clinical trial. *Multiple Sclerosis Journal, 11*, 58–68. http://dx.doi.org/10.1191/1352458505ms1118oa

Chiaravalloti, N. D., Demaree, H., Gaudino, E. A., & DeLuca, J. (2003). Can the repetition effect maximize learning in multiple sclerosis? *Clinical Rehabilitation, 17*, 58–68. http://dx.doi.org/10.1191/0269215503cr586oa

Chiaravalloti, N. D., Moore, N. B., Nikelshpur, O. M., & DeLuca, J. (2013). An RCT to treat learning impairment in multiple sclerosis: The MEMREHAB trial. *Neurology, 81*, 2066–2072. http://dx.doi.org/10.1212/01.wnl.0000437295.97946.a8

Chiaravalloti, N. D., Wylie, G., Leavitt, V., & DeLuca, J. (2012). Increased cerebral activation after behavioral treatment for memory deficits in MS. *Journal of Neurology, 259*, 1337–1346. http://dx.doi.org/10.1007/s00415-011-6353-x

das Nair, R., & Lincoln, N. B. (2012). Evaluation of rehabilitation of memory in neurological disabilities (ReMiND): A randomized controlled trial. *Clinical Rehabilitation, 26*, 894–903.

das Nair, R., Martin, K. J., & Lincoln, N. B. (2016). Memory rehabilitation for people with multiple sclerosis. Retrieved from *Cochrane Database of Systematic Reviews, 2016*(3). http://dx.doi.org/10.1002/14651858.CD008754.pub3

De Giglio, L., De Luca, F., Prosperini, L., Borriello, G., Bianchi, V., Pantano, P., & Pozzilli, C. (2015). A low-cost cognitive rehabilitation with a commercial video game improves sustained attention and executive functions in multiple sclerosis: A pilot study. *Neurorehabilitation and Neural Repair, 29*, 453–461. http://dx.doi.org/10.1177/1545968314554623

De Giglio, L., Tona, F., De Luca, F., Petsas, N., Prosperini, L., Bianchi, V., . . . Pantano, P. (2016). Multiple sclerosis: Changes in thalamic resting-state functional connectivity induced by a home-based cognitive rehabilitation program. *Radiology, 280*, 202–211. http://dx.doi.org/10.1148/radiol.2016150710

Dobryakova, E., Wylie, G. R., DeLuca, J., & Chiaravalloti, N. D. (2014). A pilot study examining functional brain activity 6 months after memory retraining in MS: The MEMREHAB trial. *Brain Imaging and Behavior, 8*, 403–406. http://dx.doi.org/10.1007/s11682-014-9309-9

Ernst, A., Blanc, F., De Seze, J., & Manning, L. (2015). Using mental visual imagery to improve autobiographical memory and episodic future thinking in relapsing-remitting multiple sclerosis patients: A randomised-controlled trial study. *Restorative Neurology and Neuroscience, 33*, 621–638. http://dx.doi.org/10.3233/RNN-140461

Ernst, A., Blanc, F., Voltzenlogel, V., de Seze, J., Chauvin, B., & Manning, L. (2013). Autobiographical memory in multiple sclerosis patients: Assessment and cognitive facilitation. *Neuropsychological Rehabilitation, 23*, 161–181. http://dx.doi.org/10.1080/09602011.2012.724355

Filippi, M., Riccitelli, G., Mattioli, F., Capra, R., Stampatori, C., Pagani, E., . . . Rocca, M. A. (2012). Multiple sclerosis: Effects of cognitive rehabilitation on structural and functional MR imaging measures—An explorative study. *Radiology, 262*, 932–940. http://dx.doi.org/10.1148/radiol.11111299

Fink, F., Rischkau, E., Butt, M., Klein, J., Eling, P., & Hildebrandt, H. (2010). Efficacy of an executive function intervention programme in MS: A placebo-controlled and pseudo-randomized trial. *Multiple Sclerosis Journal, 16*, 1148–1151. http://dx.doi.org/10.1177/1352458510375440

Foley, F. W., Dince, W. M., Bedell, J. R., LaRocca, N. G., Kalb, R., Caruso, L. S., . . . Shnek, Z. M. (1994). Psychoremediation of communication skills for cognitively impaired persons with multiple sclerosis. *Neurorehabilitation & Neural Repair, 8*(4), 165–176. http://dx.doi.org/10.1177/136140969400800401

Gentry, T. (2008). PDAs as cognitive aids for people with multiple sclerosis. *American Journal of Occupational Therapy, 62*, 18–27. http://dx.doi.org/10.5014/ajot.62.1.18

Gich, J., Freixanet, J., García, R., Vilanova, J. C., Genís, D., Silva, Y., . . . Ramió-Torrentà, L. (2015). A randomized, controlled, single-blind, 6-month pilot study to evaluate the efficacy of MS-Line! A cognitive rehabilitation programme for patients with multiple sclerosis. *Multiple Sclerosis Journal*, *21*, 1332–1343. http://dx.doi.org/10.1177/1352458515572405

Goverover, Y., Basso, M., Wood, H., Chiaravalloti, N., & DeLuca, J. (2011). Examining the benefits of combining two learning strategies on recall of functional information in persons with multiple sclerosis. *Multiple Sclerosis Journal*, *17*, 1488–1497. http://dx.doi.org/10.1177/1352458511406310

Goverover, Y., Chiaravalloti, N., & DeLuca, J. (2008). Self-generation to improve learning and memory of functional activities in persons with multiple sclerosis: Meal preparation and managing finances. *Archives of Physical Medicine and Rehabilitation*, *89*, 1514–1521. http://dx.doi.org/10.1016/j.apmr.2007.11.059

Goverover, Y., Chiaravalloti, N. D., & DeLuca, J. (2014). Task meaningfulness and degree of cognitive impairment: Do they affect self-generated learning in persons with multiple sclerosis? *Neuropsychological Rehabilitation*, *24*, 155–171. http://dx.doi.org/10.1080/09602011.2013.868815

Goverover, Y., Genova, H. M., Hillary, F. G., & DeLuca, J. (2007). The relationship between neuropsychological measures and the Timed Instrumental Activities of Daily Living task in multiple sclerosis. *Multiple Sclerosis Journal*, *13*, 636–644. http://dx.doi.org/10.1177/1352458506072984

Goverover, Y., Hillary, F. G., Chiaravalloti, N., Arango-Lasprilla, J. C., & DeLuca, J. (2009). A functional application of the spacing effect to improve learning and memory in persons with multiple sclerosis. *Journal of Clinical and Experimental Neuropsychology*, *31*, 513–522. http://dx.doi.org/10.1080/13803390802287042

Hancock, L. M., Bruce, J. M., Bruce, A. S., & Lynch, S. G. (2015). Processing speed and working memory training in multiple sclerosis: A double-blind randomized controlled pilot study. *Journal of Clinical and Experimental Neuropsychology*, *37*, 113–127. http://dx.doi.org/10.1080/13803395.2014.989818

Hanssen, K. T., Beiske, A. G., Landrø, N. I., Hofoss, D., & Hessen, E. (2016). Cognitive rehabilitation in multiple sclerosis: A randomized controlled trial. *Acta Neurologica Scandinavica*, *133*, 30–40. http://dx.doi.org/10.1111/ane.12420

Hanssen, K. T., Šaltytė Benth, J., Beiske, A. G., Landrø, N. I., & Hessen, E. (2015). Goal attainment in cognitive rehabilitation in MS patients. *Neuropsychological Rehabilitation*, *25*, 137–154. http://dx.doi.org/10.1080/09602011.2014.971818

Hildebrandt, H., Lanz, M., Hahn, H. K., Hoffmann, E., Schwarze, B., Schwendemann, G., & Kraus, J. A. (2007). Cognitive training in MS: Effects and relation to brain atrophy. *Restorative Neurology and Neuroscience*, *25*, 33–43.

Hubacher, M., Kappos, L., Weier, K., Stöcklin, M., Opwis, K., & Penner, I. K. (2015). Case-based fMRI analysis after cognitive rehabilitation in MS: A novel approach. *Frontiers in Neurology*, *6*, 78. http://dx.doi.org/10.3389/fneur.2015.00078

Janssen, A., Boster, A., Lee, H., Patterson, B., & Prakash, R. S. (2015). The effects of video-game training on broad cognitive transfer in multiple sclerosis: A pilot randomized controlled trial. *Journal of Clinical and Experimental Neuropsychology*, *37*, 285–302. http://dx.doi.org/10.1080/13803395.2015.1009366

Jønsson, A., Korfitzen, E. M., Heltberg, A., Ravnborg, M. H., & Byskov-Ottosen, E. (1993). Effects of neuropsychological treatment in patients with multiple sclerosis. *Acta Neurologica Scandinavica*, *88*, 394–400. http://dx.doi.org/10.1111/j.1600-0404.1993.tb05366.x

Leavitt, V. M., Cirnigliaro, C., Cohen, A., Farag, A., Brooks, M., Wecht, J. M., . . . Sumowski, J. F. (2014). Aerobic exercise increases hippocampal volume and improves memory in multiple sclerosis: Preliminary findings. *Neurocase*, *20*, 695–697. http://dx.doi.org/10.1080/13554794.2013.841951

Leavitt, V. M., Lengenfelder, J., Moore, N. B., Chiaravalloti, N. D., & DeLuca, J. (2011). The relative contributions of processing speed and cognitive load to working memory accuracy in multiple sclerosis. *Journal of Clinical and Experimental Neuropsychology*, *33*, 580–586. http://dx.doi.org/10.1080/13803395.2010.541427

Leavitt, V. M., Wylie, G. R., Girgis, P. A., DeLuca, J., & Chiaravalloti, N. D. (2014). Increased functional connectivity within memory networks following memory rehabilitation in multiple sclerosis. *Brain Imaging and Behavior*, *8*, 394–402. http://dx.doi.org/10.1007/s11682-012-9183-2

Lengenfelder, J., Bryant, D., Diamond, B. J., Kalmar, J. H., Moore, N. B., & DeLuca, J. (2006). Processing speed interacts with working memory efficiency in multiple sclerosis. *Archives of Clinical Neuropsychology*, *21*, 229–238. http://dx.doi.org/10.1016/j.acn.2005.12.001

Lincoln, N. B., Dent, A., & Harding, J. (2003). Treatment of cognitive problems for people with multiple sclerosis. *International Journal of Therapy and Rehabilitation*, *10*, 412–416. http://dx.doi.org/10.12968/bjtr.2003.10.9.13495

Lincoln, N. B., Dent, A., Harding, J., Weyman, N., Nicholl, C., Blumhardt, L. D., & Playford, E. D. (2002). Evaluation of cognitive assessment and cognitive intervention for people with multiple sclerosis. *Journal of Neurology, Neurosurgery, & Psychiatry*, *72*, 93–98. http://dx.doi.org/10.1136/jnnp.72.1.93

Lumos Labs, Inc. (2015). Lumosity [Computer software]. San Francisco, CA: Author.

Mäntynen, A., Rosti-Otajärvi, E., Koivisto, K., Lilja, A., Huhtala, H., & Hämäläinen, P. (2014). Neuropsychological rehabilitation does not improve cognitive performance but reduces perceived cognitive deficits in patients with multiple sclerosis: A randomised, controlled, multi-centre trial. *Multiple Sclerosis Journal*, *20*, 99–107. http://dx.doi.org/10.1177/1352458513494487

Martínez-González, A. E., & Piqueras, J. A. (2015). Long-term effectiveness of combined cognitive-behavioral and neuropsychological intervention in a case of multiple sclerosis. *Neurocase*, *21*, 584–591. http://dx.doi.org/10.1080/13554794.2014.960425

Mattioli, F., Bellomi, F., Stampatori, C., Capra, R., & Miniussi, C. (2016). Neuro-enhancement through cognitive training and anodal tDCS in multiple sclerosis. *Multiple Sclerosis Journal, 22,* 222–230. http://dx.doi.org/10.1177/1352458515587597

Mattioli, F., Bellomi, F., Stampatori, C., Provinciali, L., Compagnucci, L., Uccelli, A., . . . Capra, R. (2016). Two years follow up of domain specific cognitive training in relapsing remitting multiple sclerosis: A randomized clinical trial. *Frontiers in Behavioral Neuroscience, 10,* 28. http://dx.doi.org/10.3389/fnbeh.2016.00028

Mattioli, F., Stampatori, C., Bellomi, F., Danni, M., Compagnucci, L., Uccelli, A., . . . Capra, R. (2014). A RCT comparing specific intensive cognitive training to aspecific psychological intervention in RRMS: The SMICT study. *Frontiers in Neurology, 5,* 278. http://dx.doi.org/10.3389/fneur.2014.00278

Mattioli, F., Stampatori, C., Scarpazza, C., Parrinello, G., & Capra, R. (2012). Persistence of the effects of attention and executive functions intensive rehabilitation in relapsing remitting multiple sclerosis. *Multiple Sclerosis and Related Disorders, 1,* 168–173. http://dx.doi.org/10.1016/j.msard.2012.06.004

Mattioli, F., Stampatori, C., Zanotti, D., Parrinello, G., & Capra, R. (2010). Efficacy and specificity of intensive cognitive rehabilitation of attention and executive functions in multiple sclerosis. *Journal of the Neurological Sciences, 288,* 101–105. http://dx.doi.org/10.1016/j.jns.2009.09.024

Mendoza, R. J., Pittenger, D. J., & Weinstein, C. S. (2001). Unit management of depression of patients with multiple sclerosis using cognitive remediation strategies: A preliminary study. *Neurorehabilitation and Neural Repair, 15,* 9–14. http://dx.doi.org/10.1177/154596830101500102

Mendozzi, L., Pugnetti, L., Motta, A., Barbieri, E., Gambini, A., & Cazzullo, C. L. (1998). Computer-assisted memory retraining of patients with multiple sclerosis. *Italian Journal of Neurological Sciences, 19,* S431–S438. http://dx.doi.org/10.1007/BF00539601

Mitolo, M., Venneri, A., Wilkinson, I. D., & Sharrack, B. (2015). Cognitive rehabilitation in multiple sclerosis: A systematic review. *Journal of the Neurological Sciences, 354,* 1–9. http://dx.doi.org/10.1016/j.jns.2015.05.004

Moore, K. S., Peterson, D. A., O'Shea, G., McIntosh, G. C., & Thaut, M. H. (2008). The effectiveness of music as a mnemonic device on recognition memory for people with multiple sclerosis. *Journal of Music Therapy, 45,* 307–329. http://dx.doi.org/10.1093/jmt/45.3.307

Motl, R. W., Sandroff, B. M., & DeLuca, J. (2016). Exercise training and cognitive rehabilitation: A symbiotic approach for rehabilitating walking and cognitive functions in multiple sclerosis? *Neurorehabilitation and Neural Repair, 30,* 499–511. http://dx.doi.org/10.1177/1545968315606993

National Institutes of Health. (1998). Rehabilitation of persons with traumatic brain injury. *NIH Consensus Statement, 16,* 1–41.

O'Brien, A., Chiaravalloti, N., Arango-Lasprilla, J. C., Lengenfelder, J., & DeLuca, J. (2007). An investigation of the differential effect of self-generation to improve learning and memory in multiple sclerosis and traumatic brain injury. *Neuropsychological Rehabilitation, 17*, 273–292. http://dx.doi.org/10.1080/09602010600751160

O'Brien, A. R., Chiaravalloti, N., Goverover, Y., & DeLuca, J. (2008). Evidenced-based cognitive rehabilitation for persons with multiple sclerosis: A review of the literature. *Archives of Physical Medicine and Rehabilitation, 89*, 761–769. http://dx.doi.org/10.1016/j.apmr.2007.10.019

Parisi, L., Rocca, M. A., Mattioli, F., Copetti, M., Capra, R., Valsasina, P., . . . Filippi, M. (2014). Changes of brain resting state functional connectivity predict the persistence of cognitive rehabilitation effects in patients with multiple sclerosis. *Multiple Sclerosis Journal, 20*, 686–694. http://dx.doi.org/10.1177/1352458513505692

Parisi, L., Rocca, M. A., Valsasina, P., Panicari, L., Mattioli, F., & Filippi, M. (2014). Cognitive rehabilitation correlates with the functional connectivity of the anterior cingulate cortex in patients with multiple sclerosis. *Brain Imaging and Behavior, 8*, 387–393. http://dx.doi.org/10.1007/s11682-012-9160-9

Plohmann, A. M., Kappos, L., Ammann, W., Thordai, A., Wittwer, A., Huber, S., . . . Lechner-Scott, J. (1998). Computer assisted retraining of attentional impairments in patients with multiple sclerosis. *Journal of Neurology, Neurosurgery, and Psychiatry, 64*, 455–462. http://dx.doi.org/10.1136/jnnp.64.4.455

Plohmann, A., Kappos, L., & Brunnschweiler, H. (1994). Evaluation of a computer-based attention retraining program for patients with multiple sclerosis. *Schweizer Archiv für Neurologie und Psychiatrie, 145*(3), 35–36.

Pöttgen, J., Lau, S., Penner, I., Heesen, C., & Moritz, S. (2015). Managing neuropsychological impairment in multiple sclerosis: Pilot study on a standardized metacognitive intervention. *International Journal of MS Care, 17*, 130–137. http://dx.doi.org/10.7224/1537-2073.2014-015

Pusswald, G., Mildner, C., Zebenholzer, K., Auff, E., & Lehrner, J. (2014). A neuropsychological rehabilitation program for patients with multiple sclerosis based on the model of the ICF. *NeuroRehabilitation, 35*, 519–527. http://dx.doi.org/10.3233/NRE-141145

Rilo, O., Peña, J., Ojeda, N., Rodriguez-Antigüedad, A., Mendibe-Bilbao, M., Gómez-Gastiasoro, A., . . . Ibarretxe-Bilbao, N. (2016). Integrative group-based cognitive rehabilitation efficacy in multiple sclerosis: A randomized clinical trial. *Disability and Rehabilitation, 40*, 208–216.

Rosti-Otajärvi, E., Mäntynen, A., Koivisto, K., Huhtala, H., & Hämäläinen, P. (2013a). Neuropsychological rehabilitation has beneficial effects on perceived cognitive deficits in multiple sclerosis during nine-month follow-up. *Journal of the Neurological Sciences, 334*, 154–160. http://dx.doi.org/10.1016/j.jns.2013.08.017

Rosti-Otajärvi, E., Mäntynen, A., Koivisto, K., Huhtala, H., & Hämäläinen, P. (2013b). Patient-related factors may affect the outcome of neuropsychological rehabilitation in multiple sclerosis. *Journal of the Neurological Sciences, 334,* 106–111. http://dx.doi.org/10.1016/j.jns.2013.07.2520

Rosti-Otajärvi, E., Mäntynen, A., Koivisto, K., Huhtala, H., & Hämäläinen, P. (2014). Predictors and impact of the working alliance in the neuropsychological rehabilitation of patients with multiple sclerosis. *Journal of the Neurological Sciences, 338,* 156–161. http://dx.doi.org/10.1016/j.jns.2013.12.039

Sastre-Garriga, J., Alonso, J., Renom, M., Arévalo, M. J., González, I., Galán, I., . . . Rovira, A. (2011). A functional magnetic resonance proof of concept pilot trial of cognitive rehabilitation in multiple sclerosis. *Multiple Sclerosis Journal, 17,* 457–467. http://dx.doi.org/10.1177/1352458510389219

Shatil, E., Metzer, A., Horvitz, O., & Miller, A. (2010). Home-based personalized cognitive training in MS patients: A study of adherence and cognitive performance. *NeuroRehabilitation, 26,* 143–153.

Shevil, E., & Finlayson, M. (2010). Pilot study of a cognitive intervention program for persons with multiple sclerosis. *Health Education Research, 25,* 41–53. http://dx.doi.org/10.1093/her/cyp037

Solari, A., Motta, A., Mendozzi, L., Pucci, E., Forni, M., Mancardi, G., & Pozzilli, C. (2004). Computer-aided retraining of memory and attention in people with multiple sclerosis: A randomized, double-blind controlled trial. *Journal of the Neurological Sciences, 222,* 99–104. http://dx.doi.org/10.1016/j.jns.2004.04.027

Stuifbergen, A. K., Becker, H., Perez, F., Morison, J., Kullberg, V., & Todd, A. (2012). A randomized controlled trial of a cognitive rehabilitation intervention for persons with multiple sclerosis. *Clinical Rehabilitation, 26,* 882–893. http://dx.doi.org/10.1177/0269215511434997

Sumowski, J. F., Chiaravalloti, N., & DeLuca, J. (2010). Retrieval practice improves memory in multiple sclerosis: Clinical application of the testing effect. *Neuropsychology, 24,* 267–272. http://dx.doi.org/10.1037/a0017533

Sumowski, J. F., Leavitt, V. M., Cohen, A., Paxton, J., Chiaravalloti, N. D., & DeLuca, J. (2013). Retrieval practice is a robust memory aid for memory-impaired patients with MS. *Multiple Sclerosis Journal, 19,* 1943–1946. http://dx.doi.org/10.1177/1352458513485980

Thaut, M. H., Peterson, D. A., McIntosh, G. C., & Hoemberg, V. (2014). Music mnemonics aid verbal memory and induce learning-related brain plasticity in multiple sclerosis. *Frontiers in Human Neuroscience, 8,* 395. http://dx.doi.org/10.3389/fnhum.2014.00395

Vogt, A., Kappos, L., Calabrese, P., Stöcklin, M., Gschwind, L., Opwis, K., & Penner, I. K. (2009). Working memory training in patients with multiple sclerosis— Comparison of two different training schedules. *Restorative Neurology and Neuroscience, 27,* 225–235.

14

EXERCISE, PHYSICAL ACTIVITY, PHYSICAL FITNESS, AND COGNITION IN MULTIPLE SCLEROSIS

BRIAN M. SANDROFF AND ROBERT W. MOTL

Exercise training represents a promising behavioral approach for managing cognitive dysfunction in persons with multiple sclerosis (MS), but this area has been understudied (Motl, Sandroff, & Benedict, 2011; Sandroff, 2015). There is emerging interest by researchers and clinicians in the effects of exercise, physical activity, and physical fitness (see Table 14.1) on cognition in individuals with MS, in part, based on the concept of cognitive-motor coupling (i.e., co-occurring cognitive and motor dysfunction) in MS (Benedict et al. 2011; Motl, Sandroff, & DeLuca, 2016). Of note, this body of literature is smaller than that of cognitive rehabilitation in MS (Motl et al., 2016; see also Chapter 11, this volume). The examination of exercise, physical activity, and physical fitness effects of cognition in MS further is based on the well-established body of literature in the general population across the life span (i.e., in healthy children, young adults, and older adults). Such literature supports robust, beneficial effects of exercise, physical activity, and

http://dx.doi.org/10.1037/0000097-015
Cognition and Behavior in Multiple Sclerosis, J. DeLuca and B. M. Sandroff (Editors)
Copyright © 2018 by the American Psychological Association. All rights reserved.

TABLE 14.1
American College of Sports Medicine Definitions of Exercise, Physical Activity, and Physical Fitness

Construct	Definition
Exercise	Physical activity that is planned, structured, and repetitive for the purpose of improving or maintaining one or more components of physical fitness
Physical activity	Bodily movement produced by contraction of skeletal muscle that increases energy expenditure above basal level
Physical fitness	An attained set of attributes (e.g., cardiorespiratory capacity and endurance, flexibility, body composition, skeletal muscle strength and endurance) that relates to the ability to perform physical activity

Note. Data from American College of Sports Medicine (2013).

physical fitness on cognitive functioning and its underlying neural substrates (Voss, Nagamatsu, Liu-Ambrose, & Kramer, 2011). The body of literature on exercise, physical activity, and physical fitness effects on cognition in MS is substantially smaller than that in the general population (Sandroff, 2015).

Of the existing studies in this area involving MS, most are not randomized controlled trials (RCTs), and further suffer from significant methodological flaws, including small sample sizes, poorly defined interventions, lack of adequate control groups, and inclusion of cognition as a non-primary outcome (Sandroff, 2015; Sandroff, Motl, Scudder, & DeLuca, 2016). Such concerns highlight that the MS studies are not on par with the methodological rigor of studies of exercise training on cognition in the general population (Motl, Sandroff, et al., 2011). In addition, the constructs of exercise, physical activity, and physical fitness are oftentimes considered to be single construct of "exercise" in the MS literature, when, by definition, these are related but separate constructs (American College of Sports Medicine [ACSM], 2013; Bouchard & Shephard, 1994; Sandroff, 2015; see Table 14.1). Overall, researchers and clinicians experience difficulty drawing firm conclusions regarding the efficacy of exercise, physical activity, and physical fitness effects on cognition in MS (Sandroff, 2015). For example, reviews have highlighted that research on exercise effects on cognition primarily involves intervention-based approaches, whereas studies of physical activity and physical fitness effects on cognition are generally observational and might be important for informing the development of exercise training interventions (Sandroff, 2015; Sandroff, Motl, Scudder, et al., 2016). Given the distinction between exercise, physical activity, and physical fitness, those constructs might have differential effects on cognition in MS (Motl, Sandroff, et al., 2011; Sandroff, 2015). Another observation is that within each construct, some individual studies have reported beneficial effects of exercise, physical activity, and physical fitness on cognition in MS, and others have reported null results (Sandroff, Motl, Scudder, et al., 2016).

This chapter comprehensively reviews the evidence of exercise, physical activity, and physical fitness effects, respectively (i.e., as three separate constructs), on cognition specifically in persons with MS. This provides an updated snapshot of the state of the field regarding those behavioral approaches for improving cognition in MS, considering the seemingly heterogeneous results of Class I–IV studies (Sandroff, Motl, Scudder, et al., 2016). The current chapter then presents future directions for consideration for systematically designing studies of exercise and physical activity on cognition in this population.

EXERCISE AND COGNITION IN MS

Comprehensive Review of Evidence

To date, there are nine published studies on the effects of chronic exercise training on cognition; four additional studies examined the effects of acute exercise (i.e., single bouts of exercise) on cognition. Based on American Academy of Neurology (AAN; Gross & Johnston, 2009) criteria for rating levels of evidence, of the 13 total studies in this area, there is one Class I study (chronic exercise), two Class II studies (both chronic exercise), six Class III studies (three chronic exercise, three acute exercise), and four Class IV studies (three chronic exercise, one acute exercise). This section first reviews the experimental details of each study; discussions pertaining to each study are presented in the following section.

Chronic Exercise Training

The single Class I study (Oken et al., 2004) examined the effects of (chronic) exercise training on tests of attention, executive function, learning and memory, and processing speed in 57 persons with MS. This study involved 6 months of a once-weekly yoga class, once-weekly aerobic exercise class, or wait-list control condition using an RCT design. The yoga class consisted of a 90-minute session of Iyengar yoga (adapted for persons with MS). The aerobic exercise intervention involved mainly group exercise on a stationary bicycle at a very light intensity. Alternatively, participants had the option to exercise on a Swiss ball instead; home exercise was encouraged. Following the completion of the intervention, neither the yoga group nor the exercise group demonstrated significant improvements in any cognitive measure (e.g., Stroop Color–Word Interference Test, Paced Auditory Serial Addition Test [PASAT]) compared with the wait-list control group.

Two published Class II studies (Carter et al., 2014; Hoang, Schoene, Gandevia, Smith, & Lord, 2016) examined the effects of exercise training on cognition. The first study (Carter et al., 2014) involved an RCT on the effects of 12 weeks of a practically implemented exercise program compared with a usual-care control group on processing speed (i.e., PASAT performance) in 99 persons with MS. The exercise intervention consisted of primarily aerobic exercise (i.e., light-to-moderate intensity arm ergometry and stepping exercise) with some strength exercise. The intervention was partially supervised. During the first half of the intervention, participants engaged in supervised exercise 2 days/week and home-based exercise once per week. During the second half of the intervention, participants engaged in supervised exercise once per week and home-based exercise twice per week. Although there were significant intervention effects on self-reported exercise behavior (i.e., the primary study outcome), there were no reported intervention effects on PASAT scores ($p = .17$).

The second Class II study (Hoang et al., 2016) involved a comparison of 12 weeks of home-based step-training (i.e., exergaming) with a wait-list control condition on processing speed (i.e., Symbol Digit Modalities Test [SDMT] performance) and executive function (i.e., Trail Making Test [TMT] performance) in 44 persons with MS using an RCT design. Home-based step-training sessions took place twice per week for 30 minutes. This study did not report on the intensity of step-training sessions. Cognition was not a primary study outcome, and accordingly, there were no intervention effects on SDMT performance ($p = .38$) or TMT performance ($p = .49$).

There are three published Class III studies on chronic exercise training effects on cognition (Briken et al., 2014; Romberg, Virtanen, & Ruutiainen, 2005; Velikonja, Ćurić, Ožura, & Jazbec, 2010). One Class III study reported nonsignificant effects of 26 weeks of combined aerobic and resistance exercise training compared with a wait-list control group on processing speed (i.e., PASAT performance; Romberg et al., 2005) using an RCT design in 91 persons with MS. The exercise training intervention consisted of five resistance training sessions and five aerobic training sessions in the first 3 weeks of the intervention, followed by 23 weeks of a prescribed home exercise regimen. This part of the program involved primarily resistance exercise (i.e., suggested to take place three to four times per week) with additional sessions of aerobic exercise (i.e., suggested to take place once per week). Participants were encouraged via phone to adhere to the home exercise program on four separate occasions over the 26-week intervention. The primary study outcomes involved measures of functional impairment in MS; the 3' PASAT was included as a secondary outcome of processing speed. Accordingly, 3' PASAT performance did not significantly improve in persons with MS who underwent the exercise intervention ($p = .38$).

The second Class III exercise training study (Velikonja et al., 2010) was a prospective, randomized comparison of the effects of 10 weeks of sports climbing and yoga on cognition (i.e., attention and executive function) in 20 persons with MS using a prospective, randomized design (Velikonja et al., 2010). There was no control condition included in this study. The sports climbing condition involved participants climbing on a 90-degree climbing wall once per week, and the yoga condition consisted of once-weekly Hatha yoga (adapted for persons with MS). Those who underwent the yoga condition demonstrated improvements in selective attention based on Brickenkamp d2 test performance ($p < .01$). There were no significant effects of either intervention on executive function (i.e., Tower of London test performance). Of note, it is unclear if spasticity, fatigue, or cognition represented the primary study outcome.

The third Class III exercise training study (Briken et al., 2014) involved an RCT design and examined the effects of a supervised, 8–10 week aerobic exercise training intervention on fitness and cognition in 42 persons with progressive MS. Participants were randomly assigned to one of three aerobic exercise training conditions (i.e., arm ergometry, rowing, cycle ergometry) or a wait-list control condition. The exercise training sessions took place two to three times per week for 15–45 minutes per session at a moderate intensity. Verbal memory (i.e., Verbal Learning and Memory Test performance) improved for all three exercise conditions relative to the wait-list control group ($p = .01$). However, aspects of attention/alertness (i.e., Test Battery of Attention performance) improved in the cycle ergometry and arm ergometry but not rowing group relative to the control group. There were no intervention effects in processing speed (SDMT), executive function (Achievement Testing System), or verbal fluency (Regensburg Verbal Fluency Test). Cardiorespiratory fitness improved in those who underwent the cycle ergometry but not rowing or arm ergometry group relative to the control group. Furthermore, change in fitness explained ~16% of variance in changes in verbal memory and alertness within the cycle ergometry group.

There are three published Class IV studies on chronic exercise training effects on cognition (Leavitt et al., 2014; Pilutti et al., 2011; Sangelaji et al., 2015). One Class IV study examined the effects of 12 weeks of body weight-supported treadmill training on processing speed (i.e., PASAT) in six persons with progressive MS using a longitudinal pre-post design. There was no control condition, and cognition was not a primary outcome. Body weight-supported treadmill training took place three times per week for 30 minutes per session. Exercise progression was based on first increasing speed, followed by decreases in percent body weight support. Although there were improvements in quality of life, there were no significant effects on processing speed (i.e., 3' PASAT performance; $d = 0.12$).

The second Class IV study on exercise training (Leavitt et al., 2014) involved a case study design that collected data on hippocampal volume and resting-state functional connectivity and cognitive functioning from two ambulatory, memory-impaired persons with MS who were randomly assigned into 12 weeks of aerobic exercise training (i.e., stationary cycling) or stretching and toning. Both conditions took place three times per week for 30 minutes per session. The intensity of stationary cycling gradually progressed over the 12-week intervention. Aerobic exercise training resulted in a 16.5% increase in hippocampal volume, 55.9% increase in verbal memory (i.e., California Verbal Learning Test-II [CVLT-II] performance), and 53.7% increase in nonverbal memory (i.e., Brief Visuospatial Memory Test-Revised [BVMT-R] performance), as well as increased hippocampal resting-state functional connectivity. There were no changes in processing speed (i.e., PASAT, SDMT), executive function (i.e., Stroop Test), or working memory (i.e., Digit Span), overall cerebral gray matter, or nonhippocampal deep gray matter structures. Furthermore, there were no changes in cognitive or neuroimaging outcomes for the participant who underwent stretching and toning.

The third Class IV study on exercise training (Sangelaji et al., 2015) involved a quasi-experimental pre-post design that examined the effects of an 8-week combined exercise training program on cognition in 17 persons with MS. There was no control condition. The exercise training program took place three times per week for 8 weeks. The training sessions consisted of aerobic exercise (i.e., treadmill walking/cycle ergometry) for 20 minutes, balance exercises (i.e., trampoline, tilt board) for 30 minutes, and lower limb stretching exercises (twice per week) for 15 minutes. There were apparent intervention effects on long-term memory based on the Selective Reminding Task (SRT), although the exact outcomes were unclear. Furthermore, there were improvements in processing speed based on PASAT and SDMT performance. There were no effects on visuospatial memory (i.e., 10/36 Spatial Recall Test [SPART]) or verbal fluency (Word List Generation [WLG]).

Acute Exercise

There are three published Class III studies (Sandroff, Hillman, Benedict, & Motl, 2015; Sandroff, Hillman, Benedict, & Motl, 2016; Sandroff, Motl, & Davis, 2016) and one Class IV study (Skjerbæk et al., 2013) on acute exercise effects on cognition in this population. One Class III study of acute exercise on cognition (Sandroff, Hillman, Benedict, et al., 2015) involved an examination of the acute effects of different modalities of exercise on aspects of processing speed and executive function (i.e., inhibitory control) relative to a quiet rest control condition in 24 persons with mild MS disability using a within-subjects, repeated measures design. Participants completed four experimental conditions that consisted of 20 minutes of quiet rest, moderate intensity treadmill walking exercise, moderate intensity cycle ergometer exercise, and guided yoga that was adapted for persons with MS. There were general pre-to-post improvements in processing speed (i.e., generalized reaction time [RT] on the modified flanker task) for all three exercise modalities compared with quiet rest (all $\eta_p^2 > .24$). Of note, there were pre-to-post improvements in inhibitory control (i.e., reductions in the cost of interfering stimuli on RT on the modified flanker task) for treadmill walking but not cycle ergometry or yoga relative to quiet rest ($\eta_p^2 = .17$).

A follow-up (Class III) study (Sandroff, Hillman, et al., 2016) examined the effects of 20-minute bouts of light, moderate, and vigorous intensity treadmill walking exercise compared with a quiet rest control condition on processing speed and inhibitory control in 24 fully ambulatory persons with MS, again using a within-subjects, repeated-measures design. There were statistically significant pre-to-post improvements in processing speed (i.e., reductions in generalized RT on the modified flanker task) and inhibitory control (i.e., reductions in the cost of interfering stimuli on RT on the modified flanker task) for light, moderate, and vigorous intensity exercise compared with quiet rest ($\eta_p^2 = .16$) that were similar in magnitude.

Similarly, another follow-up (Class III) study (Sandroff, Motl, & Davis, 2016) examined the effects of 20 minutes of vigorous intensity treadmill walking exercise compared with seated quiet rest on processing speed, inhibitory control, and core body temperature in 14 thermosensitive persons with MS using a within-subjects, repeated-measures design. This study addressed a growing concern that elevations in core body temperature might result in deleterious effects on cognitive performance in persons with MS (Hämäläinen, Ikonen, Romberg, Helenius, & Ruutiainen, 2012) and hypothesized that exercise-related increases in core body temperature would nullify acute improvements in cognitive performance. However, that study reported that despite large exercise-related increases in core body temperature, there were acute pre-to-post improvements in processing speed and inhibitory control for vigorous intensity treadmill walking exercise relative to quiet rest ($\eta_p^2 > .29$) in thermosensitive persons with MS that were large in magnitude.

The Class IV study on acute exercise (Skjerbæk et al., 2013) compared the acute effects of aerobic and resistance exercise on processing speed (i.e., PASAT performance) in 16 persons with MS using a within-subjects, repeated-measures design. The primary outcomes were core body temperature and symptom intensity; the PASAT was included as a secondary exploratory outcome. Participants underwent a 30-minute bout of moderate intensity cycle ergometry exercise and a 30-minute bout of moderate intensity upper and lower extremity resistance exercise. There were no changes in processing speed (i.e., 3' PASAT performance) from before to after exercise for either aerobic or resistance exercise.

Discussion

Overall, examination of the effects of exercise, either chronic or acute, on cognition in MS involves studies of relatively weak methodological quality (i.e., only one Class I study, two Class II studies, and 10 Class III or IV studies). Based on results from Class I and II studies, there is no support for the clinical utility of exercise for improving cognition at this time. More support may be garnered from Class III and IV studies of both chronic and acute exercise, although based on AAN guidelines (Gross & Johnston, 2009), such studies involved weaker experimental designs. To that end, studies with stronger methodological quality according to AAN guidelines (i.e., Class I or II studies) reported null (nonsignificant) effects on cognition, whereas five Class III and two Class IV studies reported positive, beneficial effects on cognition (see Figure 14.1). Evidence from five of nine studies (i.e., one Class I study, two Class II studies, one Class III, and one Class IV study) does not support the efficacy of chronic exercise for improving cognition in persons with MS (i.e., non-statistically significant results). However, evidence from four of

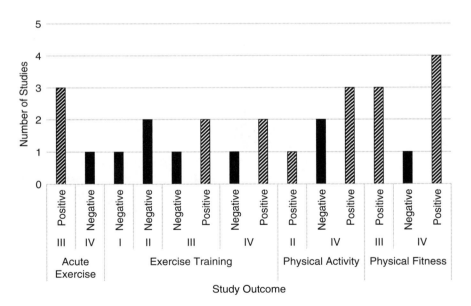

Figure 14.1. Summary of exercise, physical activity, and physical fitness effects on cognition in persons with multiple sclerosis, based on class of evidence.

nine studies (i.e., two Class III studies and two Class IV studies) does support the efficacy of chronic exercise for improving cognition in this population. Evidence from three Class III studies supports acute exercise for improving cognition in persons with MS, whereas one Class IV study did not. Such conflicting evidence might have to do with the inclusion of cognition as a primary study outcome. With the exception of the Class I study, each of the studies that reported nonsignificant results of chronic exercise training on cognition (Carter et al., 2014; Hoang et al., 2016; Pilutti et al., 2011; Romberg et al., 2005) did not include cognition as a primary outcome. However, each of the two Class III (Briken et al., 2014; Velikonja et al., 2010) and two Class IV studies (Leavitt et al., 2014; Sangelaji et al., 2015) that reported significant, beneficial effects of exercise training did include cognition as a primary or a priori secondary outcome (see Figure 14.2). Among acute exercise studies, the three positive Class III studies (i.e., Sandroff, Hillman, Benedict, et al., 2015; Sandroff, Hillman, et al., 2016; Sandroff, Motl, & Davis, 2016) focused on cognition as a primary outcome, whereas the Class IV study (Skjerbæk et al., 2013) did not.

Strong methodological quality according to AAN is based on criteria, such as having random assignment with concealed allocation, blinding of outcome assessors, defining a primary study outcome, defining inclusion/exclusion criteria, and adequate accounting of dropouts. However, despite

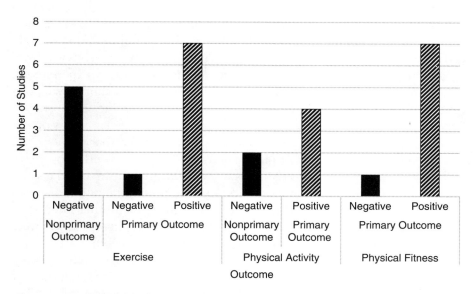

Figure 14.2. Summary of exercise, physical activity, and physical fitness effects on cognition in persons with multiple sclerosis, based on inclusion of cognition as a primary or non-primary outcome.

satisfying AAN criteria for a Class I or II study, there are a number of noteworthy limitations that might have resulted in such null effects. First, those Class I and II studies on exercise did not involve cognitively impaired persons with MS. Importantly, only one of 13 studies (Leavitt et al., 2014) recruited participants based on having cognitive impairment. This greatly limits the impact of the findings such that the interventions were not tested in those who presumably have the most need for such an intervention and introduces the possibility of ceiling effects for the potential improvement in cognition. There were other concerns from an exercise prescription standpoint. For example, in the Class I study (Oken et al., 2004), the aerobic exercise stimulus was not frequent or intense enough such that the maximal benefits of exercise training on cognition could not be realized (i.e., exercise prescription insufficient to meet public health guidelines; ACSM, 2013). Adherence to both the aerobic exercise and yoga interventions was low (i.e., participation in ~65% of sessions), and a portion of the aerobic exercise intervention was unsupervised, further reducing the chances of intervention effects on cognition. Importantly, none of the Class I (Oken et al., 2004) or Class II (Carter et al., 2014; Hoang et al., 2016) studies included a physical fitness outcome measure for documenting the success of the exercise training conditions. This too reduces the impact of the primary results, as, by definition, exercise training is planned, structured, and repetitive bodily movement done to improve or maintain one or more components of physical fitness (ACSM, 2013). Perhaps most important, both Class II studies did not clearly include cognition as a primary outcome. As such, neither intervention (i.e., combined exercise training (Carter et al., 2014) and step-training (Hoang et al., 2016) were specifically designed for improving cognition in persons with MS.

On the other hand, there is weaker evidence from an experimental design perspective (e.g., Class III and IV evidence) that seemingly supports exercise training for improving cognition in persons with MS. For instance, one Class III RCT (Briken et al., 2014) did report beneficial effects of aerobic exercise training on cardiorespiratory fitness and verbal memory and alertness (i.e., as an a priori secondary outcome) in persons with progressive MS. Although this study involved concealed allocation, it involved a small sample of persons with progressive MS (i.e., ~10 persons randomly assigned to each condition) who were not cognitively impaired. Another interesting aspect of that study was that improvements in cardiorespiratory fitness were associated with improvements in verbal memory (Briken et al., 2014). This is consistent with evidence in older adults, whereby aerobic exercise training improves both fitness and memory (Erickson et al., 2011). Such results further provide preliminary experimental evidence, whereby improvements in cardiorespiratory fitness might be a mechanism for improved cognition in MS. This hypothesis is consistent with cross-sectional evidence of associations between cardiorespiratory fitness and processing speed in persons with MS that are reviewed in a later section of this chapter (e.g., Prakash, Snook, Motl, & Kramer, 2010; Sandroff & Motl, 2012; Sandroff, Hillman, & Motl, 2015; Sandroff, Pilutti, Benedict, & Motl, 2015).

The Class IV evidence that described beneficial effects of exercise on cognition involved a case study/pilot RCT (Leavitt et al., 2014) and a quasi-experimental pre-post design (Sangelaji et al., 2015), respectively. Despite relatively weak experimental designs, both of those studies reported beneficial effects of exercise training on aspects of learning and memory. Although the case study did not involve a representative, highly generalizable sample based on the sample size, this is the only study of exercise, physical activity, or physical fitness effects on cognition in persons with MS that recruited participants based on cognitive impairment (Leavitt et al., 2014).

Acute exercise studies that reported statistically significant beneficial effects on cognition included cognition as a primary outcome, and this is consistent with the pattern of results from chronic exercise training studies in MS. Those studies involved within-subjects, repeated-measures designs, whereby participants served as their own controls (Sandroff, Hillman, Benedict, et al., 2015; Sandroff, Hillman, et al., 2016; Sandroff, Motl, & Davis, 2016). Collectively, those studies reported that treadmill walking exercise, perhaps at light, moderate, and vigorous intensities, was associated with improved processing speed and inhibitory control relative to quiet rest, even among thermosensitive persons with MS (Sandroff, Hillman, Benedict, et al., 2015; Sandroff, Hillman, et al., 2016; Sandroff, Motl, & Davis, 2016). However, none of those studies involved cognitively impaired MS samples, limiting the impact of the results.

One important aspect of the body of literature on the effects of exercise on cognition in MS involves the inconsistency in study characteristics. This includes heterogeneity in exercise prescription (i.e., modality, frequency, intensity, duration), measurement of physical fitness as a manipulation check, the nature of the control comparison condition, and domains of cognitive domains/neuropsychological tests. In fact, no two exercise studies involved identical exercise stimuli. Such heterogeneous study characteristics create difficulty in evaluating the overall effectiveness of exercise on cognition in this population. Indeed, there has been no true replication of studies, which creates considerable difficulty in making definitive overall recommendations for clinical research and practice. One consistent methodological weakness across the chronic exercise studies was the absence of active control groups (i.e., stretching and toning). Rather, RCTs included wait-list control conditions that did not account for attention/social interaction that are normally associated with exercise training. From an outcomes perspective, many of the reviewed studies did not include comprehensive neuropsychological batteries that are well established in persons with MS (e.g., Minimal Assessment of Cognitive Function in Multiple Sclerosis [MACFIMS]). Rather, many of those studies included only one or two neuropsychological outcomes as measures of cognitive performance. This was either due to cognition being included as a non-primary outcome or an a priori investigation on exercise effects on a certain cognitive domain (e.g., Sandroff, Hillman, Benedict, et al., 2015; Sandroff, Hillman, et al., 2016; Sandroff, Motl, & Davis, 2016). Participant-specific characteristics also might explain the overall conflicting evidence for exercise effects on cognition in persons with MS. For example, it is possible that exercise training might have differential effects on cognition, based on the severity of MS-related disability, as has been reported in studies of physical activity (Sandroff, Pilutti, Dlugonski, & Motl, 2013; Sandroff, Klaren, et al., 2014) and physical fitness (Sandroff, Pilutti, et al., 2015) on cognition in this population. In addition, exercise studies that recruit low-fit/relatively sedentary samples of persons with MS are advantageous as this avoids potential ceiling effects, whereby exercise training may not result in substantial improvements in fitness and/or cognition. In summary, the body of literature on the effects of exercise on cognition in persons with MS is clearly in its infancy. Despite the lack of evidence from Class I and II studies, future research might consider the more promising evidence from Class III and IV studies for informing the development of better exercise training interventions for improving cognition in MS (Sandroff, 2015).

PHYSICAL ACTIVITY AND COGNITION IN MS

Comprehensive Review of Evidence

Six studies focused on the effects of physical activity on cognition. Of the six studies, there is one Class II study (Sandroff, Klaren, et al., 2014) and five Class IV studies (Motl, Gappmaier, Nelson, & Benedict, 2011; Prakash, Patterson, Janssen, Abduljalil, & Boster, 2011; Sandroff et al., 2013; Sandroff, Dlugonski, et al., 2014; Waschbisch et al., 2012). The Class II study (Sandroff, Klaren, et al., 2014) involved an RCT design to examine the effects of a 6-month Internet-based behavioral physical activity intervention compared with a wait-list control group on processing speed in 76 persons with mild and moderate MS ambulatory disability. The intervention condition involved visiting a study website that was based on social cognitive theory; wearing a pedometer, completing a logbook, and using computerized software for guiding goal-setting and attainment; and participating in one-on-one video chat sessions with a behavior-change coach. There were statistically significant improvements in processing speed (i.e., SDMT performance) for persons with mild but not moderate MS ambulatory disability who underwent the intervention compared with persons who underwent the wait-list control condition ($\eta_p^2 = .08$). Among persons in the intervention condition, changes in objectively measured physical activity were associated with changes in SDMT scores in persons with mild but not moderate MS ambulatory disability.

The first Class IV study (Motl, Gappmaier, et al., 2011) involved a cross-sectional examination on the effects of objectively measured, free-living physical activity on processing speed and learning and memory in 33 older persons with MS. Participants wore a StepWatch activity monitor for 7 days for measurement of average steps per day. Persons with MS demonstrated moderately impaired processing speed but not learning and memory, based on neuropsychological test performance. After controlling for age, sex, and education, physical activity was significantly associated with a composite measure of processing speed (i.e., PASAT, SDMT scores; $pr = .39$), but not learning and memory (i.e., SRT, BVMT-R scores; $pr = .20$), such that greater steps per day was associated with faster processing speed.

The second Class IV study (Prakash et al., 2011) involved a cross-sectional design and examined the effects of objective, free-living physical activity on hippocampal resting-state functional connectivity and episodic memory in 45 persons with MS. Participants wore an ActiGraph accelerometer for a 7-day period for measurement of average activity counts per day. Participants further underwent an fMRI scan, where participants performed a behavioral task of episodic memory (i.e., encoding of faces, scenes, and face–scene pairings), and underwent measurement of hippocampal resting-state functional connectivity. Although physical activity was associated with increased resting-state functional connectivity, which in turn was associated with better episodic memory, average activity counts per day were not directly associated with episodic memory performance ($p > .05$).

The third cross-sectional Class IV study (Waschbisch et al., 2012) examined differences in several cognitive domains in 42 physically active and physically inactive persons with relapsing–remitting MS. The primary study outcomes involved measures of brain-derived neurotrophic factor, vitamin D, cardiorespiratory fitness, and immune parameters; cognition was included as a secondary outcome. Participants were classified as physically active or physically inactive based on self-report (i.e., Baecke questionnaire). There were no significant differences between groups in processing speed (i.e., PASAT performance; $p = .11$) and short- and long-term memory, attention, and fatigue (i.e., MUSIC neuropsychological battery performance; $p = .07$). This study did not report correlations between physical activity level and cognitive performance or between cardiorespiratory fitness and cognitive performance.

The fourth Class IV study (Sandroff et al., 2013) involved a prospective examination of objectively measured, free-living physical activity and processing speed in 78 persons with mild and moderate MS ambulatory disability. Participants wore an ActiGraph accelerometer for 7 days for measurement of physical activity, expressed as average steps per day. After a 6-month period without intervention, participants underwent neuropsychological assessments of processing speed (i.e., PASAT, SDMT). After controlling for age, sex, and self-reported ambulatory disability status in the overall sample, steps per day were significantly associated with processing speed based on oral and written SDMT scores (pr_s = .25–.29); steps per day were not significantly associated with performance on the PASAT (pr_s = .12). After controlling for age, steps per day were associated with SDMT performance in persons with mild (pr_s = .35–.36) but not moderate MS ambulatory disability (pr_s = .24–.27).

The fifth Class IV study (Sandroff, Dlugonski, et al., 2014) involved a cross-sectional examination on the effects of objectively measured, free-living physical activity on measures of processing speed in a large sample of 212 persons with MS. Participants wore an ActiGraph accelerometer for 7 days for measurement of average steps per day. After controlling for age, sex, and education, physical activity was significantly associated with a composite measure of processing speed (i.e., mean z-scores for PASAT and SDMT; pr = .26). This association was attenuated but remained statistically significant after further controlling for ambulatory status (pr = .13).

Discussion

Overall, the evidence for the effects of physical activity on cognition is generally positive, although not definitive or extensive. This is based on one Class II study and three Class IV studies that reported beneficial effects of physical activity on cognition, whereas two Class IV studies reported null effects (see Figure 14.1). No studies reported harmful effects. This seemingly indicates that taking more steps per day is associated with better processing speed in persons with MS. Similar to the literature on exercise effects on cognition in MS, physical activity studies that included cognition as a primary outcome (e.g., Motl, Gappmaier, et al., 2011; Sandroff et al., 2013; Sandroff, Dlugonski, et al., 2014; Sandroff, Klaren, et al., 2014) generally reported positive beneficial effects, whereas the studies that did not (e.g., Prakash et al., 2011; Waschbisch et al., 2012), reported null results (see Figure 14.2). However, given the absence of a Class I study, and the vast majority of studies classified as Class IV evidence, at this time, there is not enough evidence to definitively support the clinical utility of physical activity for selectively improving cognition in persons with MS.

Collectively, studies of physical activity included neurocognitive tests of attention, aspects of learning and memory, and processing speed. Importantly, no physical activity study included measures of executive function, the third most commonly impaired cognitive domain in MS (Chiaravalloti & DeLuca, 2008). To that end, no physical activity studies included any MS-specific neuropsychological batteries (e.g., Brief Repeatable Battery of Neuropsychological Tests [BRB-N]; see Rao, 1990; MACFIMS; see Benedict et al., 2006; Brief International Cognitive Assessment for Multiple Sclerosis; see Langdon et al., 2012) as outcome measures. Five of the six studies included measures of processing speed that involved either the SDMT or PASAT (Motl, Gappmaier, et al., 2011; Sandroff et al., 2013; Sandroff, Dlugonski, et al., 2014; Sandroff, Klaren, et al., 2014; Waschbisch et al., 2012), whereas only three involved measures of learning and memory (Motl, Gappmaier, et al., 2011; Prakash et al., 2011; Waschbisch et al., 2012), and one involved measures of attention (Waschbisch et al., 2012). Importantly, given that only one study involved an intervention approach, processing speed represents the only domain of cognition that was reported to have improved over time, based on engaging in more physical activity behavior (Sandroff, Klaren, et al., 2014).

To that end, one limitation of this body of work is that only one study involved an intervention approach that could be classified as a Class II study (Sandroff, Klaren, et al., 2014). That study had several methodological limitations (e.g., outcome assessors were not treatment blinded, sample did not involve persons with impaired processing speed), but it represents the strongest evidence to date for increased participation in physical activity improving processing speed in persons with MS. To better classify the overall effectiveness of physical activity on cognition in MS, replication of this intervention approach is necessary. Among observational studies with weaker experimental designs (i.e., Class IV evidence), most reported beneficial effects on cognition and involved objective measures of physical activity (e.g., accelerometer-measured average steps per day). Collectively, although some of these studies involved samples of persons with MS who demonstrated poor cognitive performance (e.g., Motl, Gappmaier, et al., 2011), none of the physical activity studies involved cognitive impairment as an a priori inclusion criterion. Furthermore, there is a pattern of results among the physical activity literature, whereby engaging in more physical activity behavior is associated with better cognitive performance in persons with mild but not moderate MS ambulatory disability (Sandroff et al., 2013; Sandroff, Klaren, et al., 2014). However, examining disability status as a moderator of the physical activity–cognition relationship has not been fully explored and should be replicated for better defining target populations for physical activity interventions on cognition in persons with MS.

Comprehensive Review of Evidence

Eight studies focused on physical fitness and cognition in MS. Of the eight published studies in this area, there are three Class III studies (Prakash et al., 2010; Sandroff & Motl, 2012; Sandroff, Hillman, & Motl, 2015) and five Class IV studies (Batista et al., 2012; Beier, Bombardier, Hartoonian, Motl, & Kraft, 2014; Prakash et al., 2007; Sandroff, Hubbard, Pilutti, & Motl, 2015; Sandroff, Pilutti, et al., 2015). The primary difference between the Class III and Class IV studies is that the Class III studies involved healthy control comparison groups, whereas the Class IV studies did not.

The first Class III study (Prakash et al., 2010) involved a cross-sectional examination of the relationship between cardiorespiratory fitness, structural MRI outcomes, and cognition in a sample of 21 persons with MS and 15 healthy controls. Participants underwent an incremental exercise test (IET) to exhaustion on a cycle ergometer for determination of cardiorespiratory fitness (i.e., VO_{2peak}), Rao's BRB-N, and an MRI for measurement of grey matter volume and white matter integrity. There were significant differences between persons with MS and controls in cardiorespiratory fitness, processing speed (i.e., PASAT, SDMT), grey matter volume, and white matter integrity (i.e., $d > 0.67$). In the MS subsample, higher cardiorespiratory fitness was associated with better performance on a composite measure of processing speed ($pr = .46$), but not in learning and memory (i.e., SRT, 10/36 SPART), executive function (Wisconsin Card Sort Test), or verbal fluency (WLG).

The second Class III study (Sandroff & Motl, 2012) examined the relationships among multiple domains of physical fitness (e.g., cardiorespiratory fitness, lower extremity muscular strength, balance) and processing speed in 31 persons with MS and 31 matched controls. Participants underwent maximal exercise tests of cardiorespiratory fitness for measurement of VO_{2peak}, muscular strength for measurement of lower limb muscular strength asymmetry (i.e., relative difference in strength of a particular muscle group between strong and weak limbs), and static posturography for measurement of balance. Participants further underwent neuropsychological tests of processing speed (i.e., PASAT, SDMT). There were significant differences in measures of fitness and processing speed between persons with MS and matched controls (i.e., $d > 0.46$). In the MS subsample, cardiorespiratory fitness (i.e., higher VO_{2peak}; $r = .44$), lower limb muscular strength (i.e., lower knee extensor peak torque asymmetry; $r = -.39$), and balance (i.e., less postural sway; $r = -.39$) were significantly associated with processing speed, and that those three domains of fitness accounted for group differences (between persons with

MS and controls) in processing speed and explained a statistically significant amount of variance in processing speed ($R^2 = .39$) in the MS subsample.

The third Class III study (Sandroff, Hillman & Motl, 2015) examined the relationship between cardiorespiratory fitness and inhibitory control in 28 persons with MS and 28 matched controls. Participants underwent an IET to exhaustion on a cycle ergometer for measurement of VO_{2peak} and underwent the modified flanker task for measurement of processing speed and inhibitory control. Persons with MS demonstrated worse cardiorespiratory fitness, as well as slower processing speed (i.e., generalized RT on the modified flanker task) and inhibitory control (i.e., worse accuracy on the modified flanker task), compared with controls. In the MS subsample, higher cardiorespiratory fitness was significantly associated with faster processing speed ($\rho > 0.48$) but not better inhibitory control. Post hoc analyses revealed that there were no differences in processing speed on this task between higher fit persons with MS and matched controls.

The first Class IV study (Prakash et al., 2007) involved a cross-sectional examination on the effects of cardiorespiratory fitness and cortical activation in 24 persons with MS. Participants underwent an IET to exhaustion on a cycle ergometer for measurement of VO_{2peak}, cognitive measures of processing speed (i.e., PASAT, SDMT), learning and memory (i.e., SRT, 10/36 SPART), and verbal fluency (WLG), and a task-based fMRI paradigm that involved a modified version of the PASAT. After controlling for age, education, and disease duration, higher cardiorespiratory fitness was significantly correlated with faster processing speed (i.e., better PASAT performance; $pr = .42$), but not other cognitive domains. In addition, higher cardiorespiratory fitness was associated with better behavioral performance and greater activation of the right inferior frontal gyrus and middle frontal gyrus, and less activation of the anterior cingulate cortex during the fMRI task.

The second Class IV study (Batista et al., 2012) involved a retrospective, cross-sectional investigation on the effects of bone mineral density on cognitive performance in 58 persons with MS. Participants underwent dual-energy x-ray absorptiometry (DEXA) for measurement of femur bone mineral density (i.e., a marker for osteopenia/osteoporosis) and the MACFIMS neuropsychological battery, consisting of tests of executive function (Delis-Kaplan Executive Function System (sorting task), learning and memory (CVLT-II, BVMT-R), processing speed (PASAT, SDMT), spatial perception (Judgement of Line Orientation), and verbal fluency (Controlled Oral Word Association Test). Based on neuropsychological performance, the sample was classified into cognitively impaired and cognitively preserved groups. Cognitively impaired persons with MS had lower femur bone mineral density than the cognitively preserved group ($d = -0.68$). Furthermore, after controlling for age, sex, and disability status, BVMT-R total learning score predicted

32% of the variance in femur bone mineral density, such that those with worse visuospatial learning had lower femoral bone mineral density.

The third Class IV study (Beier et al., 2014) involved a retrospective, longitudinal examination on the effects of changes in physical fitness and cognition in 82 persons with MS. This study involved a secondary analysis of the results of a behavioral intervention that involved a 12-week telephone-based health promotion program. This secondary analysis was performed in persons who chose exercise as a health behavior that they wanted help with. There was not a control comparison group. Participants underwent measurements of physical fitness before and after the 12-week period that included cardiorespiratory fitness (i.e., cycling time to exhaustion based on an IET on a cycle ergometer) and lower limb muscular strength based on a 10-repetition maximum for knee extensors and knee flexors. Participants further underwent neuropsychological tests of processing speed (i.e., PASAT) and executive function (i.e., TMT). Those who demonstrated improved physical fitness over the 12-week period (based on a z-score composite of both cardiorespiratory and muscular fitness) demonstrated improvements in executive function (i.e., TMT performance) but not processing speed (i.e., PASAT performance), relative to those who did not demonstrate improved fitness ($d = 0.58$).

The fourth Class IV study (Sandroff, Pilutti, et al., 2015) involved a cross-sectional examination of multiple domains of physical fitness and multiple domains of cognition in 62 persons with mild, moderate, and severe MS disability. Cardiorespiratory fitness was measured as VO_{2peak} from an IET to exhaustion on a recumbent stepper, and lower limb muscle strength was expressed as peak torque of knee extensors and flexors, as well as asymmetry scores based on a maximal isometric muscle strength protocol on an isokinetic dynamometer. Participants also underwent the SDMT as a measure of processing speed and the CVLT-II and BVMT-R as measures of learning and memory. In the overall sample, higher cardiorespiratory fitness and greater lower limb muscle strength were associated with better processing speed ($r = .35–.41$), but learning and memory were not ($r < .19$). Furthermore, higher cardiorespiratory fitness and greater muscle strength were associated with faster processing speed in persons with mild ($r = .39–.53$), but moderate or severe MS disability were not ($r < .21$).

The fifth Class IV study (Sandroff, Hubbard, et al., 2015) involved a cross-sectional examination of aspects of body composition (i.e., bone mineral density and measures of body fat) based on DEXA and cognition in 60 persons with MS. Briefly, objective measures of body fat were not associated with processing speed (i.e., SDMT performance) or learning and memory (i.e., CVLT-II, BVMT-R performance). Higher lean body mass was associated with faster processing speed, and higher whole-body bone mineral density was associated with both faster processing speed and better learning and memory. However, those associations were attenuated and nonsignificant after controlling for age and disability status. This study was a different analysis from the same dataset as Sandroff, Pilutti, et al. (2015).

Discussion

Overall, the evidence from three Class III studies and four Class IV studies support better physical fitness as being associated with better cognitive performance in persons with MS, whereas only one Class IV study did not report positive effects (Sandroff, Hubbard, et al., 2015; see Figure 14.1). Of note, in this area, there are no RCTs (i.e., Class I or II evidence) examining the effects of physical fitness on cognition. To that end, it is difficult to recommend the clinical utility of physical fitness for improving cognition in persons with MS based on the preceding studies alone. However, by definition, an RCT examining improvements in physical fitness is classified as an exercise training intervention (Bouchard & Shephard, 1994), thus it was expected that the studies examining the effects of physical fitness on cognition in MS would only involve Class III and IV evidence. Consequently, the Class III and IV studies reporting relatively consistent associations between better physical fitness and cognitive functioning might offer a partial explanation for the null results of Class I and II studies of exercise training on cognition in MS, considering that none of those studies reported fitness improvements (Sandroff, Motl, Scudder, et al., 2016).

Importantly, all of the studies of physical fitness included cognition as a primary outcome (Figure 14.2), but none of these studies involved the a priori recruitment of cognitively impaired persons with MS. Nevertheless, the literature on physical fitness effects on cognition in MS seemingly suggests that better cardiorespiratory fitness, muscular strength, balance, and perhaps femur bone mineral density might be associated with better performance on several domains of cognition (e.g., processing speed, learning and memory, executive function). The associations between domains of physical fitness and cognition further might depend on the ambulatory status of the sample (Sandroff, Pilutti, et al., 2015), based on cognitive-motor coupling (Benedict et al., 2011; Motl et al., 2016) and associations between fitness and ambulation in MS (Motl, 2010).

Briefly, the most commonly measured domain of physical fitness included cardiorespiratory fitness (i.e., six of eight studies). Furthermore, in all six of those studies, cardiorespiratory fitness was measured based on VO_{2peak} (i.e., the gold-standard for measuring cardiorespiratory fitness; ACSM, 2013), using an IET to exhaustion. All of those studies consistently reported significant associations between aspects of fitness and cognition (Beier et al.,

2014; Prakash et al., 2007; Prakash et al., 2010; Sandroff, Hillman, & Motl, 2015; Sandroff & Motl, 2012; Sandroff, Pilutti, et al., 2015). Other studies measured lower extremity muscular strength and reported statistically significant associations between better fitness and better cognition (Beier et al., 2014; Sandroff & Motl, 2012; Sandroff, Pilutti, et al., 2015). The two studies that measured body composition based on DEXA were conflicting, as one reported significant associations between femur bone mineral density and learning and memory (Batista et al., 2012), and the other did not (Sandroff, Hubbard, et al., 2015). Finally, physical fitness studies included neurocognitive tests of executive function, learning and memory, processing speed, spatial perception, and verbal fluency. All eight studies included at least one measure of processing speed, with seven of the eight studies including either the PASAT or SDMT; one study included the modified flanker task as a measure of both executive function and processing speed (Sandroff, Hillman, & Motl, 2015). To that end, most studies in this area reported significant associations between measures of physical fitness and processing speed (Prakash et al., 2007, 2010; Sandroff & Motl, 2012; Sandroff, Hillman, & Motl, 2015; Sandroff, Pilutti, et al., 2015).

CONCLUSIONS AND FUTURE DIRECTIONS

Although the overall data on the effects of exercise, physical activity, and physical fitness on cognition in MS do hold some promise, such behavioral approaches for improving cognition are not yet ready for clinical application in this population. Although there have been 27 total studies on the effects of exercise, physical activity, and physical fitness on cognition in persons with MS, there are several overarching limitations that are important for guiding future research. First and foremost, there is a substantial proportion of the literature that did not examine cognition as a primary outcome. This is particularly evident for exercise training studies (i.e., only 44% included cognition as a primary outcome), and is especially troubling given the high prevalence and impact of cognitive dysfunction in this population. As there is increasing emphasis on developing behavioral, intervention-based approaches for managing MS-related cognitive impairment, more research on exercise, physical activity, and physical fitness that selectively targets cognitive functioning is necessary. Such studies should be systematically performed to first identify features of an optimal exercise training intervention (i.e., domains of exercise/fitness, domains of cognition, clinical characteristics) for improving cognition using non-RCT designs prior to initiating RCTs (Sandroff, 2015). This presumably increases the potential for the realization of meaningful cognitive improvements over time. Such an approach is consistent with research in older adults that documents robust, beneficial effects of exercise, physical activity, and physical fitness on cognition and brain structure/function (Colcombe & Kramer, 2003; Heyn, Abreu, & Ottenbacher, 2004; Kelly et al., 2014).

Within the context of this approach, five different cross-sectional studies reported that cardiorespiratory fitness is associated with processing speed—the most commonly impaired domain of cognition in MS. Such consistent evidence suggests that improved cardiorespiratory fitness might result in improved processing speed over time. Yet as a whole, there have been no highly developed Class I or Class II aerobic exercise training interventions for selectively improving aspects of processing speed while concurrently improving cardiorespiratory fitness in persons with MS. Moreover, this research should include cognitively impaired persons with MS for better determining the efficacy of exercise for managing MS-related cognitive impairment. To that end, another troubling observation is that, of the 27 reviewed studies, only *one* specifically recruited persons with cognitive impairment (Leavitt et al., 2014); this includes both developmental and intervention studies. This is problematic, considering that those individuals presumably have the greatest need for interventions that target cognition. Although studies involving non-cognitively impaired persons with MS might provide proof-of-concept data for the effects of exercise, physical activity, and/or physical fitness on cognition in MS, to maximize the impact of intervention research and suggest possible treatment approaches for MS-related cognitive impairment, studies must include cognitively impaired samples.

Another issue for consideration is that the classification of a study based on established criteria (i.e., AAN evidence) alone might not be sufficient for determining its impact. For example, four studies can be characterized as Class I or Class II evidence based on methodological features, such as an RCT design, blinded/objective outcome assessment, equivalent baseline characteristics between groups, concealed allocation, clear identification of a primary outcome and inclusion/exclusion criteria, and adequate accounting for dropout. However, all four of those studies had major methodological limitations, including lack of inclusion of cognitively impaired samples, cognition not being a primary outcome, lack of treatment-blinded outcome assessors, no manipulation check for documenting success of intervention, poorly designed exercise intervention, and poor adherence to the intervention. Although having high internal validity from a methodological standpoint is advantageous for reducing Type I error, these studies might not actually provide high-quality evidence on the efficacy of exercise and physical activity for improving cognition in MS. This again highlights the importance of developing better interventions based on results from studies using non-RCT designs. For example, an optimal exercise training intervention should include a systematically developed exercise stimulus (i.e., method of delivery, modality, intensity, frequency, duration) based on cross-sectional studies that report positive associations between physical fitness and cognition. Such an intervention should choose cognitive outcomes and patient samples based on cross-sectional results. Indeed, researchers and clinicians should carefully consider methodological aspects of studies (i.e., study characteristics and participant-specific characteristics) that have been classified as Class I or Class II before making recommendations for practice.

Another interesting issue related to the effects of exercise and physical activity on cognition in MS involves the role of sedentary behavior. By definition, sedentary behavior is not merely engaging in insufficient physical activity behavior (Pate, O'Neill, & Lobelo, 2008) but, rather, refers to engaging in prolonged, wakeful bouts of inactivity (i.e., sitting or lying down), whereby energy expenditure is below 1.5 metabolic equivalents (Pate et al., 2008). In the general population, across the life span, engaging in more sedentary behavior is associated with worse cognitive functioning (Middleton et al., 2011). However, only one study has examined this issue in persons with MS (Hubbard & Motl, 2015) and reported that engaging in more sedentary behavior was not associated with processing speed in this population based on SDMT performance. More research is clearly needed for fully exploring the complex relationship between physical activity, sedentary behavior, and cognition in those with MS.

Overall, research on the effects of exercise, physical activity, and physical fitness on cognition in persons with MS is in its infancy. Although there are a few Class I and Class II studies from which to consider, there is insufficient well-designed research to definitively conclude that exercise, physical activity, and physical fitness are effective for improving cognition in persons with MS. Thus, at this time, it is premature to definitively support the clinical application of those approaches for improving cognition in this population. However, there is promising evidence from Class III and Class IV studies that might inform the development of better intervention research. This should eventually result in higher quality (i.e., Class I or II) RCT evidence. Collectively, we recommend that future exercise, physical activity, and physical fitness research focus on cognition as a primary outcome, increase methodological rigor with regard to exercise interventions in particular, and include samples of cognitively impaired persons with MS.

REFERENCES

American College of Sports Medicine. (2013). *ACSM's resource manual for guidelines for exercise testing and prescription* (7th ed.). Philadelphia, PA: Lippincott Williams & Wilkins.

Batista, S., Teter, B., Sequeira, K., Josyula, S., Hoogs, M., Ramanathan, M., . . . Weinstock-Guttman, B. (2012). Cognitive impairment is associated with reduced bone mass in multiple sclerosis. *Multiple Sclerosis Journal, 18*, 1459–1465. http://dx.doi.org/10.1177/1352458512440206

Beier, M., Bombardier, C. H., Hartoonian, N., Motl, R. W., & Kraft, G. H. (2014). Improved physical fitness correlates with improved cognition in multiple sclerosis. *Archives of Physical Medicine and Rehabilitation, 95*, 1328–1334. http://dx.doi.org/10.1016/j.apmr.2014.02.017

Benedict, R. H. B., Cookfair, D., Gavett, R., Gunther, M., Munschauer, F., Garg, N., & Weinstock-Guttman, B. (2006). Validity of the Minimal Assessment of Cognitive Function in Multiple Sclerosis (MACFIMS). *Journal of the International Neuropsychological Society, 12*, 549–558. http://dx.doi.org/10.1017/S1355617706060723

Benedict, R. H. B., Holtzer, R., Motl, R. W., Foley, F. W., Kaur, S., Hojnacki, D., & Weinstock-Guttman, B. (2011). Upper and lower extremity motor function and cognitive impairment in multiple sclerosis. *Journal of the International Neuropsychological Society, 17*, 643–653. http://dx.doi.org/10.1017/S1355617711000403

Bouchard, C., & Shephard, R. J. (1994). *Physical activity, fitness, and health: international proceedings and consensus statement.* Champaign, IL: Human Kinetics.

Briken, S., Gold, S. M., Patra, S., Vettorazzi, E., Harbs, D., Tallner, A., . . . Heesen, C. (2014). Effects of exercise on fitness and cognition in progressive MS: A randomized, controlled pilot trial. *Multiple Sclerosis Journal, 20*, 382–390. http://dx.doi.org/10.1177/1352458513507358

Carter, A., Daley, A., Humphreys, L., Snowdon, N., Woodroofe, N., Petty, J., . . . Saxton, J. M. (2014). Pragmatic intervention for increasing self-directed exercise behaviour and improving important health outcomes in people with multiple sclerosis: A randomised controlled trial. *Multiple Sclerosis Journal, 20*, 1112–1122. http://dx.doi.org/10.1177/1352458513519354

Chiaravalloti, N. D., & DeLuca, J. (2008). Cognitive impairment in multiple sclerosis. *Lancet Neurology, 7*, 1139–1151. http://dx.doi.org/10.1016/S1474-4422(08)70259-X

Colcombe, S., & Kramer, A. F. (2003). Fitness effects on the cognitive function of older adults: A meta-analytic study. *Psychological Science, 14*, 125–130. http://dx.doi.org/10.1111/1467-9280.t01-1-01430

Editor's note to authors and readers: Levels of evidence coming to Neurology®. (2010). Retrieved from https://pdfs.semanticscholar.org/c130/341c8c5c6c07014e7c885c85fb82ad18ecb7.pdf

Erickson, K. I., Voss, M. W., Prakash, R. S., Basak, C., Szabo, A., Chaddock, L., . . . Kramer, A. F. (2011). Exercise training increases size of hippocampus and improves memory. *Proceedings of the National Academy of Sciences, 108*, 3017–3022. http://dx.doi.org/10.1073/pnas.1015950108

Gross, R. A., & Johnston, K. C. (2009). Levels of evidence Taking Neurology® to the next level. *Neurology, 72*(1), 8–10.

Hämäläinen, P., Ikonen, A., Romberg, A., Helenius, H., & Ruutiainen, J. (2012). The effects of heat stress on cognition in persons with multiple sclerosis. *Multiple Sclerosis Journal, 18,* 489–497. http://dx.doi.org/10.1177/1352458511422926

Heyn, P., Abreu, B. C., & Ottenbacher, K. J. (2004). The effects of exercise training on elderly persons with cognitive impairment and dementia: A meta-analysis. *Archives of Physical Medicine and Rehabilitation, 85,* 1694–1704. http://dx.doi.org/10.1016/j.apmr.2004.03.019

Hoang, P., Schoene, D., Gandevia, S., Smith, S., & Lord, S. R. (2016). Effects of a home-based step training programme on balance, stepping, cognition and functional performance in people with multiple sclerosis—A randomized controlled trial. *Multiple Sclerosis Journal, 22,* 94–103. http://dx.doi.org/10.1177/1352458515579442

Hubbard, E. A., & Motl, R. W. (2015). Sedentary behavior is associated with disability status and walking performance, but not cognitive function, in multiple sclerosis. *Applied Physiology, Nutrition, and Metabolism, 40,* 203–206. http://dx.doi.org/10.1139/apnm-2014-0271

Kelly, M. E., Loughrey, D., Lawlor, B. A., Robertson, I. H., Walsh, C., & Brennan, S. (2014). The impact of exercise on the cognitive functioning of healthy older adults: A systematic review and meta-analysis. *Ageing Research Reviews, 16,* 12–31. http://dx.doi.org/10.1016/j.arr.2014.05.002

Langdon, D. W., Amato, M. P., Boringa, J., Brochet, B., Foley, F., Fredrikson, S., . . . Benedict, R. H. B. (2012). Recommendations for a Brief International Cognitive Assessment for Multiple Sclerosis (BICAMS). *Multiple Sclerosis Journal, 18,* 891–898. http://dx.doi.org/10.1177/1352458511431076

Leavitt, V. M., Cirnigliaro, C., Cohen, A., Farag, A., Brooks, M., Wecht, J. M., . . . Sumowski, J. F. (2014). Aerobic exercise increases hippocampal volume and improves memory in multiple sclerosis: Preliminary findings. *Neurocase, 20,* 695–697. http://dx.doi.org/10.1080/13554794.2013.841951

Middleton, L. E., Manini, T. M., Simonsick, E. M., Harris, T. B., Barnes, D. E., Tylavsky, F., . . . Yaffe, K. (2011). Activity energy expenditure and incident cognitive impairment in older adults. *Archives of Internal Medicine, 171,* 1251–1257. http://dx.doi.org/10.1001/archinternmed.2011.277

Motl, R. W. (2010). Physical activity and irreversible disability in multiple sclerosis. *Exercise and Sport Sciences Reviews, 38,* 186–191. http://dx.doi.org/10.1097/JES.0b013e3181f44fab

Motl, R. W., Gappmaier, E., Nelson, K., & Benedict, R. H. B. (2011). Physical activity and cognitive function in multiple sclerosis. *Journal of Sport & Exercise Psychology, 33,* 734–741. http://dx.doi.org/10.1123/jsep.33.5.734

Motl, R. W., Sandroff, B. M., & Benedict, R. H. B. (2011). Cognitive dysfunction and multiple sclerosis: Developing a rationale for considering the efficacy of exercise training. *Multiple Sclerosis Journal, 17,* 1034–1040. http://dx.doi.org/10.1177/1352458511409612

Motl, R. W., Sandroff, B. M., & DeLuca, J. (2016). Exercise training and cognitive rehabilitation: A symbiotic approach for rehabilitating walking and cognitive functions in multiple sclerosis? *Neurorehabilitation and Neural Repair, 30,* 499–511. http://dx.doi.org/10.1177/1545968315606993

Oken, B. S., Kishiyama, S., Zajdel, D., Bourdette, D., Carlsen, J., Haas, M., . . . Mass, M. (2004). Randomized controlled trial of yoga and exercise in multiple sclerosis. *Neurology, 62,* 2058–2064. http://dx.doi.org/10.1212/01.WNL.0000129534.88602.5C

Pate, R. R., O'Neill, J. R., & Lobelo, F. (2008). The evolving definition of "sedentary". *Exercise and Sport Sciences Reviews, 36,* 173–178. http://dx.doi.org/10.1097/JES.0b013e3181877d1a

Pilutti, L. A., Lelli, D. A., Paulseth, J. E., Crome, M., Jiang, S., Rathbone, M. P., & Hicks, A. L. (2011). Effects of 12 weeks of supported treadmill training on functional ability and quality of life in progressive multiple sclerosis: A pilot study. *Archives of Physical Medicine and Rehabilitation, 92,* 31–36. http://dx.doi.org/10.1016/j.apmr.2010.08.027

Prakash, R. S., Patterson, B., Janssen, A., Abduljalil, A., & Boster, A. (2011). Physical activity associated with increased resting-state functional connectivity in multiple sclerosis. *Journal of the International Neuropsychological Society, 17,* 986–997. http://dx.doi.org/10.1017/S1355617711001093

Prakash, R. S., Snook, E. M., Erickson, K. I., Colcombe, S. J., Voss, M. W., Motl, R. W., & Kramer, A. F. (2007). Cardiorespiratory fitness: A predictor of cortical plasticity in multiple sclerosis. *NeuroImage, 34,* 1238–1244. http://dx.doi.org/10.1016/j.neuroimage.2006.10.003

Prakash, R. S., Snook, E. M., Motl, R. W., & Kramer, A. F. (2010). Aerobic fitness is associated with gray matter volume and white matter integrity in multiple sclerosis. *Brain Research, 1341,* 41–51. http://dx.doi.org/10.1016/j.brainres.2009.06.063

Rao, S. (1990). *A manual for the Brief Repeatable Battery of Neuropsychological Tests in multiple sclerosis.* Milwaukee: Medical College of Wisconsin.

Romberg, A., Virtanen, A., & Ruutiainen, J. (2005). Long-term exercise improves functional impairment but not quality of life in multiple sclerosis. *Journal of Neurology, 252,* 839–845. http://dx.doi.org/10.1007/s00415-005-0759-2

Sandroff, B. M. (2015). Exercise and cognition in multiple sclerosis: The importance of acute exercise for developing better interventions. *Neuroscience and Biobehavioral Reviews, 59,* 173–183. http://dx.doi.org/10.1016/j.neubiorev.2015.10.012

Sandroff, B. M., Dlugonski, D., Pilutti, L. A., Pula, J. H., Benedict, R. H. B., & Motl, R. W. (2014). Physical activity is associated with cognitive processing speed in persons with multiple sclerosis. *Multiple Sclerosis and Related Disorders, 3,* 123–128. http://dx.doi.org/10.1016/j.msard.2013.04.003

Sandroff, B. M., Hillman, C. H., Benedict, R. H. B., & Motl, R. W. (2015). Acute effects of walking, cycling, and yoga exercise on cognition in persons with relapsing-remitting multiple sclerosis without impaired cognitive processing speed. *Journal of Clinical and Experimental Neuropsychology, 37*, 209–219. http://dx.doi.org/10.1080/13803395.2014.1001723

Sandroff, B. M., Hillman, C. H., Benedict, R. H. B., & Motl, R. W. (2016). Acute effects of varying intensities of treadmill walking exercise on inhibitory control in persons with multiple sclerosis: A pilot investigation. *Physiology & Behavior, 154*, 20–27. http://dx.doi.org/10.1016/j.physbeh.2015.11.008

Sandroff, B. M., Hillman, C. H., & Motl, R. W. (2015). Aerobic fitness is associated with inhibitory control in persons with multiple sclerosis. *Archives of Clinical Neuropsychology, 30*, 329–340. http://dx.doi.org/10.1093/arclin/acv022

Sandroff, B. M., Hubbard, E. A., Pilutti, L. A., & Motl, R. W. (2015). No association between body composition and cognition in ambulatory persons with multiple sclerosis: A brief report. *Journal of Rehabilitation Research and Development, 52*, 301–308. http://dx.doi.org/10.1682/JRRD.2014.09.0208

Sandroff, B. M., Klaren, R. E., Pilutti, L. A., Dlugonski, D., Benedict, R. H. B., & Motl, R. W. (2014). Randomized controlled trial of physical activity, cognition, and walking in multiple sclerosis. *Journal of Neurology, 261*, 363–372. http://dx.doi.org/10.1007/s00415-013-7204-8

Sandroff, B. M., & Motl, R. W. (2012). Fitness and cognitive processing speed in persons with multiple sclerosis: A cross-sectional investigation. *Journal of Clinical and Experimental Neuropsychology, 34*, 1041–1052. http://dx.doi.org/10.1080/13803395.2012.715144

Sandroff, B. M., Motl, R. W., & Davis, S. L. (2016). Effects of vigorous walking exercise on core body temperature and inhibitory control in thermosensitive persons with multiple sclerosis. *Neurodegenerative Disease Management, 6*, 13–21. http://dx.doi.org/10.2217/nmt.15.69

Sandroff, B. M., Motl, R. W., Scudder, M. R., & DeLuca, J. (2016). Systematic, evidence-based review of exercise, physical activity, and physical fitness effects on cognition in persons with multiple sclerosis. *Neuropsychology Review, 26*, 271–294. http://dx.doi.org/10.1007/s11065-016-9324-2

Sandroff, B. M., Pilutti, L. A., Benedict, R. H. B., & Motl, R. W. (2015). Association between physical fitness and cognitive function in multiple sclerosis: Does disability status matter? *Neurorehabilitation and Neural Repair, 29*, 214–223. http://dx.doi.org/10.1177/1545968314541331

Sandroff, B. M., Pilutti, L. A., Dlugonski, D., & Motl, R. W. (2013). Physical activity and information processing speed in persons with multiple sclerosis: A prospective study. *Mental Health and Physical Activity, 6*, 205–211. http://dx.doi.org/10.1016/j.mhpa.2013.08.001

Sangelaji, B., Estebsari, F., Nabavi, S. M., Jamshidi, E., Morsali, D., & Dastoorpoor, M. (2015). The effect of exercise therapy on cognitive functions in multiple sclerosis patients: A pilot study. *Medical Journal of the Islamic Republic of Iran, 29*, 205–213.

Skjerbæk, A. G., Møller, A. B., Jensen, E., Vissing, K., Sørensen, H., Nybo, L., . . . Dalgas, U. (2013). Heat sensitive persons with multiple sclerosis are more tolerant to resistance exercise than to endurance exercise. *Multiple Sclerosis Journal*, *19*, 932–940. http://dx.doi.org/10.1177/1352458512463765

Velikonja, O., Čurić, K., Ožura, A., & Jazbec, S. S. (2010). Influence of sports climbing and yoga on spasticity, cognitive function, mood and fatigue in patients with multiple sclerosis. *Clinical Neurology and Neurosurgery, 112*, 597–601. http://dx.doi.org/10.1016/j.clineuro.2010.03.006

Voss, M. W., Nagamatsu, L. S., Liu-Ambrose, T., & Kramer, A. F. (2011). Exercise, brain, and cognition across the life span. *Journal of Applied Physiology, 111*, 1505–1513. http://dx.doi.org/10.1152/japplphysiol.00210.2011

Waschbisch, A., Wenny, I., Tallner, A., Schwab, S., Pfeifer, K., & Mäurer, M. (2012). Physical activity in multiple sclerosis: A comparative study of vitamin D, brain-derived neurotrophic factor and regulatory T cell populations. *European Neurology, 68*, 122–128. http://dx.doi.org/10.1159/000337904

15

NEUROPROTECTION AND COGNITION IN MULTIPLE SCLEROSIS: EFFECTS OF COGNITIVE AND BRAIN RESERVE

BRUNO BROCHET

Multiple sclerosis (MS) is a chronic inflammatory autoimmune disease of the central nervous system (CNS) characterized by perivascular infiltration of lymphocytes and macrophages, which in turn promote demyelination and axonal injuries disseminated within the CNS (Brochet, 2015). Although MS has been classically thought of as a typical white matter (WM) disorder, the involvement of gray matter (GM) has (re)emerged as an important target of the disease that contributes significantly to clinical symptoms (Geurts, Calabrese, Fisher, & Rudick, 2012). Among them, cognitive impairment (CI) associated with MS (CIAMS) is a disabling manifestation that is frequently observed from the early stages of the disease with significant impact in terms of quality of life, vocational status, and compliance to therapy (Ruet, 2015). Focal and diffuse brain damage, including WM and GM, explain the occurrence of CIAMS (Rocca et al., 2015). However, although some correlations have been shown between the extent and severity of brain damage, and

http://dx.doi.org/10.1037/0000097-016
Cognition and Behavior in Multiple Sclerosis, J. DeLuca and B. M. Sandroff (Editors)
Copyright © 2018 by the American Psychological Association. All rights reserved.

both the presence and the severity of CIAMS, such correlations are relatively weak (Rocca et al., 2015). MRI findings, including lesion load and atrophy measures, cannot fully account for the extent and severity of CIAMS (Rocca et al., 2015). The severity of CI could vary between patients with the same level of brain damage (Bonnet et al., 2006). One possible explanation for this so-called clinical-radiological paradox is based on the concept of reserve. The theory of cognitive reserve (CR) has been proposed by Stern and colleagues after studies on Alzheimer's disease (AD; Stern, 2009; Stern et al., 1994). It has been described as spare cognitive capacity available to buffer the effects of brain damage induced by disease or trauma (Stern, 2009). It is based on observations showing that subjects with greater CR were less likely to show CI as pathology accumulated. The CR theory has been supported typically by studies showing that subjects with a high level of background education were less frequently and less severely affected by the disease or at a later age (Amieva et al., 2014; Stern et al., 1994; Stern, 2009). CR is assessed using proxy variables associated with lifetime intellectual enrichment, such as education, which is the most frequently used variable; occupational attainment; reading tests; vocabulary; premorbid IQ; and participation in cognitively stimulating activities (e.g., hobbies, reading). CR has been studied in several other populations, including traumatic brain injury (Mathias & Wheaton, 2015; Nunnari, Bramanti, & Marino, 2014), stroke (Nunnari et al, 2014), Parkinson's disease (Hindle, Martyr, & Clare, 2014), and HIV-related dementias (Cody & Vance, 2016). Most of these studies have suggested a protective effect of CR—frequently assessed by educational level—on the severity of CI. In normal aging, it also has been observed that engagement in socially, mentally, and physically stimulating leisure activities is predictive of change in cognitive speed with age (Lövdén, Ghisletta, & Lindenberger, 2005).

Since the early description of CR, the concept of reserve has evolved toward a differentiation between a *functional reserve*, defined as active reserve by Stern (2009), which is built up by education and cognitive functioning, and could be improved by current intellectual enrichment, and an *inborn fixed reserve* or *brain reserve (BR)*, which is determined mainly by genetics and corresponds to the inborn brain capacity (Schofield, Logroscino, Andrews, Albert, & Stern, 1997; Sumowski, 2015; Sumowski et al., 2013). This differentiation has been summarized by Sumowski et al. (2013) as "What you've got (BR) and how you use it (CR)." CR is assessed using proxy variables associated with lifetime intellectual enrichment, as just described (see Table 15.1). CR is considered to accumulate based on previous and current engagement in CR-building pursuits (Schwartz et al., 2015). BR is considered as a function of brain size or neuronal count, and is usually assessed by intracranial volume (ICV) or head size as an estimate of the larger maximal lifetime brain

TABLE 15.1
Main Proxies of Reserve

Concept	Proxies	Comment
CR	Education	Years of education
	Premorbid intelligence	Verbal intelligence (vocabulary or reading tests)
	Premorbid cognitive leisure	Cognitive leisure activities questionnaire
	Occupational attainment	Occupational categories
	CRI	Integrates years of education, premorbid verbal intelligence, and premorbid cognitive leisure
	Ongoing reserve-building activities	Current cognitive activity
Brain reserve	Intracranial volume	Estimate of the larger MLBV

Note. CR = cognitive reserve; CRI = Cognitive Reserve Index; MLBV = maximal lifetime brain volume.

volume (MLBV; Schofield et al., 1997; Sumowski, 2015; Sumowski et al., 2013). Smaller head circumference has been shown to be associated with an increased risk of developing AD (Schofield et al., 1997).

However, the independence of these measures is questionable. It is likely that the inborn brain capacity influences the learning capacities of an individual and therefore education level and IQ. Indeed, small head circumference in students has been associated lower IQ (Ivanovic et al., 2004). In other words, the proxies used for CR might be influenced by BR. The main determinants of head size in children are socioeconomic status, head size of the parents, and prenatal nutritional indicators, suggesting that a mix of environmental and genetic factors is involved (Ivanovic et al., 2004). Conversely, it also is possible that intellectual activity in early life could influence brain development. For example, studies of brain plasticity in healthy adults showed that some intense cognitive activity could modify volume in some parts of the brain (May, 2011). For example, changes in GM morphology have been observed after motor learning and the acquisition of abstract knowledge in early adulthood (Draganski et al., 2004, 2006). A protective effect of spatial navigation training has been reported against age-related decline of hippocampal volume in both young and older adults (Lövdén et al., 2012). An illustration of the variability of the interaction between education and brain development is given by the correlation observed in 62 MS patients between years of education and ICV (Sumowski et al., 2013), although no correlation was found in another study of 71 MS patients (Modica et al., 2016).

It is probably more relevant to describe reserve at a given time. For example, inborn fixed reserve (i.e., BR), mainly determined by genetics and prenatal environmental factors (Ivanovic et al., 2004), corresponds to the brain capacity and potential at birth and could be considered as a baseline characteristic. CR is the net consequence on brain structure and brain function of past and current reserve-building activities and also environmental factors, lifestyle, and pathological conditions (Reuter-Lorenz & Park, 2014). CR, therefore, could be considered as a mix of structural and functional reserve. CR-building activities modify the inborn brain status but also are, in part, dependent on it.

Higher reserve at a given moment of life could be defined not only by a greater number of neurons, synapses, and networks, as determined by genes, environment, and brain functioning, but also by a better brain functional organization and efficiency (Reuter-Lorenz & Park, 2014). MLBV is likely to be a measure of BR at the end of brain development.

The mechanisms by which CR and BR preserve cognitive performance are thought to be via the maintenance of better compensatory mechanisms. Neural resources could be enriched during a lifetime by CR-building activities, such as education and cognitive leisure activities, but also could be decreased due to the disease process. The effect of age could be positive (i.e., brain maturation) or negative (i.e., brain aging) on neural resources. Brain structure and brain function, which are closely related, depend on neural resources enrichment or deterioration. Cognitive performance at a given point in time, or over time, is controlled by brain resources. However, it can be enhanced or preserved by compensatory mechanisms after specific interventions (e.g., cognitive training or rehabilitation) or lifetime adjustments for increasing engagement in reserve-building activities.

Another important parameter is the effect of MS on the maintenance of brain capacities (Nyberg, Lövdén, Riklund, Lindenberger, & Bäckman, 2012; Reuter-Lorenz & Park, 2014). For example, in many cases, the disease process is known to begin several months to years before the clinical onset of the disease (Lebrun, 2015) and could start during adolescence before the end of the brain maturation (Renoux et al., 2007). This is particularly relevant in pediatric onset MS (POMS; Renoux et al., 2007). This early pathological process could limit the protective effect of reserve and also could induce bias by using some CR proxies, which can have been influenced by the disease process, such as education and IQ.

EVIDENCE OF CR IN MS

Since the first study (Bonnet et al., 2006), showing a protective effect of education on cognitive performance in patients with relapsing–remitting MS (RRMS), several studies have shown the importance of CR in MS. Most of these concerned education (Benedict, Morrow, Weinstock Guttman,

Cookfair, & Schretlen, 2010; Bonnet et al., 2006; Luerding, Gebel, Gebel, Schwab-Malek, & Weissert, 2016; Martins Da Silva et al., 2015; Modica et al., 2016; Pinter et al., 2014; Scarpazza et al., 2013), premorbid intelligence (Benedict et al., 2010; Feinstein, Lapshin, O'Connor, & Lanctôt, 2013; Ghaffar, Fiati, & Feinstein, 2012; Sandry & Sumowski, 2014; Sumowski, Chiaravalloti, & DeLuca, 2009; Sumowski, Chiaravalloti, Leavitt, & DeLuca, 2012; Sumowski, Chiaravalloti, Wylie, & DeLuca, 2009; Sumowski, Wylie, Chiaravalloti, & DeLuca, 2010; Sumowski, Wylie, DeLuca, & Chiaravalloti, 2010), or premorbid cognitive leisure activity (Sumowski et al., 2013; Sumowski, Rocca, Leavitt, Riccitelli, Meani, et al., 2016; Sumowski, Wylie, Gonnella, Chiaravalloti, & DeLuca, 2010). Few studies have concerned ongoing CR-building activities (Schwartz et al., 2015; Schwartz, Snook, Quaranto, Benedict, Rapkin, et al., 2013). Interestingly, MS patients seem to have less CR-building activities than healthy subjects (HS; Schwartz et al., 2015). Next is a discussion of various CR proxies in more detail, organized based on studies with/without neuroimaging outcomes.

Education as a Proxy for CR and CIAMS

First Study

In the first study demonstrating the effect of past education on cognition in MS, 43 consecutive patients diagnosed with RRMS in the previous 6 months and 43 HS matched on sex, age, and educational levels were classified according to years of education: low educational level (LEL; no schooling or less than 12 years of schooling without obtaining any secondary level diploma) and high educational level (HEL; secondary education lasting 12 years or more, leading to a diploma and university level; Bonnet et al., 2006). This resulted in 19 RRMS and 19 HS with LEL and 24 RRMS patients and 24 HS with HEL, respectively (Bonnet et al., 2006). All patients had detailed neuropsychological (NP) evaluation and MRI scans. LEL patients had lower performance than LEL HS in all but two cognitive tests (13 out of 15 scores). The most significantly altered cognitive tests were the Symbol Digit Modalities Test (SDMT), a test of information processing speed (IPS); Selective Reminding Test (SRT), a test of verbal memory; and similarities subtest of the Wechsler Adult Intelligence Scale–Revised, assessing verbal conceptualization. Two tests of executive functions, the Go/No-Go, a test for inhibition, and the Word List Generation, a test for verbal fluency, did not differ between LEL RRMS patients and matched HS. On the contrary, cognitive performance of HEL patients differed significantly from those of HEL HS on only three NP scores out of 15: the SDMT; Paced Auditory Serial Addition Test (PASAT) at 2s, a test of working memory and IPS; and the

Stroop test, a test for executive inhibitory control. For all the other NP tests, no difference was observed between HEL RRMS patients and HEL HS. CI (defined by the presence of two scores less than the 5th percentile of controls) was more frequent in LEL MS patients than in HEL MS patients (CI in 84% of RRMS patients with LEL and 42% of RRMS patients with HEL). Interestingly, cognitive scores of LEL HS did not differ significantly from those of HEL HS. In this study, the protective effect of CR (i.e., education) was limited or absent against IPS impairment, in particular, because HEL RRMS patients had lower scores at the SDMT and the PASAT than HS.

This study, performed at the very early stages of the disease, provided the opportunity to examine two groups of MS patients (i.e., LEL and HEL) with a similar burden of the disease. Indeed, the two groups did not differ according to demographics (i.e., age, gender), disease course (i.e., same disease duration), clinical variables (i.e., Expanded Disability Status Scale [EDSS], depressive scores at the Montgomery and Asberg Depression Rating Scale, and fatigue score), and treatment (almost all patients were not on disease-modifying therapy). Moreover, all patients were extensively studied by MRI with measures of lesion load, brain atrophy measured by the ventricular fraction (VF) and the brain parenchymal fraction (BPF), but also measures of mean magnetization transfer ratio in the lesion mask and in normal-appearing brain tissue. None of these parameters differed significantly between HEL and LEL RRMS patients, demonstrating that the differences in cognitive performance between the two groups were not explained by a different degree in disease severity. These results illustrate the clinical–radiological paradox: two groups of patients with the same disease severity on MRI and with marked differences in cognitive scores.

In the same study, it was observed that deep brain atrophy (i.e., VF) correlated only with one NP score of visual memory (spatial recall test) in RRMS with LEL, although in RRMS with HEL (and very few CI), several NP scores correlated with BPF. This could suggest that in HEL RRMS patients, CI was only present in those with severe disease burden, that is, resulting in a stronger correlation.

Numerous other studies have used education as a proxy for CR in MS.

Clinical Studies Without Imaging Outcomes

Three clinical studies without imaging provided converging results (Benedict et al., 2010; Luerding et al., 2016; Martins Da Silva et al., 2015). A longitudinal retrospective study was performed in 91 MS patients with various clinical phenotypes assessed twice by the SDMT, roughly five years apart (Benedict et al., 2010). In this study, years of education was used as CR proxy together with the North American Adult Reading Test (NAART), a measure of premorbid verbal intellectual ability. After controlling for baseline characteristics, both CR proxies were associated with lesser cognitive decline in regression models. SDMT scores were stable in MS patients with HEL (more than 14 years of education), whereas they declined significantly in patients with LEL. Therefore, that study showed a protective effect of education on IPS decline in MS. A more recent study in a large sample of 419 MS patients with various phenotypes confirmed the protective effect of education on cognition (Martins Da Silva et al., 2015). Patients were classified in two groups, patients with LEL and HEL, according to the number of years of education (less than or equal to and more than 9 years, respectively). The groups differed according to age and disease severity measured by the EDSS and the Multiple Sclerosis Severity Score (MSSS), with LEL MS patients having worse EDSS. A linear regression model showed an independent effect of past education on cognitive deficits for psychomotor speed, visual exploration, verbal memory, and executive functions when taking into account age, EDSS, and MSSS, suggesting a protective effect of education against CI. A third, recent, cross-sectional study concerned 128 MS patients with various clinical phenotypes and with a subjective cognitive complaint (Luerding et al, 2016). Patients were divided in three groups according to years of education and were evaluated using a large NP battery. The study confirmed that patients with HEL had better test results for all cognitive domains than those with an LEL. However, the demographics and clinical characteristics of the three groups were not compared and taken into account. Interestingly, the authors studied the influence of past education on the effect of other current reserve-building activities on cognition. Unexpectedly, enrichment by reading, physical activities, and challenging vocational practices were more effective in patients with LEL than those with HEL. Also retrospective and cross sectional, this study suggested that the effect of past education can be explained by intensive CR-building activities, and this is a very encouraging result for cognitive reeducation in patients with MS. These results need to be reproduced in a homogeneous sample, according to demographics and clinical and imaging characteristics.

Clinical Studies With Imaging Outcomes

In a study of 137 patients with different phenotypes of MS, it was observed that the number of years of education predicted better cognition, assessed by the Brief Repeatable Battery of Neuropsychological Tests (BRB-N; Pinter et al., 2014). The negative effects of T2 lesion load and third ventricle width (an indicator of deep brain atrophy) but not normalized brain volume (NBV) were moderated by education. Education did not moderate the negative effects of global atrophy on cognitive function in this sample possibly because the effect of deep brain structures pathology on CIAMS could precede the effect of cortical structures.

Another study focused on deep GM atrophy (Modica et al., 2016). In this 3-year longitudinal controlled study, 71 MS patients with various phenotypes and 23 HS were studied by the Brief International Cognitive Assessment for Multiple Sclerosis (BICAMS) and by MRI twice, 3 years apart. SDMT decline was observed, again only in patients with the lowest years of education tertile (LEL). Subcortical GM change predicted SDMT decline MS with LEL but not with HEL. There was no effect on memory. However, other parameters that could influence the cognitive outcome, such as disease severity and age, were not entered into the model. The reason for the discrepancy between these results in HEL with the study by Bonnet et al. (2006) is not clear, but the populations studied are clearly different (i.e., early RRMS against various phenotypes at later stages).

Taken together, these studies, despite important methodological differences concerning the clinical phenotypes included, the type and duration of education that vary according to countries, and the consideration or not of important confounding factors, such as clinical or imaging markers of disease severity, consistently showed that educational level has a protective effect against CIAMS in different cognitive domains and a protective effect against IPS decline in longitudinal studies. Imaging data are limited so far but have suggested that deep GM structures seem to be involved in the interaction.

Premorbid Intelligence As a Proxy for CR and CIAMS

Several studies have used premorbid intelligence, particularly verbal intelligence, either alone or in combination with other measures, as a proxy for CR in MS (Benedict et al., 2010; Feinstein et al., 2013; Ghaffar et al., 2012; Sandry & Sumowski, 2014; Sumowski, Chiaravalloti, & DeLuca, 2009; Sumowski et al., 2012; Sumowski, Chiaravalloti, Wylie, et al., 2009; Sumowski, Wylie, Chiaravalloti, et al., 2010; Sumowski, Wylie, DeLuca, et al., 2010).

Clinical Studies Without Imaging Outcomes

Using the Wide Range Achievement Test reading subtest as a proxy of premorbid intelligence in 58 MS patients with various clinical phenotypes, Sumowski and colleagues observed that patients performed worse than controls in complex information processing efficiency and verbal learning and memory at lower, but not higher, levels of CR, based on premorbid intelligence (Sumowski, Chiaravalloti, & DeLuca, 2009).

In the longitudinal study described previously (Benedict et al., 2010), the NAART was used in addition to education. As mentioned, both measures were similarly protective against cognitive decline. However, no interaction effects of NAART score on IPS were observed, suggesting that education might be a stronger proxy of CR.

In the only CR study focusing only on secondary progressive MS (SPMS), the authors combined verbal intelligence (i.e., vocabulary subtest of the Wechsler Abbreviated Scale of Intelligence) and education as a composite index (i.e., the mean sample-based z-score for vocabulary knowledge and educational attainment; Sumowski et al., 2012). These authors assessed IPS and verbal memory in 25 SPMS patients. SPMS patients with low CR had lower performances for IPS and memory compared with a group of HS; SPMS patients with high CR had similar IPS performance as HS. It is likely that these authors used this composite index for overcoming the limitations of each individual proxy. However, its superiority to individual measures of CR has not been tested.

Feinstein and colleagues studied 144 MS patients with various clinical phenotypes with the Minimal Assessment of Cognitive Function in Multiple Sclerosis (MACFIMS; Feinstein et al., 2013). Verbal intelligence was measured by the American National Adult Reading Test (AMNART), a previous version of the NAART. The AMNART score and the EDSS predicted CI in multivariate analysis. These authors calculated a projected score for the Controlled Oral Word Association Test (COWAT), a test of verbal fluency, based on AMNART scores. A significant number of patients (31%) who were not cognitively impaired according to the MACFIMS had actual COWAT scores that were below their projected COWAT score. The AMNART score for these patients did not differ from patients who were not cognitively impaired according to the MACFIMS but had actual COWAT scores above their projected COWAT score. The AMNART scores of these two groups of patients were significantly superior to those of the CI patients. This elegant study suggested that a continuum exists between preserved and impaired cognitive functioning that is possible to observe in patients with high CR. CR mainly delays the occurrence of CI in patients with high CR, rather than decreases the frequency of CI, as it has been suggested by longitudinal studies in AD at the premorbid stage (Amieva et al., 2014). In the Paquid longitudinal study, Amieva and colleagues compared the pattern and duration of clinical trajectories before AD in subjects with low and high education, and found that early cognitive symptoms may precede up to 16 years before dementia in HEL subjects and up to 7 years in LEL individuals (Amieva et al., 2014). This suggests that the initial decline in cognition occurs at the onset of comparable pathology in both groups but is followed by immediate decline to dementia in subjects with low CR and is slower in individuals with higher CR (Amieva et al., 2014).

Clinical Studies With Imaging Outcomes

One early study using verbal intelligence (Wechsler Vocabulary) as a proxy of CR in MS assessed IPS in 38 MS patients with various clinical phenotypes (Sumowski, Chiaravalloti, Wylie, et al., 2009). A composite score of IPS was used, based on the SDMT and the PASAT. Worse IPS composite score was predicted by third-ventricle width, a measure of deep brain atrophy, and better IPS was predicted by CR. However, the negative effect of atrophy on IPS was attenuated by higher levels of CR. In another study by this group, the same methodology was used to evaluate the effect of CR on learning and memory, using the SRT in 44 MS patients with various clinical phenotypes (Sumowski, Wylie, Chiaravalloti, et al., 2010). Again, the third ventricle width predicted worse cognitive outcome (here, SRT scores) and higher CR moderated this negative impact of brain atrophy on both learning and memory. They also observed a correlation between third ventricle width and cognition only in patients with low intellectual enrichment. The same group used verbal intelligence as a proxy of CR in a functional MRI (fMRI) study (see text that follows; Sumowski, Wylie, DeLuca, et al., 2010).

Altogether, studies using premorbid intelligence as a CR proxy gave consistent results on the effect of CR on CIAMS, such that higher premorbid intelligence was associated with less severe CI. Furthermore, neuroimaging studies have suggested that the negative effects of brain atrophy on cognitive performance is attenuated by higher verbal intelligence.

Occupational Attainment As a Proxy for CR and CIAMS

Occupational attainment has been proposed as a proxy for CR that reflects lifetime experience/intellectual enrichment, but studies have reported contradictory results. In a first study, verbal intelligence as a proxy for CR was compared with two other measures of CR, education and occupational attainment, in a study in 72 MS patients with various clinical phenotypes (Ghaffar et al., 2012). Verbal intelligence was measured by the AMNART. Occupational attainment was divided into high or low attainment, based on occupational category: *High occupational attainment* was defined as professional, technical, and managerial occupations, and *low occupational attainment* was defined as clerical/sales, agricultural/fishery/forestry, processing, machine trades, benchwork, and structural occupations. Cognitive performance was measured using the MACFIMS, and BPF was used as a marker of global brain atrophy. Patients with higher occupational attainment had greater AMNART scores and higher educational attainment. Verbal intelligence was significantly associated with the number of years of education. Occupational attainment was a significant predictor of IPS, memory, and executive function in hierarchical linear regressions after accounting for BPF and verbal intelligence. However, the frequency of overall CI was not predicted by occupational attainment. Interestingly, AMNART predicted performance on all cognitive tests, but occupation accounted for additional variance in almost all tests except the SDMT. Past education did not predict any cognitive outcome, but the statistical significance of occupation was lost for executive functions when education was included. It is unclear why education did not predict cognitive outcomes in that study, contrary to results from previous studies. However, these results were not confirmed by another study using occupational attainment and education as CR proxies in a sample of 50 patients with RRMS (Scarpazza et al., 2013). IPS was assessed by the PASAT alone. RRMS patients with HEL performed normally at the PASAT, although LEL RRMS patients performed worse at faster PASAT speeds than HS, as expected. Contrary to the previous study, occupational attainment did not influence cognitive performance of RRMS patients. Indeed, the role of occupational attainment in CR in persons with MS is unclear and needs to be reassessed in further studies, in particular, in a longitudinal way.

Premorbid Cognitive Leisure Activity
As a Proxy for CR and CIAMS

Cognitive leisure activities, including games, hobbies, reading, and artistic activities, have been used as CR proxy in CIAMS, as has been done in the AD literature. In one study, premorbid leisure activities were assessed in 36 MS patients with various phenotypes by a questionnaire asking patients about the frequency and types of activities (i.e., reading books or newspapers, nonartistic writing, artistic production, other hobbies like gardening) they performed during their early 20s (i.e., before they developed MS; Sumowski, Wylie, Gonnella, et al., 2010). This Cognitive Reserve Index (CRI) based on this questionnaire was positively associated with cognitive performance, measured by a composite score of IPS and memory, controlling for third ventricle width and education (Sumowski, Wylie, Gonnella, et al., 2010). Another study compared the effect of this CR proxy to education and ICV and is discussed later in the BR section (Sumowski et al., 2013).

In another recent study, premorbid cognitive leisure was assessed with the same questionnaire as a proxy of CR in 187 relapse-onset MS patients (i.e., RRMS and SPMS), in which total brain, GM and thalamus, caudate, putamen, pallidum, amygdala, and hippocampus volumes were measured

(Sumowski, Rocca, Leavitt, Riccitelli, Sandry, et al., 2016). The cognitive leisure index was positively correlated with hippocampal volume in MS patients, and this was interpreted as greater impact of life experience and cognitive activities on hippocampal volume relative to other brain regions. Data in HS would be useful to confirm this hypothesis. Moreover, greater cognitive leisure and larger hippocampal volume were associated with better memory, and larger hippocampal volume partially mediated the relationship between greater cognitive leisure and better memory. These results were extended in another study, which showed that reading–writing was predictive of hippocampal but not the other cognitive leisure activities (Sumowski, Rocca, Leavitt, Riccitelli, Meani, et al., 2016). These results suggested certain specificity between a type of cognitive activity and the building of a CR, which selectively protects against deficits in a given cognitive domain; here, memory that is typically associated with hippocampal atrophy. Another study showing the protective effect of General Mathematical Ability on PASAT performance in 45 MS patients suggested that a domain specific CR could exist (Sandry, Paxton, & Sumowski, 2016). It is also possible that the PASAT is confounded by mathematical ability.

A limitation could be discussed about studies using the cognitive leisure index as a proxy for CR. Although only patients who were diagnosed after the age of 25 were enrolled, it cannot be excluded that the pathological process began earlier during a preclinical stage in some of them and overlapped with the period studied for cognitive leisure, which cannot be considered strictly as premorbid. It could be a limitation as compared with other CR proxies: education and premorbid verbal intelligence.

CRI As a Proxy for CR and CIAMS

Amato et al. (2013) introduced a CRI, which was calculated based on years of education, premorbid verbal intelligence, and premorbid leisure activities. A mean of z-scores of the three CR indices was calculated (global CRI). This study followed 35 RRMS patients over an average of 1.6 years. Although the follow-up was relatively short, a significant cognitive decline was observed over time. In the regression analyses at baseline, higher CRI was an independent predictor of better performance on most of the BRB-N tests, including tests of verbal memory, IPS, and verbal fluency. However, at the follow-up evaluation, the CRI was not related to cognitive decline and did not attenuate the effects of progressing cortical atrophy on this decline. This suggested that extent of tissue damage and atrophy is a limiting factor for compensatory capacities of CR against cognitive decline. This is in agreement with the study by Bonnet et al. (2006), discussed earlier, on the effect of education on cognition. In that study, the poor correlation of MR markers of diffuse pathology with cognitive performance in RRMS with LEL, contrasting with the correlation observed between several NP scores and brain atrophy in HEL RRMS patients, suggested that, above a certain extent, brain atrophy limits the effect of CR.

Recently, Nunnari et al. (2016) used a CRI based on education, work activity, and leisure times, based on a mixed estimation of participation in current activities versus past/premorbid activities, in a cross-sectional study in 72 MS patients who were assessed by the BRB-N. The total score of CRI had effect on sustained attention, concentration, IPS, and verbal learning; higher CR was associated with better performances. Among the three components of the CRI, education and working activity had the largest influence. However, here, the CR indexes did not moderate the negative influence of atrophy on cognitive status.

ICV As a Proxy for CR and CIAMS (BR)

The studies about the effect of ICV as a marker of MLBV and BR on CIAMS have yielded contradictory results. The first study was performed in 62 MS patients with various phenotypes and showed a correlation of ICV with CI, assessed by measures of IPS (i.e., SDMT and PASAT) and memory (i.e., SRT; Sumowski et al., 2013). A greater ICV decreased the negative impact of T2 lesion load on cognitive status. This effect was driven by an effect of ICV on IPS. No effect of ICV was observed on memory. In the same sample, the effect of education and cognitive leisure on cognition was measured. Cognitive leisure was measured by the index previously described (Sumowski, Wylie, Gonnella, et al., 2010). After controlling for ICV, there was a positive correlation between cognitive performance and education, which was driven only by memory (no effect of education on IPS). There also was an effect of cognitive leisure on cognitive performance (both on IPS and memory). Cognitive leisure moderated the effect of T2 lesion load on memory but not IPS after controlling for ICV. Sumowski et al. (2014) extended their analysis on the effect of ICV by conducting a longitudinal study in 40 MS patients with various phenotypes over a 4.5-year period. Over this time period, IPS and memory performance declined significantly and MRI markers showed also a progression of disease burden (T2 lesion load and NBV). Baseline ICV moderated the effect of lesion burden on IPS decline but not on memory. These studies suggested a selective effect of BR on IPS performances.

A recent study did not replicate the previous findings (Modica et al., 2016). A sample of 71 MS patients with various clinical phenotypes and 23 matched HS were studied twice over a 3-year period. As described previously, a decline for the SDMT was observed only in patients with LEL.

In that sample, there was no global cognitive worsening, although deep GM volume decreased over time. However, ICV had no effect on cognitive change. In summary, education (i.e., CR) but not ICV (i.e., BR) contributed to IPS decline.

Effect of Current CR Activities on Symptom Experience

The effect of CR on symptom experience has been studied in an epidemiological register study (Schwartz, Quaranto, Healy, Benedict, & Vollmer, 2013). These authors performed a secondary analysis of longitudinal data from the North American Research Committee on Multiple Sclerosis (NARCOMS) registry. Passive CR (i.e., previous participation in CR-building activities) was measured using the Sole-Padulles Childhood Enrichment measure, and active CR (i.e., current participation in CR-building activities) was measured by the Stern Leisure Activities Measure. Longitudinal modeling revealed a significant interaction of active CR and time in mobility, fatigue, and overall disability. Moreover, active CR was associated with less deterioration, but passive CR was not. The same group reported studies from the NARCOMS registry that showed that MS patients with high CR reported lower levels of perceived disability and perceived cognitive deficits, and higher levels of physical health, mental health, and well-being and quality of life (Schwartz, Snook, Quaranto, Benedict, Rapkin, et al., 2013; Schwartz, Snook, Quaranto, Benedict, & Vollmer, 2013). However, the data were not adjusted on neurological disability, and this could be a limitation.

CR in POMS

The study of CR in POMS is complex because the early disease process can interfere with the CR-building activities, thus confounding some CR proxies. A few studies have examined this question, with contradictory results (Hosseini, Flora, Banwell, & Till, 2014; Pastò et al., 2016; Till et al., 2013).

A recent study in 48 POMS patients, followed up over a mean of 4.7 years, examined the effect of CR estimated by the Wechsler Intelligence Scale for Children—Revised (Pastò et al., 2016). At baseline, 29.2% of POMS patients had CI, as defined by failure on three tests on an NP battery. Cognitive decline from baseline was observed in 37.6% of patients using the reliable change index, based on differences in tests scores over time. Among the 34 cases that were cognitively preserved at baseline, a higher CR predicted stable or improving performance at follow-up (odds ratio = 1.11; 95% CI [1.03, 1.20]; $p = 0.006$). Although the intelligence quotient might have been affected by the disease process, the size of and the robustness of the effect (not affected by disease duration) suggested a meaningful effect of CR. To avoid these possible limitations, the educational level of the parents of the children affected by MS has been proposed as a CR proxy. Till et al. (2013) studied change in cognitive performance in 28 patients with POMS and 26 age-matched HS over a 1-year period. Seven of 28 patients (25%) showed cognitive deterioration compared with only one of 26 controls (3.8%). Interestingly, those whose cognitive performance remained stable or improved were more likely to have higher educated parents compared with subjects with deteriorating performance.

Another study used both types of CR proxies (i.e., baseline intelligence and parental social status) in 35 POMS patients, 28 out of them having at least two NP assessments (Hosseini et al., 2014). This study did not show any effect of CR on cognitive longitudinal trajectories. Baseline intelligence and parental social status did not moderate any of the cognitive changes.

MECHANISMS AND IMPLICATIONS

The mechanisms of CR are not well understood. The cognitive mechanisms have been poorly studied. The relationship between CR, estimated with the Wechsler Test of Adult Reading and Peabody Picture Vocabulary Test. and verbal memory impairment in MS could be mediated by working memory, as suggested by a recent study (Sandry & Sumowski, 2014). Alternatively, fMRI studies could help to study network adaptations associated with CR. In one study, a test of working memory was used, the n-back task, with three levels of complexity in fMRI in 18 MS patients with various clinical phenotypes (Sumowski, Wylie, DeLuca, et al., 2010). CR was measured using verbal intelligence (Wechsler Abbreviated Scale of Intelligence). Lower performance was observed for the more complex n-back condition only. For all conditions of the task, higher CR was associated with less activation of the prefrontal cortex and greater activation of the anterior cingulate cortex. The task performances were improved for the more complex level with higher CR. Interestingly, the brain regions activated in relation to the effect of CR are part of the default mode network (DMN), suggesting that MS patients with high CR were able to better maintain resting-state activity during cognitive processing. Resting-state fMRI studies of the DMN produced contradictory results in MS, according to CI showing either increased or decreased connectivity in this network in MS patients (Schoonheim, Meijer, & Geurts, 2015). It has been suggested that the current interpretation of functional reorganization processes in MS are too simplistic. Longitudinal studies, associating connectivity studies in rest, and activation fMRI are necessary for a better understanding of brain adaptive mechanisms.

A study in young HS, at the same age range of MS patients, examined the effect of education on cognition and brain activity (Bonnet et al., 2009). Using a test of executive function of increasing complexity (Go/No-Go) during fMRI, the authors showed an effect of education on IPS (i.e., reaction times during the test). HS with HEL exhibited higher activity in the cerebellum and lower activity in medial prefrontal and inferior parietal cortices compared with LEL HS during the task. These results suggest that a high level of education enhances automation capacity of the cerebellum, leading to better cognitive performances. Interestingly, it has been shown that cerebellum connectivity is decreased in cognitively preserved RRMS patients and that this disconnection is associated with the increase of compensatory mechanisms, as shown by the activation of medial prefrontal cortex (Bonnet et al., 2010). Taken together, these studies suggest that education can promote better cognitive performances by enhancing automatic processes in the cerebellum and that these mechanisms could be altered in MS patients. Another study showed that MS patients with various clinical phenotypes have different abnormalities in activation and effective connectivity between the right cerebellum and frontoparietal cortices, with increasing cognitive load (Rocca et al., 2012). This likely contributes to inefficient cortical reorganization. These results suggest that the effect of education on cerebellum activity observed in HS could not be maintained in MS. Indeed, several studies have showed that cerebellum dysfunction or damage is associated with CI in MS, especially concerning IPS (Ruet et al., 2014), and an association between cerebellar atrophy and IPS and working memory impairment have been shown in MS (Moroso et al., 2016). Interestingly, cognitive rehabilitation could restore some cerebellum activity in MS patients while improving cognitive performance (Sastre-Garriga et al., 2011).

The CR theory has important implications for therapeutic strategies in MS patients based on active intellectual enrichment and potentiation of passive individual reserve. A cross-sectional study measured the effect of change in active reserve-building activities (i.e., recreational activities) on the correlation between brain atrophy and neurocognitive performance in 57 RRMS patients and 27 HS (Booth et al., 2013). Indeed, brain atrophy (i.e., third ventricle width) was negatively associated with cognition assessed by the PASAT and the SDMT in patients reporting current declines in recreational activities. On the contrary, there was not a correlation in patients reporting stable participation in these activities. Because MS patients seem to develop fewer current reserve-building activities than HS, longitudinal studies are needed to test the beneficial effect of lifestyle adaptation in MS.

CONCLUSIONS AND FUTURE DIRECTIONS

Altogether, these studies suggest that CR significantly affects cognitive functioning in persons with MS. However, there are some discrepancies in the results among studies, and more work is needed to determine the respective contribution of different reserve-building activities, such as education and cognitive leisure, to better analyze the effect of CR on different cognitive domains. It further is necessary to determine the natural course of decline over time of the CR effect after the onset of the disease process.

Some other important points of future studies are as follows:

- Longitudinal studies are necessary to demonstrate the effect of CR on cognitive decline.
- Longitudinal studies are needed for analyzing the effect of active CR on cognitive status.
- A cognitive assessment encompassing several cognitive domains (at least IPS, episodic memory, working memory, executive function, and attention) is necessary to study the differential effect of CR on these domains. So far, most of the studies have focused on a few tests and a few cognitive domains; this is a limitation to our current knowledge.
- The baseline severity of the disease has to be taken into account when analyzing the effect of CR on cognitive status. Longitudinal studies in patients with low and high CR but similar burden of the disease at baseline are necessary.
- Interventional longitudinal studies on lifestyle adaptation are necessary to show the ability of active CR to influence cognitive decline.
- Longitudinal imaging studies should associate morphological parameters, including volumetry and diffusion tensor imaging, functional connectivity at rest, and fMRI activation during task performance.

REFERENCES

Amato, M. P., Razzolini, L., Goretti, B., Stromillo, M. L., Rossi, F., Giorgio, A., . . . De Stefano, N. (2013). Cognitive reserve and cortical atrophy in multiple sclerosis: A longitudinal study. *Neurology*, 80, 1728–1733. http://dx.doi.org/10.1212/WNL.0b013e3182918c6f

Amieva, H., Mokri, H., Le Goff, M., Meillon, C., Jacqmin-Gadda, H., Foubert-Samier, A., . . . Dartigues, J. F. (2014). Compensatory mechanisms in higher-educated subjects with Alzheimer's disease: A study of 20 years of cognitive decline. *Brain: A Journal of Neurology, 137,* 1167–1175. http://dx.doi.org/10.1093/brain/awu035

Benedict, R. H. B., Morrow, S. A., Weinstock Guttman, B., Cookfair, D., & Schretlen, D. J. (2010). Cognitive reserve moderates decline in information processing speed in multiple sclerosis patients. *Journal of the International Neuropsychological Society, 16,* 829–835. http://dx.doi.org/10.1017/S1355617710000688

Bonnet, M. C., Allard, M., Dilharreguy, B., Deloire, M., Petry, K. G., & Brochet, B. (2010). Cognitive compensation failure in multiple sclerosis. *Neurology, 75,* 1241–1248. http://dx.doi.org/10.1212/WNL.0b013e3181f612e3

Bonnet, M. C., Deloire, M. S., Salort, E., Dousset, V., Petry, K. G., & Brochet, B., & AQUISEP Study Group. (2006). Evidence of cognitive compensation associated with educational level in early relapsing-remitting multiple sclerosis. *Journal of the Neurological Sciences, 251,* 23–28. http://dx.doi.org/10.1016/j.jns.2006.08.002

Bonnet, M. C., Dilharreguy, B., Allard, M., Deloire, M. S., Petry, K. G., & Brochet, B. (2009). Differential cerebellar and cortical involvement according to various attentional load: Role of educational level. *Human Brain Mapping, 30,* 1133–1143. http://dx.doi.org/10.1002/hbm.20575

Booth, A. J., Rodgers, J. D., Schwartz, C. E., Quaranto, B. R., Weinstock-Guttman, B., Zivadinov, R., & Benedict, R. H. (2013). Active cognitive reserve influences the regional atrophy to cognition link in multiple sclerosis. *Journal of the International Neuropsychological Society, 19,* 1128–1133. http://dx.doi.org/10.1017/S1355617713001082

Brochet, B. (2015). The spectrum of demyelinating inflammatory diseases of the central nervous system. In B. Brochet (Ed.), *Neuropsychiatric symptoms of inflammatory demyelinating disease* (pp. 3–15). Cham, Switzerland: Springer. http://dx.doi.org/10.1007/978-3-319-18464-7_1

Cody, S. L., & Vance, D. E. (2016). The neurobiology of HIV and its impact on cognitive reserve: A review of cognitive interventions for an aging population. *Neurobiology of Disease, 92,* 144–156. http://dx.doi.org/10.1016/j.nbd.2016.01.011

Draganski, B., Gaser, C., Busch, V., Schuierer, G., Bogdahn, U., & May, A. (2004). Neuroplasticity: Changes in grey matter induced by training. *Nature, 427,* 311–312. http://dx.doi.org/10.1038/427311a

Draganski, B., Gaser, C., Kempermann, G., Kuhn, H. G., Winkler, J., Büchel, C., & May, A. (2006). Temporal and spatial dynamics of brain structure changes during extensive learning. *Journal of Neuroscience, 26,* 6314–6317. http://dx.doi.org/10.1523/JNEUROSCI.4628-05.2006

Feinstein, A., Lapshin, H., O'Connor, P., & Lanctôt, K. L. (2013). Sub-threshold cognitive impairment in multiple sclerosis: The association with cognitive reserve. *Journal of Neurology, 260,* 2256–2261. http://dx.doi.org/10.1007/s00415-013-6952-9

Geurts, J. J., Calabrese, M., Fisher, E., & Rudick, R. A. (2012). Measurement and clinical effect of grey matter pathology in multiple sclerosis. *The Lancet Neurology, 11*, 1082–1092. http://dx.doi.org/10.1016/S1474-4422(12)70230-2

Ghaffar, O., Fiati, M., & Feinstein, A. (2012). Occupational attainment as a marker of cognitive reserve in multiple sclerosis. *PLoS ONE, 7*, e47206. http://dx.doi.org/10.1371/journal.pone.0047206

Hindle, J. V., Martyr, A., & Clare, L. (2014). Cognitive reserve in Parkinson's disease: A systematic review and meta-analysis. *Parkinsonism & Related Disorders, 20*, 1–7. http://dx.doi.org/10.1016/j.parkreldis.2013.08.010

Hosseini, B., Flora, D. B., Banwell, B. L., & Till, C. (2014). Age of onset as a moderator of cognitive decline in pediatric-onset multiple sclerosis. *Journal of the International Neuropsychological Society, 20*, 796–804. http://dx.doi.org/10.1017/S1355617714000642

Ivanovic, D. M., Leiva, B. P., Pérez, H. T., Olivares, M. G., Díaz, N. S., Urrutia, M. S., . . . Larraín, C. G. (2004). Head size and intelligence, learning, nutritional status and brain development: Head, IQ, learning, nutrition and brain. *Neuropsychologia, 42*, 1118–1131. http://dx.doi.org/10.1016/j.neuropsychologia.2003.11.022

Lebrun, C. (2015). The radiologically isolated syndrome. *Revue Neurologique, 171*, 698–706. http://dx.doi.org/10.1016/j.neurol.2015.05.001

Lövdén, M., Ghisletta, P., & Lindenberger, U. (2005). Social participation attenuates decline in perceptual speed in old and very old age. *Psychology and Aging, 20*, 423–434. http://dx.doi.org/10.1037/0882-7974.20.3.423

Lövdén, M., Schaefer, S., Noack, H., Bodammer, N. C., Kühn, S., Heinze, H. J., . . . Lindenberger, U. (2012). Spatial navigation training protects the hippocampus against age-related changes during early and late adulthood. *Neurobiology of Aging, 33*, 620.e9–620.e22. http://dx.doi.org/10.1016/j.neurobiolaging.2011.02.013

Luerding, R., Gebel, S., Gebel, E. M., Schwab-Malek, S., & Weissert, R. (2016). Influence of Formal education on cognitive reserve in patients with multiple sclerosis. *Frontiers in Neurology, 7*, 46. http://dx.doi.org/10.3389/fneur.2016.00046

Martins Da Silva, A., Cavaco, S., Moreira, I., Bettencourt, A., Santos, E., Pinto, C., . . . Montalban, X. (2015). Cognitive reserve in multiple sclerosis: Protective effects of education. *Multiple Sclerosis, 21*, 1312–1321. http://dx.doi.org/10.1177/1352458515581874

Mathias, J. L., & Wheaton, P. (2015). Contribution of brain or biological reserve and cognitive or neural reserve to outcome after TBI: A meta-analysis (prior to 2015). *Neuroscience and Biobehavioral Reviews, 55*, 573–593. http://dx.doi.org/10.1016/j.neubiorev.2015.06.001

May, A. (2011). Experience-dependent structural plasticity in the adult human brain. *Trends in Cognitive Sciences, 15*, 475–482. http://dx.doi.org/10.1016/j.tics.2011.08.002

Modica, C. M., Bergsland, N., Dwyer, M. G., Ramasamy, D. P., Carl, E., Zivadinov, R., & Benedict, R. H. B. (2016). Cognitive reserve moderates the impact of sub-cortical gray matter atrophy on neuropsychological status in multiple sclerosis. *Multiple Sclerosis, 22*, 36–42. http://dx.doi.org/10.1177/1352458515579443

Moroso, A., Ruet, A., Lamargue-Hamel, D., Munsch, F., Deloire, M., Coupé, P., . . . Brochet, B. (2016). Posterior lobules of the cerebellum and information pro-cessing speed at various stages of multiple sclerosis. *Journal of Neurology, Neuro-surgery, & Psychiatry.* Advance online publication. http://dx.doi.org/10.1136/jnnp-2016-313867

Nunnari, D., Bramanti, P., & Marino, S. (2014). Cognitive reserve in stroke and traumatic brain injury patients. *Neurological Sciences, 35*, 1513–1518. http://dx.doi.org/10.1007/s10072-014-1897-z

Nunnari, D., De Cola, M. C., Costa, A., Rifici, C., Bramanti, P., & Marino, S. (2016). Exploring cognitive reserve in multiple sclerosis: New findings from a cross-sectional study. *Journal of Clinical and Experimental Neuropsychology, 38*, 1158–1167. http://dx.doi.org/10.1080/13803395.2016.1200538

Nyberg, L., Lövdén, M., Riklund, K., Lindenberger, U., & Bäckman, L. (2012). Memory aging and brain maintenance. *Trends in Cognitive Sciences, 16*, 292–305. http://dx.doi.org/10.1016/j.tics.2012.04.005

Pastò, L., Portaccio, E., Goretti, B., Ghezzi, A., Lori, S., Hakiki, B., . . . MS Study Group of the Italian Neurological Society. (2016). The cognitive reserve theory in the setting of pediatric-onset multiple sclerosis. *Multiple Sclerosis, 22*, 1741–1749. http://dx.doi.org/10.1177/1352458516629559

Pinter, D., Sumowski, J., DeLuca, J., Fazekas, F., Pichler, A., Khalil, M., . . . Enzinger, C. (2014). Higher education moderates the effect of T2 lesion load and third ventricle width on cognition in multiple sclerosis. *PLoS ONE, 9*, e87567. http://dx.doi.org/10.1371/journal.pone.0087567

Renoux, C., Vukusic, S., Mikaeloff, Y., Edan, G., Clanet, M., Dubois, B., . . . Adult Neurology Departments KIDMUS Study Group. (2007). Natural history of multiple sclerosis with childhood onset. *The New England Journal of Medicine, 356*, 2603–2613. http://dx.doi.org/10.1056/NEJMoa067597

Reuter-Lorenz, P. A., & Park, D. C. (2014). How does it STAC up? Revisiting the scaffolding theory of aging and cognition. *Neuropsychology Review, 24*, 355–370. http://dx.doi.org/10.1007/s11065-014-9270-9

Rocca, M. A., Amato, M. P., De Stefano, N., Enzinger, C., Geurts, J. J., Penner, I. K., . . . MAGNIMS Study Group. (2015). Clinical and imaging assess-ment of cognitive dysfunction in multiple sclerosis. *The Lancet Neurology, 14*, 302–317. http://dx.doi.org/10.1016/S1474-4422(14)70250-9

Rocca, M. A., Bonnet, M. C., Meani, A., Valsasina, P., Colombo, B., Comi, G., & Filippi, M. (2012). Differential cerebellar functional interactions during an interference task across multiple sclerosis phenotypes. *Radiology, 265*, 864–873. http://dx.doi.org/10.1148/radiol.12120216

Ruet, A. (2015). Cognitive impairment in multiple sclerosis. In B. Brochet (Ed), *Neuropsychiatric symptoms of inflammatory demyelinating disease* (pp. 227–247). Cham, Switzerland: Springer. http://dx.doi.org/10.1007/978-3-319-18464-7_16

Ruet, A., Hamel, D., Deloire, M. S. A., Charré-Morin, J., Saubusse, A., & Brochet, B. (2014). Information processing speed impairment and cerebellar dysfunction in relapsing-remitting multiple sclerosis. *Journal of the Neurological Sciences, 347,* 246–250. http://dx.doi.org/10.1016/j.jns.2014.10.008

Sandry, J., Paxton, J., & Sumowski, J. F. (2016). General mathematical ability predicts PASAT performance in MS patients: Implications for clinical interpretation and cognitive reserve. *Journal of the International Neuropsychological Society, 22,* 375–378. http://dx.doi.org/10.1017/S1355617715001307

Sandry, J., & Sumowski, J. F. (2014). Working memory mediates the relationship between intellectual enrichment and long-term memory in multiple sclerosis: An exploratory analysis of cognitive reserve. *Journal of the International Neuropsychological Society, 20,* 868–872. http://dx.doi.org/10.1017/S1355617714000630

Sastre-Garriga, J., Alonso, J., Renom, M., Arévalo, M. J., González, I., Galán, I., . . . Rovira, A. (2011). A functional magnetic resonance proof of concept pilot trial of cognitive rehabilitation in multiple sclerosis. *Multiple Sclerosis, 17,* 457–467. http://dx.doi.org/10.1177/1352458510389219

Scarpazza, C., Braghittoni, D., Casale, B., Malagú, S., Mattioli, F., di Pellegrino, G., & Ladavas, E. (2013). Education protects against cognitive changes associated with multiple sclerosis. *Restorative Neurology and Neuroscience, 31,* 619–631.

Schofield, P. W., Logroscino, G., Andrews, H. F., Albert, S., & Stern, Y. (1997). An association between head circumference and Alzheimer's disease in a population-based study of aging and dementia. *Neurology, 49,* 30–37. http://dx.doi.org/10.1212/WNL.49.1.30

Schoonheim, M. M., Meijer, K. A., & Geurts, J. J. (2015). Network collapse and cognitive impairment in multiple sclerosis. *Frontiers in Neurology, 6,* 82. http://dx.doi.org/10.3389/fneur.2015.00082

Schwartz, C. E., Ayandeh, A., Ramanathan, M., Benedict, R., Dwyer, M. G., Weinstock-Guttman, B., & Zivadinov, R. (2015). Reserve-building activities in multiple sclerosis patients and healthy controls: A descriptive study. *BMC Neurology, 15,* 135. http://dx.doi.org/10.1186/s12883-015-0395-0

Schwartz, C. E., Quaranto, B. R., Healy, B. C., Benedict, R. H., & Vollmer, T. L. (2013). Cognitive reserve and symptom experience in multiple sclerosis: A buffer to disability progression over time? *Archives of Physical Medicine and Rehabilitation, 94,* 1971–1981. http://dx.doi.org/10.1016/j.apmr.2013.05.009

Schwartz, C. E., Snook, E., Quaranto, B., Benedict, R. H. B., Rapkin, B. D., & Vollmer, T. (2013). Cognitive reserve and appraisal in multiple sclerosis. *Multiple Sclerosis and Related Disorders, 2,* 36–44. http://dx.doi.org/10.1016/j.msard.2012.07.006

Schwartz, C. E., Snook, E., Quaranto, B., Benedict, R. H. B., & Vollmer, T. (2013). Cognitive reserve and patient-reported outcomes in multiple sclerosis. *Multiple Sclerosis, 19,* 87–105. http://dx.doi.org/10.1177/1352458512444914

Stern, Y. (2009). Cognitive reserve. *Neuropsychologia, 47,* 2015–2028. http://dx.doi.org/10.1016/j.neuropsychologia.2009.03.004

Stern, Y., Gurland, B., Tatemichi, T. K., Tang, M. X., Wilder, D., & Mayeux, R. (1994). Influence of education and occupation on the incidence of Alzheimer's disease. *JAMA, 271,* 1004–1010. http://dx.doi.org/10.1001/jama.1994.03510370056032

Sumowski, J. F. (2015). Cognitive reserve as a useful concept for early intervention research in multiple sclerosis. *Frontiers in Neurology, 6,* 176. http://dx.doi.org/10.3389/fneur.2015.00176

Sumowski, J. F., Chiaravalloti, N., & DeLuca, J. (2009). Cognitive reserve protects against cognitive dysfunction in multiple sclerosis. *Journal of Clinical and Experimental Neuropsychology, 31,* 913–926. http://dx.doi.org/10.1080/13803390902740643

Sumowski, J. F., Chiaravalloti, N., Leavitt, V. M., & DeLuca, J. (2012). Cognitive reserve in secondary progressive multiple sclerosis. *Multiple Sclerosis, 18,* 1454–1458. http://dx.doi.org/10.1177/1352458512440205

Sumowski, J. F., Chiaravalloti, N., Wylie, G., & DeLuca, J. (2009). Cognitive reserve moderates the negative effect of brain atrophy on cognitive efficiency in multiple sclerosis. *Journal of the International Neuropsychological Society, 15,* 606–612. http://dx.doi.org/10.1017/S1355617709090912

Sumowski, J. F., Rocca, M. A., Leavitt, V. M., Dackovic, J., Mesaros, S., Drulovic, J., . . . Filippi, M. (2014). Brain reserve and cognitive reserve protect against cognitive decline over 4.5 years in MS. *Neurology, 82,* 1776–1783. http://dx.doi.org/10.1212/WNL.0000000000000433

Sumowski, J. F., Rocca, M. A., Leavitt, V. M., Riccitelli, G., Comi, G., DeLuca, J., & Filippi, M. (2013). Brain reserve and cognitive reserve in multiple sclerosis: What you've got and how you use it. *Neurology, 80,* 2186–2193. http://dx.doi.org/10.1212/WNL.0b013e318296e98b (Erratum published 2013, *Neurology, 81,* 604. http://dx.doi.org/10.1212/WNL.0b013e3182a0ef3d)

Sumowski, J. F., Rocca, M. A., Leavitt, V. M., Riccitelli, G., Meani, A., Comi, G., & Filippi, M. (2016). Reading, writing, and reserve: Literacy activities are linked to hippocampal volume and memory in multiple sclerosis. *Multiple Sclerosis, 22,* 1621–1625. http://dx.doi.org/10.1177/1352458516630822

Sumowski, J. F., Rocca, M. A., Leavitt, V. M., Riccitelli, G., Sandry, J., DeLuca, J., . . . Filippi, M. (2016). Searching for the neural basis of reserve against memory decline: Intellectual enrichment linked to larger hippocampal volume in multiple sclerosis. *European Journal of Neurology, 23,* 39–44. http://dx.doi.org/10.1111/ene.12662

Sumowski, J. F., Wylie, G. R., Chiaravalloti, N., & DeLuca, J. (2010). Intellectual enrichment lessens the effect of brain atrophy on learning and memory in multiple sclerosis. *Neurology, 74,* 1942–1945. http://dx.doi.org/10.1212/WNL.0b013e3181e396be

Sumowski, J. F., Wylie, G. R., DeLuca, J., & Chiaravalloti, N. (2010). Intellectual enrichment is linked to cerebral efficiency in multiple sclerosis: Functional magnetic resonance imaging evidence for cognitive reserve. *Brain: A Journal of Neurology, 133,* 362–374. http://dx.doi.org/10.1093/brain/awp307

Sumowski, J. F., Wylie, G. R., Gonnella, A., Chiaravalloti, N., & DeLuca, J. (2010). Premorbid cognitive leisure independently contributes to cognitive reserve in multiple sclerosis. *Neurology, 75,* 1428–1431. http://dx.doi.org/10.1212/WNL.0b013e3181f881a6

Till, C., Racine, N., Araujo, D., Narayanan, S., Collins, D. L., Aubert-Broche, B., . . . Banwell, B. (2013). Changes in cognitive performance over a 1-year period in children and adolescents with multiple sclerosis. *Neuropsychology, 27,* 210–219. http://dx.doi.org/10.1037/a0031665

INDEX

Arnett, P. A., 96–97, 99, 283
Arrondo, G., 257
Artieda, J., 257
Artistic activities, 331
Ashtari, F., 255
Assessment
    of activities of daily living, 175–184
    of anxiety, 114
    of cognitive fatigue, 129–130
    of cognitive impairment. *See*
        Assessment of cognitive
        impairment in MS
Assessment of cognitive impairment in
    MS, 7–23
    computer-assisted, 13–17
    conventional psychometric
        techniques for, 8–13
    frequency of, 21–22
    future directions in development
        of, 23
    interpretation of, 22–23
    and monitoring, 19–22
    and pediatric MS, 230–232
    screening methods in, 18–19
Assessment of Motor and Process Skills
    (AMPS), 177, 179
Assistive devices, 160
Associative memory, 278
Attention
    and activities of daily living, 180
    cognitive rehabilitation for, 265,
        266, 273–279, 281
    and depression with MS, 92–93, 99
    effects of antifatigue drugs on, 251
    effects of stimulants on, 258
    and exercise, 297
    and functional magnetic resonance
        imaging, 48
    and global brain atrophy, 39
    and gray matter atrophy, 41
    and pediatric multiple sclerosis, 226,
        233
    and physical activity, 307
    prevalence of deficits with, 208
    selective, 130, 282
    sustained, 39, 41–43
Attention-deficit/hyperactivity disorder
    (ADHD), 258
Attention Processing Training program,
    238, 274

Au Duong, M. V., 71, 72
Audoin, B., 70, 76
Autobiographical memory, 273
Automated Neuropsychological
    Assessment Metrics (ANAM),
    14–15
Avoidant personality disorder, 150
Axonal damage/loss, 69
Axonal regression, 69
Axon growth, 68–69

BADLs. *See* Basic activities of daily
    living
Bakshi, R., 77, 154
Balance, 67, 127, 196, 201, 308
Banwell, B. L., 226, 230, 236
Baruch, N. F., 237
Basak, T., 174
Basal ganglia
    and cerebral reorganization, 77
    and cognitive fatigue, 131, 134–136
    and cognitive rehabilitation, 277
    and depression with MS, 99
Basic activities of daily living (BADLs)
    assessment of, 176
    overview, 173
    research on MS and limitations with,
        174–175
Basso, M. R., 271–272
Bathing, 173
Batista, S., 77
Beck Depression Inventory—Fast
    Screen (BDI–FS), 91, 97, 101
Beck Depression Inventory—II (BDI–II),
    93, 102, 103
Beery Buktenica Development test, 227,
    229
Behan, P. O., 132
Behavioral Assessment of the
    Dysexecutive Syndrome, 175
Behavioral Assessment System for
    Children, Second Edition, 233
Behavioral interventions, 138
Behavioral issues, 130–131
Behavioral strategies, 238
Behavioral symptoms (BS), 158–162.
    See also Personality changes with
    multiple sclerosis
    anger, 159–160
    apathy. *See* Apathy

falls and accidents, 160–162
with pediatric multiple sclerosis, 232
Behavior Rating Inventory of Executive
Function, 226
Beiske, A. G., 278
Belman, A. L., 232–233
Benedict, R. H. B., 77, 99, 154
BENEFIT trial, 247
Benign multiple sclerosis (BMS), 73,
74, 76
BICAMS. *See* Brief International
Cognitive Assessment for MS
Bilateral inferior parietal cortex, 278
Bipolar affective disorder, 115–117
Bisecco, A., 133
Bladder dysfunction, 201
and domestic accidents, 161
and economic impact of cognitive
impairment in MS, 207
and employment, 196
Blood oxygen level-dependent (BOLD)
activation, 70, 71, 73
BMS (benign multiple sclerosis), 73,
74, 76
Body functions, 172
BOLD (blood oxygen level-dependent)
activation, 70, 71, 73
Bonavita, S., 278
Bonnet, M. C., 79, 328, 332
Bonzano, L., 76
Borderline personality disorder, 150
Bornstein, R. A., 271
Boster, A., 278
Bowel dysfunction, 161, 196, 201
BPF (brain parenchymal fraction), 99,
326
BR (brain reserve), 322
Brain atrophy
and cognitive rehabilitation,
279–280
and cognitive reserve, 326
and depression with MS, 99
global, 39
gray matter, 39–43
and magnetic resonance imaging,
38–39
and pediatric multiple sclerosis,
234
white matter, 39–40
Brain atrophy analysis, 68

Brain imaging. *See also* Magnetic
resonance imaging
and acetylcholinesterase inhibitors,
255
and anxiety, 114–115
and bipolar disorder, 115–116
and cerebral reorganization in MS,
67–68
of cognitive impairment in pediatric
multiple sclerosissclerosis,
233–236
and cognitive reserve, 328–330
data on cognitive fatigue from,
131–136, 139–140
and depression with MS, 98
of effects with cognitive
rehabilitation, 277
and euphoria, 118
Brain integrity, 96
Brain network efficiency, 52–53
Brain parenchymal fraction (BPF), 99,
326
Brain reserve (BR), 322
Brain reserve capacity (BRC), 94–96
BrainStim program, 274
Brain Twister n-back task, 275
BRB. *See* Brief Repeatable Battery
BRB-N (Brief Repeatable Battery of
Neuropsychological Tests), 327
BRC (brain reserve capacity), 94–96
Brenk, A., 281
Brief International Cognitive
Assessment for MS (BICAMS)
and activities of daily living, 182
and cognitive reserve, 328
interpretation of, 22, 23
overview, 19–21
and pediatric multiple sclerosis,
231
Brief Neuropsychological Battery for
Children (BNBC), 230–231
Brief Repeatable Battery (BRB)
assessment of cognitive impairment
with, 9–11
and cerebral reorganization in MS,
77
limitations of, 12
Brief Repeatable Battery of
Neuropsychological Tests
(BRB-N), 327

Brief Repeatable Neuropsychological
    Battery (BRNB)
    and acetylcholinesterase inhibitors,
        257
    and disease-modifying treatments,
        248–250
Brief Visuospatial Memory Test—
    Revised (BVMT–R)
    assessment with, 11, 12
    and depression with MS, 99, 100
    and magnetic resonance imaging,
        41, 43
    and monitoring, 19–21
    and pediatric multiple sclerosis, 231
    and physical fitness, 309, 310
Brissart, H., 278
Bruce, A. S., 275
Bruce, J. M., 254, 275
Brunnschweiler, H., 274
BS. See Behavioral symptoms
Bupropion, 137
BVMT–R. See Brief Visuospatial
    Memory Test—Revised

Caceres, F., 9
Cadden, M. H., 96–97
Cader, S., 255
Calabrese, M., 134–135
California Verbal Learning Test—
    Second Edition (CVLT–II)
    and acetylcholinesterase inhibitors,
        257
    assessment with, 11, 12
    and cognitive rehabilitation, 267
    and depression with MS, 99, 100,
        103
    and economic impact of cognitive
        impairment in MS, 215
    and employment, 197–198
    and magnetic resonance imaging, 39,
        41–43
    and monitoring, 19–20
    and pediatric multiple sclerosis, 231
    and physical fitness, 310
Cardiorespiratory fitness
    and exercise, 297, 302
    and physical activity, 305
    and physical fitness, 308, 309, 311
Caregivers, 209
Carone, D. A., 154

Caudate, 331
CDR (Cognitive Drug Research), 14, 15
Center for Neurological Study—Lability
    Scale (CNS–LS), 121
Central atrophy, 38
Central fatigue, 128
Central nervous system (CNS)
    and antifatigue drugs, 251
    effects of disease-modifying
        treatments on, 247, 248
    effects of MS on, 3–4, 321
    effects of stimulants on, 257
    and pediatric multiple sclerosis, 232
    and personality changes with MS,
        150
Cerasa, A., 275
Cerebellum
    and cerebral reorganization in MS,
        73
    and cognitive rehabilitation, 277
    and pediatric multiple sclerosis, 235
Cerebral metabolic activity, 152–153
Cerebral reorganization in multiple
    sclerosis, 67–80
    adaptive vs. maladaptive changes in,
        78–79, 132
    data on, 79–80
    future directions for research on, 80
    levels of, 68–78
Cerebrospinal fluid (CSF), 102
Cersosimo, B., 232–233
CF. See Cognitive fatigue
Chaplin, W. F., 150
Charcot, J.-M., 3, 4
Charvet, L. E., 227, 232–233, 280
Chaudhuri, A., 132
Chiaravalloti, N. D., 70, 266–267,
    270–273, 282–283
Chicago Multiscale Depression
    Inventory, 91
Chlorpromazine, 117
Chrisodoulou, C., 229
Chronic exercise training, 295–298
Chruzander, C., 174
CIAMS. See Cognitive impairment
    associated with multiple sclerosis
CII (Cognitive Impairment Index), 250
Cingulate cortex, 160
Cingulate gyrus, 132, 270
Cingulum, 133

CIS patients. *See* Clinically isolated syndrome patients

Cleary, R. E., 227

Clinically isolated syndrome (CIS) patients
    assessment of cognitive impairment in, 14
    and brain atrophy, 39
    and cerebral reorganization in MS, 76
    use of disease-modifying treatments with, 247

Cloninger, C. R., 150, 152

CMI (cognitive-motor interference), 161–162

CNAD (computerized neuropsychological assessment devices), 13

CNS. *See* Central nervous system

CNS–LS (Center for Neurological Study—Lability Scale), 121

Cochrane Review, 267

COGIMUS (Cognitive Impairment in Multiple Sclerosis) study, 248

Cognitive behavior therapy
    for anxiety, 115
    for cognitive fatigue, 138
    effects of telephone-administered, 94

Cognitive Drug Research (CDR), 14, 15

Cognitive dysfunction, 161

Cognitive fatigue (CF), 127–140
    behavioral issues with, 130–131
    brain imaging data on, 131–136, 139–140
    defined, 128
    future directions for research on, 138–140
    objective measures of, 129
    principal treatments of, 136–138
    subjective measures of, 130

Cognitive flexibility, 225

Cognitive impairment associated with multiple sclerosis (CIAMS). *See also specific headings*
    overview, 4, 321–322
    prevalence of, 4, 7

Cognitive Impairment Index (CII), 250

Cognitive Impairment in Multiple Sclerosis (COGIMUS) study, 248

Cognitive-motor interference (CMI), 161–162

Cognitive rehabilitation, 265–285
    and activities of daily living, 185
    for attention, processing speed, and working memory, 265, 266, 273–280, 283, 284
    and cerebral reorganization in MS, 77–78
    for executive function, 266, 267, 269, 276–279
    future directions for, 284–285
    home-based programs for, 279–280
    for learning and memory, 266–273, 276–279
    multimodal programs for, 266, 276–279
    nonspecific interventions for, 280–284
    overview, 265–267

Cognitive reserve (CR), 321–337
    and cognitive fatigue, 138–139
    and depression with MS, 94–98, 103
    and fatigue. *See* Cognitive fatigue
    future directions for research on, 337
    mechanisms of, 335–336
    and pediatric multiple sclerosis, 238
    proxies used in assessment of, 322–335
    theory of, 322–323

Cognitive Reserve Index (CRI), 331–333

Cognitive speed, 130

Cognitive Stability Index, 13

Cognitive therapy, 283. *See also* Cognitive behavior therapy

Cognitive training, 280–281

Combs, D., 271

Communication skills, 265

Comorbid neuropsychiatric disorders, 113–122
    anxiety disorders, 114–115
    bipolar affective disorder, 115–117
    euphoria, 117–120
    pseudobulbar affect, 119–121

Computed tomography (CT)
    and brain atrophy, 38
    and cerebral reorganization in MS, 80
    single-photon emission, 101

Computer-assisted assessment, 13–17

neural underpinnings of, 98–103
overview, 4, 90–94
and personality changes with MS,
    155–156
and prevalence of cognitive
    impairment, 90
Depressiveness, 131
De Seze, J., 273
DeSouza, J. F., 226
Deterministic tractography, 101
Devices, 209
DEXA. *See* Dual-energy x-ray
    absorptiometry
Dextromethorphan, 121
*Diagnostic and Statistical Manual of
    Mental Disorders (DSM)*, 91, 119
Didactic presentation methods, 271
Diffusion tensor imaging (DTI)
    and cerebral reorganization in MS,
        68, 76
    and cognitive fatigue, 133
    and depression with MS, 102
    overview, 35–36, 43–44
DIR. *See* Double inversion recovery
Direct medical costs, 209
Disability
    and activities of daily living, 171
    components of, 172
    and Internet technologies, 180–181
    and pediatric multiple sclerosis, 232
    and physical activity, 307
Disease burden, 96, 97
Disease-modifying treatments (DMTs),
    246–251
    future directions for research on,
        250–251
    glatiramer acetate, 248–249
    interferons beta, 246–248
    natalizumab, 249–250
Disease onset, 191
Disinhibition, 150
Dizziness, 127
DKEFS. *See* Delis–Kaplan Executive
    Functioning System Sorting Test
DMN. *See* Default mode network
DMTs. *See* Disease-modifying
    treatments
Doble, S. E., 177
Dobryakova, E., 74, 270

Domestic accidents, 160–162
Donepezil, 256
Dopamine
    and antifatigue drugs, 254
    and cerebral reorganization in MS, 79
    and medications for cognitive
        fatigue, 137
Dorsolateral prefrontal cortex, 277
Double inversion recovery (DIR)
    future uses of, 53, 54
    overview, 34–36
Dressing, 173
Driver Simulator Dual Task (DSDT), 17
Driving, 173
Driving accidents, 160–162
*DSM (Diagnostic and Statistical Manual
    of Mental Disorders)*, 91, 119
DTI. *See* Diffusion tensor imaging
D2 Alertness Test, 254
Dual-energy x-ray absorptiometry
    (DEXA), 309, 310, 312
Duloxetine, 137
Duncan, A., 118

Early retirement, 209
Eating, 173
Economic impact of cognitive
    impairment in MS, 207–219
    aspects of, 209–214
    considerations with, 216–218
    and employment, 209, 215–218
    future directions for research on,
        218–219
    overview, 207–209
EDSS. *See* Expanded Disability Status
    Scale
Educational level, 95, 97, 325–328
Education programs, 138
EF. *See* Executive functioning
Effective connectivity research, 73–76
EFPT (Executive Function Performance
    Test), 177–180
Electroencephalogram, 283
Emotional incontinence, 119
Emotional lability
    and euphoria, 117–118
    pseudobulbar affect vs., 120
Emotional processing, 90
Emotion-focused therapy, 94

Houtchens, M. K., 99
hrQoL (health-related Quality of Life), 214
Hubacher, M., 237
Huhtala, H., 275, 281
HVLT–R (Hopkins Verbal Learning Test—Revised), 269
Hypomania, 116

IADLS. *See* Instrumental activities of daily living
ICF *(International Classification of Functioning, Disability, and Health)*, 172
ICV (intracranial volume), 322–323, 333–334
IFNs (interferons beta), 246–248
Illness management, 193
Inborn fixed reserve, 323–324
Incerti, C. C., 151, 156
Inferior frontal gyrus, 102, 277
Inferior parietal cortex, 51
Inferior parietal lobe (IPL), 50
Information processing speed (IPS). *See* Processing speed
Infratentorial involvement, 234
Inhibition, 39, 155, 325
Inhibitory control, 299, 309, 326
Inpatient care, 209
Insomnia, 114
Instrumental activities of daily living (IADLs)
    assessment of, 175–178, 180–184
    overview, 173
    prevalence of impairments with, 185
    research on MS and limitations with, 174–175
Insurance, 216–217, 270
Intellectual activity, 322, 323
Intelligence
    assessment of, 8, 95
    and depression with MS, 95, 97, 98
    fluid, 97, 98
    measures of, 231
    and pediatric multiple sclerosis, 230
    premorbid, 323, 325, 328–330
    verbal, 38, 329, 330, 335
Interferons beta (IFNs), 246–248
International Classification of Functioning, Disability, and Health (ICF), 172

Internet technologies, 180–181
Interpretation (assessment), 22–23
Intracranial volume (ICV), 322–323, 333–334
Introversion, 157
iPads, 15
IPS (information processing speed). *See* Processing speed
Ipsilateral ventrolateral prefrontal cortex, 50
Irritability, 118, 150, 155
Iyengar yoga, 295

Janghorbani, M., 255
Janssen, A., 278
Jehna, M., 160
Jensen, H. B., 259
JLO (Judgment of Line Orientation Test), 12
Johansson, S., 174
Johnson, K. L., 193
Jønsson, A., 280
Judgment of Line Orientation Test (JLO), 12
Julian, L., 226–227

Kalmar, J. H., 180
Kappos, L., 78, 274
Katz Extended ADL Index, 174
Kitchen Task Assessment, 179
Kiy, G., 102–103
Koivisto, K., 275, 281
Kraft, G. H., 181, 185
Krupp, L. B., 229, 232–233, 256
Krysko, K. M., 236

Lamargue-Hamel, D., 17
L-amphetamine sulphate, 257–258
Landrø, N. I., 278
Langdon, D. W., 159
Lange, R., 254
Language ability
    on Brief Repeatable Battery, 9
    and cognitive fatigue, 130
    and cognitive rehabilitation, 279
    measures of, 231
    and pediatric multiple sclerosis, 224, 227, 233
    and synaptic pruning, 67
LaRocca, N., 195

Mood stabilizers, 116
Moore, K. S., 283
Moore, N. B., 283
Moritz, S., 282
Morrow, S. A., 257–258
Mortality, 192
Motor function
    and accidents, 162
    and antipsychotic medications, 117
    and cognitive fatigue, 130
    and economic impact of cognitive
        impairment in MS, 207
    effects of antifatigue drugs on, 251
    and employment, 215
    and pediatric multiple sclerosis,
        226–227
    and synaptic pruning, 67
Motor learning, 323
MRI. See Magnetic resonance imaging
MRS (magnetic resonance
    spectroscopy), 36
MS. See Multiple sclerosis
MS-Line!, 278
mSMT. See Modified Story Memory
    Technique
MS Neuropsychological Screening
    Questionnaire, 18
MSPT (Multiple Sclerosis Processing
    Speed Test), 15, 17
MSSS (Multiple Sclerosis Severity
    Score), 327
MT (magnetization transfer), 76, 133
Multimodal cognitive rehabilitation,
    266, 276–279
Multiple sclerosis (MS). See also specific
    headings
    onset of, 207
    overview, 3
    prevalence of, 3
Multiple Sclerosis Council for Clinical
    Practice Guidelines, 128, 155
Multiple Sclerosis Functional
    Composite (MSFC)
    and assessment of cognitive
        impairment, 15, 20, 23
    and depression with MS, 103
    and disease-modifying treatments,
        246, 247
Multiple Sclerosis Processing Speed Test
    (MSPT), 15, 17

Multiple Sclerosis Severity Score
    (MSSS), 327
Muscle weakness
    and fall risk, 160
    as symptom of MS, 95
Muscular strength, 308
Music-assisted learning, 283
Myasthenia gravis, 128

NAART (North American Adult
    Reading Test), 326–327, 329
NABT (normal-appearing brain tissue)
    injury, 76
N-acetylaspartate (NAA), 69–70
Naci, H., 214
Narcissistic personality disorder, 150
NARCOMS (North American
    Research Committee on Multiple
    Sclerosis), 334
Natalizumab, 249–250
Natalizumab Safety and Efficacy in
    Relapsing Remitting Multiple
    Sclerosis (AFFIRM) trial, 249
National Institute for Health and Care
    Excellence, 21
NBV (normalized brain volume), 327
NDMA (N-methyl-D-aspartic acid)
    receptors, 251
Neocorticol volume, 9
NEO–PI (Neuroticism Extraversion
    Openness—Personality
    Inventory), 151
Networks, 52
Neural cell elimination, 69
Neurogenesis, 68–69
Neuroimaging. See Brain imaging
Neuronal compensation, 132
Neuroplasticity
    and cerebral reorganization in
        MS, 67, 69, 77, 79. See also
        Cerebral reorganization in
        multiple sclerosis
    and cognitive fatigue, 132
    effects of cognitive rehabilitation
        on, 275
Neuroprotection. See Cognitive reserve
Neuropsychiatric disorders, comorbid.
        See Comorbid neuropsychiatric
        disorders
Neuropsychiatric Inventory, 118, 158

Posterior cingulate cortex (PCC), 51, 277, 278
Potassium channel blockers, 258–259
Pöttgen, J., 282
Prakash, R. S., 278
Precentral gyrus, 270
Precuneus, 51
Precuneus prefrontal cortex, 277
Prednisone, 116
Prefrontal cortex (PFC)
    and cognitive fatigue, 134–136
    and cognitive rehabilitation, 277, 280
Prefrontal regions, 73
Premorbid cognitive leisure activities, 325, 331–332
Premorbid intelligence, 323, 325, 328–330
Primary fatigue, 139
Primary sensory cortex, 132
Processing speed (PS)
    and activities of daily living, 171
    assessment of, 7, 8, 12
    on Brief Repeatable Battery, 9
    and cerebral reorganization in MS, 70–71, 74
    cognitive rehabilitation for, 266, 273–280, 283
    and cognitive reserve, 325
    and depression with MS, 92, 95, 99
    and driving accidents, 161
    effects of antifatigue drugs on, 254
    and employment, 197, 215
    and exercise, 296–299, 303
    and global brain atrophy, 39
    and gray matter atrophy, 41, 42
    and intracranial volume, 332–333
    and magnetic resonance spectroscopy, 43
    measures of, 231
    and monitoring, 19
    and pediatric multiple sclerosis, 226, 232, 233
    and physical activity, 304–306
    and physical fitness, 308–311
    prevalence of dysfunction in, 208
    and white matter atrophy, 40
    and white matter lesions, 37
Processing Speed Test (PST), 15

ProCogSEP program, 278
Proton magnetic resonance spectroscopy (1H-MRS), 69–70
PS. See Processing speed
Pseudobulbar affect (PBA)
    and emotional lability, 118
    overview, 119–121
PSIR. See Phase-sensitive inversion recovery
PST (Processing Speed Test), 15
Psychoeducation, 284
Psychological support, 284
Psychosis, 116, 120
Psychotherapy
    neuro-, 280–281
    and personality changes with MS, 157
Putamen, 99, 331

QALY (quality adjusted life years), 212, 214
QOL. See Quality of life
Quality adjusted life years (QALY), 212, 214
Quality of life (QOL)
    and cognitive fatigue, 138
    and cognitive rehabilitation, 266, 267, 278–281
    effects of fall risk on, 160
    and employment, 193
    and fatigue, 127
    major changes to, 4
    and personality changes with MS, 156–157
    questionnaires for assessment of, 182
Quetiapine, 117
Quinidine, 121

Rabins, P. V., 117, 118
Radial diffusivity (RD), 100
Radü, E. W., 78
Raimo, S., 158
Rao, Stephen, 8–11
Rausch, M., 78
Ravnborg, M., 259
RCBF (regional cerebral blood flow), 101
RD (radial diffusivity), 100
Reading, 331

ABOUT THE EDITORS

John DeLuca, PhD, is the senior vice president for research and training at Kessler Foundation and a professor in the Department of Physical Medicine & Rehabilitation and the Department of Neurology at Rutgers, New Jersey Medical School. He is a licensed psychologist in New Jersey and New York, and is board certified in rehabilitation psychology by the American Board of Professional Psychology. Dr. DeLuca has been involved in neuropsychology and rehabilitation research for over 25 years. He is internationally known for his research on disorders of memory and information processing in a variety of clinical populations, including multiple sclerosis, traumatic brain injury, aneurysmal subarachnoid hemorrhage, and chronic fatigue syndrome. Dr. DeLuca has published over 300 articles and chapters in these areas, has edited five books in neuropsychology, neuroimaging and rehabilitation, and is a coeditor of the *Encyclopedia of Clinical Neuropsychology*. He has received over $32 million in grant support for his research. Dr. DeLuca's most recent research ventures include the cerebral mapping of human cognitive processes using functional neuroimaging, as well as the development of research-based techniques to improve cognitive impairment. He serves as an associate editor of several journals and is on the editorial boards of many other journals. He is the recipient of several awards in recognition of his work, including the 2015 Arthur Benton Award from the International Neuropsychological Society, and 2012 Rodger G. Barker Distinguished Research Contribution Award from Division 22, Rehabilitation Psychology, of the American Psychological Association. Dr. DeLuca has been very involved for many years in the training of postdoctoral fellows in neuropsychology and rehabilitation, and has directed several advanced research and training programs sponsored by the National Institute on Disability and Rehabilitation Research, the National MS Society, and the National Institutes of Health since 1990.

Brian M. Sandroff, PhD, is an assistant professor in the Department of Physical Therapy and codirector of the Exercise Neuroscience Research Laboratory at the University of Alabama at Birmingham. Dr. Sandroff earned his PhD in kinesiology from the University of Illinois at Urbana–Champaign and further completed a postdoctoral fellowship in neuropsychology and neuroscience at the Kessler Foundation. He has focused on multiple sclerosis (MS) research for the past 9 years and is an expert on exercise/physical fitness effects on cognition in this population. Dr. Sandroff has published over 100 articles and chapters in this area and has received over $2.5 million in grant support for his research. His current foci involve systematically developed randomized controlled trials of exercise training on cognition, brain structure, and brain function in cognitively impaired persons with MS.